Pocket Guide to
Nutritional Assessment
and Care

Pocket Guide to Nutritional Assessment and Care

Mary Courtney Moore, RN, RD, PhD

Research Associate Professor
Department of Molecular Physiology and Biophysics
Vanderbilt University
School of Medicine
Nashville, Tennessee

Fifth Edition

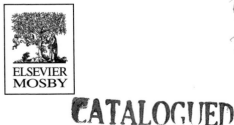

ELSEVIER
MOSBY

ELSEVIER
MOSBY

11830 Westline Industrial Drive
St. Louis, Missouri 63146

POCKET GUIDE TO NUTRITIONAL ASSESSMENT AND CARE   ISBN: 0-323-02802-0

NOTICE

Nutrition is an ever-changing field. Standard safety precautions must be followed, but as new research and clinical experience broaden our knowledge, changes in treatment and drug therapy may become necessary or appropriate. Readers are advised to check the most current product information provided by the manufacturer of each drug to be administered to verify the recommended dose, the method and duration of administration, and contraindications. It is the responsibility of the licensed prescriber, relying on experience and knowledge of the patient, to determine dosages and the best treatment for each individual patient. Neither the publisher nor the author assumes any liability for any injury and/or damage to persons or property arising from this publication.

Previous editions copyrighted 1988, 1993, 1997, and 2001

Acquisitions Editor: Yvonne Alexopoulos
Editorial Assistant: Tara Brooks
Publishing Services Manager: Catherine Jackson
Project Manager: Clay S. Broeker
Designer: Amy Buxton

Printed in the United States of America
Last digit is print number: 9 8 7 6 5 4 3 2 1

**To Bill and Evan,
the best family anywhere.**

*"I was hungry and you fed me,
thirsty and you gave me a drink ...
sick and you took care of me ..."*

Matthew 25:35-36

Reviewers

Dorothy G. Herron, PhD, RN, CS
Organizational Systems and Adult Health Department
School of Nursing
University of Maryland
Baltimore, Maryland

Paula Scharf Kohn, PhD, RN
Associate Professor
Lienhard School of Nursing
Pace University
Pleasantville, New York

Judith Fish Li, MMSc, RD, CNSD
Nutrition Consultant
Asheville, North Carolina

Jennifer M. Williams, MS, RD, LD/N, CNSD
Senior Clinical Dietitian Specialist
Clinical Nutrition Support Service
Hospital of the University of Pennsylvania
Adjunct Lecturer
School of Nursing
University of Pennsylvania
Philadelphia, Pennsylvania

Linda O. Young, MS, RD, LMNT
Director, Didactic Program in Dietetics
Department of Nutrition and Health Sciences
College of Education and Human Sciences
University of Nebraska, Lincoln
Lincoln, Nebraska

Preface

The *Pocket Guide to Nutritional Assessment and Care* is designed to be a brief, yet comprehensive resource for clinical practitioners. Many of the features of previous editions have been retained, including the emphasis on performing a thorough nutrition assessment as a basis for planning nutrition interventions and teaching, an overview of cultural impacts on nutrition, and the application of enteral and parenteral nutrition support wherever appropriate.

This edition of the book has been extensively revised to make it even more current and relevant to practice. Important changes include the incorporation of the latest additions to the Dietary Reference Intakes, expansion of the section on identification and treatment of the metabolic syndrome, an even greater emphasis on weight control and physical activity, and the expansion of the chapter on aging to include health promotion among adults of all ages.

My hope is that this fifth edition of the *Pocket Guide to Nutritional Assessment and Care* will be a timely and useful reference for health professionals and that it will serve to improve the care of their patients.

Contents

APPENDIXES

NUTRITION FOR HEALTH PROMOTION

I

The following chapters introduce normal nutrition. Included in the discussion are a summary of the required nutrients, an explanation of nutritional guidelines, an overview of digestion and absorption, a description of the process of nutritional assessment, and a discussion of nutritional needs and concerns throughout the life cycle. These chapters provide a basis for understanding the role of nutrition in health promotion and prevention of disease.

Nutrition and Health: Overview

1

More than 40 nutrients are known to be essential for human health. All of these nutrients are found in foods and beverages, but some skill and planning may be required to choose a diet adequate in all nutrients. Appendix A summarizes the roles, major food sources, and symptoms of deficiency of nutrients known to be essential.

Healthy People Initiative

Healthy People is an ongoing project aimed at increasing the years of healthy life and decreasing disparities in health care among Americans. The initiative identifies the most significant and controllable health issues for Americans and focuses on public and private sector attempts to address them. In the current summary (*Healthy People 2010;* available at http://www.health.gov/healthypeople/), the top two out of the 10 leading health indicators—physical activity and overweight/obesity—are nutrition related. Thus the need for education about nutrition and a healthy lifestyle is a high priority among Americans.

Dietary Reference Intakes

In every country it is necessary to have a careful estimate of the nutrient needs of the population in order to provide a basis for setting nutrition policy, monitoring the adequacy of the food supply, and educating the public about proper diet. Prompted by the growing recognition of the role of nutrition in health promotion and prevention of chronic diseases, U.S. and Canadian nutritionists are developing new guidelines, called the **Dietary Reference Intakes (DRIs)** (Tables 1-1a through 1-1d). The DRIs are used in regulating the

Text continued on p. 16

Table 1-1a   Criteria and Dietary Reference Intake Values for Energy by Active Individuals by Life Stage Group[a]

Life Stage Group	Criterion	Active PAL[b] EER (kcal/d)	
		Male	Female
0 through 6 mo	Energy expenditure plus energy deposition	570	520 (3 mo)
7 through 12 mo	Energy expenditure plus energy deposition	743	676 (9 mo)
1 through 2 yr	Energy expenditure plus energy deposition	1046	992 (24 mo)
3 through 8 yr	Energy expenditure plus energy deposition	1742	1642 (6 yr)
9 through 13 yr	Energy expenditure plus energy deposition	2279	2071 (11 yr)
14 through 18 yr	Energy expenditure plus energy deposition	3152	2368 (16 yr)
>18 yr	Energy expenditure	3067[c]	2403[c] (19 yr)
Pregnancy			
14 through 18 yr	Adolescent female EER plus change in TEE		
1st trimester	plus pregnancy energy deposition		2368 (16 yr)
2nd trimester			2708 (16 yr)
3rd trimester			2820 (16 yr)
19 through 50 yr	Adult female EER plus change in TEE plus		
1st trimester	pregnancy energy deposition		2403[c] (19 yr)
2nd trimester			2743[c] (19 yr)
3rd trimester			2855[c] (19 yr)

31-50 yr	700	75	5*	15	90*	1.1
51-70 yr	700	75	10*	15	90*	1.1
>70 yr	700	75	15*	15	90*	1.1
Pregnancy						
≤18 yr	750	80	5*	15	75*	1.4
19-30 yr	770	85	5*	15	90*	1.4
31-50 yr	770	85	5*	15	90*	1.4
Lactation						
≤18 yr	1200	115	5*	19	75*	1.4
19-30 yr	1300	120	5*	19	90*	1.4
31-50 yr	1300	120	5*	19	90*	1.4

Note: Tables 1-1c and 1-1d (taken from the DRI reports at www.nap.edu) present Recommended Dietary Allowances (RDAs) in bold type and Adequate Intakes (AIs) in ordinary type followed by an asterisk (*). RDAs and AIs may both be used as goals for individual intake. RDAs are likely to meet the needs of almost all (97 to 98 percent) individuals in a group. For healthy breastfed infants, the AI is the mean intake. The AI for other life stage and gender groups is believed to cover needs of all individuals in the group, but lack of data or uncertainty in the data prevent being able to specify with confidence the percentage of individuals covered by this intake.

[a] As retinol activity equivalents (RAEs). 1 RAE = 1 μg retinol, 12 μg β-carotene, 24 μg β-carotene, or 24 μg β-cryptoxanthin. To calculate RAEs from REs of provitamin A carotenoids in foods, divide the REs by 2. For preformed vitamin A in foods or supplements and for provitamin A carotenoids in supplements, 1 RE = 1 RAE.

[b] Calciferol. 1 μg calciferol = 40 IU vitamin D.

[c] In the absence of adequate exposure to sunlight.

From *Dietary reference intakes for vitamin A, vitamin K, arsenic, boron, chromium, copper, iodine, iron, manganese, molybdenum, nickel, silicon, vanadium, and zinc,* Washington, DC, 2000, National Academy Press. Used with permission.

Continued

Table 1-1c   Food and Nutrition Board, Institute of Medicine—National Academy of Sciences Dietary Reference Intakes: Recommended Intakes for Individuals, Vitamins—cont'd

Life Stage Group	Riboflavin (mg/day)	Niacin (mg/day)[e]	Vitamin B_6 (mg/day)	Folate (µg/day)[f,g,b]	Vitamin B_{12} (µg/day)[b]	Pantothenic Acid (mg/day)	Biotin (µg/day)
Infants							
0-6 mo	0.3*	2*	0.1*	65*	0.4*	1.7*	5*
7-12 mo	0.4*	4*	0.3*	80*	0.5*	1.8*	6*
Children							
1-3 yr	0.5	6	0.5	150	0.9	2*	8*
4-8 yr	0.6	8	0.6	200	1.2	3*	12*
Males							
9-13 yr	0.9	12	1.0	300	1.8	4*	20*
14-18 yr	1.3	16	1.3	400	2.4	5*	25*
19-30 yr	1.3	16	1.3	400	2.4	5*	30*
31-50 yr	1.3	16	1.3	400	2.4	5*	30*
51-70 yr	1.3	16	1.7	400	2.4[g]	5*	30*
>70 yr	1.3	16	1.7	400	2.4[g]	5*	30*
Females							
9-13 yr	0.9	12	1.0	300	1.8	4*	20*
14-18 yr	1.0	14	1.2	400[h]	2.4	5*	25*
19-30 yr	1.1	14	1.3	400[h]	2.4	5*	30*
31-50 yr	1.1	14	1.3	400[h]	2.4	5*	30*

51-70 yr	1.1	14	1.5	400	2.4[g]	5*	30*
>70 yr	1.1	14	1.5	400	2.4[g]	5*	30*
Pregnancy							
≤18 yr	1.4	18	1.9	600[i]	2.6	6*	30*
19-30 yr	1.4	18	1.9	600[i]	2.6	6*	30*
31-50 yr	1.4	18	1.9	600[i]	2.6	6*	30*
Lactation							
≤18 yr	1.6	17	2.0	500	2.8	7*	35*
19-30 yr	1.6	17	2.0	500	2.8	7*	35*
31-50 yr	1.6	17	2.0	500	2.8	7*	35*

[d] As α-Tocopherol. α-Tocopherol includes RRR-α-tocopherol, the only form of α-tocopherol that occurs naturally in foods, and the 2R-stereoisomeric forms of α-tocopherol (RRR-, RSR-, RRS-, and RSS-α-tocopherol) that occur in fortified foods and supplements. It does not include the 2S-stereoisomeric forms of α-tocopherol (SRR-, SSR-, SRS-, and SSS-α-tocopherol), also found in fortified foods and supplements.

[e] As niacin equivalents (NE). 1 mg of niacin = 60 mg of tryptophan; 0 to 6 months = preformed niacin (not NE).

[f] As dietary folate equivalents (DFE). 1 DFE = 1 μg food folate = 0.6 μg of folic acid from fortified food or as a supplement consumed with food = 0.5 μg of a supplement taken on an empty stomach.

[g] Because 10% to 30 % of older people may malabsorb food-bound B₁₂, it is advisable for those older than 50 years to meet their RDA mainly by consuming foods fortified with B₁₂ or a supplement containing B₁₂.

[h] In view of evidence linking folate intake with neural tube defects in the fetus, it is recommended that all women capable of becoming pregnant consume 400 μg from supplements or fortified foods in addition to intake of food folate from a varied diet.

[i] It is assumed that women will continue consuming 400 μg from supplements or fortified food until their pregnancy is confirmed and they enter prenatal care, which ordinarily occurs after the end of the periconceptional period—the critical time for formation of the neural tube.

From *Dietary reference intakes: applications in dietary assessment*, Washington, DC, 2002, National Academy Press. Used with permission.

Table 1-1d   Food and Nutrition Board, Institute of Medicine—National Academy of Sciences Dietary Reference Intakes: Recommended Intakes for Individuals, Elements

Life Stage Group	Calcium (mg/day)	Chromium (µg/day)	Copper (µg/day)	Fluoride (mg/day)	Iodine (µg/day)	Iron (mg/day)
Infants						
0-6 mo	210*	0.2*	200*	0.01*	110*	0.27*
7-12 mo	270*	5.5*	220*	0.5*	130*	11
Children						
1-3 yr	500*	11*	340	0.7*	90	7
4-8 yr	800*	15*	440	1*	90	10
Males						
9-13 yr	1300*	25*	700	2*	120	8
14-18 yr	1300*	35*	890	3*	150	11
19-30 yr	1000*	35*	900	4*	150	8
31-50 yr	1000*	35*	900	4*	150	8
51-70 yr	1200*	30*	900	4*	150	8
>70 yr	1200*	30*	900	4*	150	8

Females						
9-13 yr	1300*	21*	700	2*	120	8
14-18 yr	1300*	24*	890	3*	150	15
19-30 yr	1000*	25*	900	3*	150	18
31-50 yr	1000*	25*	900	3*	150	18
51-70 yr	1200*	20*	900	3*	150	8
>70 yr	1200*	20*	900	3*	150	8
Pregnancy						
≤18 yr	1300*	29*	1000	3*	220	27
19-30 yr	1000*	30*	1000	3*	220	27
31-50 yr	1000*	30*	1000	3*	220	27
Lactation						
≤18 yr	1300*	44*	1300	3*	290	10
19-30 yr	1000*	15*	1300	3*	290	9
31-50 yr	1000*	45*	1300	3*	290	9

Table 1-1d   Food and Nutrition Board, Institute of Medicine—National Academy of Sciences Dietary Reference Intakes: Recommended Intakes for Individuals, Elements—cont'd

Life Stage Group	Magnesium (mg/day)	Manganese (mg/day)	Molybdenum (µg/day)	Phosphorus (mg/day)	Selenium (µg/day)	Zinc (mg/day)
Infants						
0-6 mo	30*	0.003*	2*	100*	15*	2*
7-12 mo	75*	0.6*	3*	275*	20*	3
Children						
1-3 yr	80	1.2*	17	460	20	3
4-8 yr	130	1.5*	22	500	30	5
Males						
9-13 yr	240	1.9*	34	1250	40	8
14-18 yr	410	2.2*	43	1250	55	11
19-30 yr	400	2.3*	45	700	55	11
31-50 yr	420	2.3*	45	700	55	11
51-70 yr	420	2.3*	45	700	55	11
>70 yr	420	2.3*	45	700	55	11
Females						
9-13 yr	240	1.6*	34	1250	40	8
14-18 yr	360	1.6*	43	1250	55	9
19-30 yr	310	1.8*	45	700	55	8

31-50 yr	320	1.8*	45	700	55	8
51-70 yr	320	1.8*	45	700	55	8
>70 yr	320	1.8*	45	700	55	8
Pregnancy						
≤18 yr	400	2.0*	50	1250	60	12
19-30 yr	350	2.0*	50	700	60	11
31-50 yr	360	2.0*	50	700	60	11
Lactation						
≤18 yr	360	2.6*	50	1250	70	13
19-30 yr	310	2.6*	50	700	70	12
31-50 yr	320	2.6*	50	700	70	12

Sources: Dietary reference intakes for calcium, phosphorus, magnesium, vitamin D, and fluoride (1997); Dietary reference intakes for thiamin, riboflavin, niacin, vitamin B_6, folate, vitamin B_{12}, pantothenic acid, biotin, and choline (1998); Dietary reference intakes for vitamin C, vitamin E, selenium, and carotenoids (2000); and Dietary reference intakes for vitamin A, vitamin K, arsenic, boron, chromium, copper, iodine, iron, manganese, molybdenum, nickel, silicon, vanadium, and zinc (2001). These reports may be accessed via www.nap.edu.

fortification of foods (addition of nutrients, as in vitamin D fortification of milk) and the composition of diet supplements; setting goals and budgets for food assistance programs for low-income families, schools, and the elderly; planning menus for individuals in the military and in many institutions; determining what nutrition information should be supplied on food labels; and similar purposes.

Various types of guidelines have been set, depending on the nutrient. First, either a **Recommended Dietary Allowance (RDA)** or an **Adequate Intake (AI)** is specified, and second, a **Tolerable Upper Intake Level (UL)** is given for most nutrients. The RDA, which is estimated to meet the needs of almost all (97% to 98%) of the healthy population, is assigned where nutrient needs are well established. An AI is assigned when nutrient needs cannot be quantified as precisely, but the recommendation is believed to cover the needs of the population. When nutrient needs are less clear, an **Estimated Average Requirement (EAR)** is given; the EAR is the average daily nutrient intake that is believed to meet the requirements of half the healthy individuals in a life stage or gender group. The UL is defined as the upper limit of intake associated with a low risk of adverse effects in almost all members of a population.

Guides for Wise Food Choices

The DRIs are useful for health care professionals, the food industry, and government agencies involved in food and health policy, but most individuals would find them hard to translate into appropriate food choices. The *Dietary Guidelines for Americans* and the **Food Guide Pyramid** have been developed to help the public choose foods wisely. Nutritional labeling on foods is designed to make it easier to know what nutrients are in foods. At the time of this writing, both the *Guidelines* and the Food Guide Pyramid are under revision (Dietary Guidelines Advisory Committee, 2003; Center for Nutrition Policy and Promotion [CNPP], 2003). The exact form they will take is not yet apparent, but it is clear that fitness and healthy body weight will be top nutrition priorities for years to come.

Dietary Guidelines for Americans

The *Dietary Guidelines for Americans* (U.S. Department of Agriculture [USDA] & U.S. Department of Health and Human Services [USDHHS], 2000) are intended to help Americans optimize their health and reduce nutrition-related health risks. The guidelines are summarized as follows:

Aim for Fitness

Aim for a healthy weight

Numerous health problems—including hypertension, heart disease, stroke, type 2 diabetes, arthritis, pulmonary problems, and breast cancer and certain other cancers—are associated with being overweight. Avoiding weight gain or losing excess weight involves lifestyle changes that require specific choices, such as increasing physical activity and choosing a variety of healthful foods low in fat and added sugars.

Individuals who are overweight need to lose the excess weight gradually. A loss of 5% to 15% of body weight, even if that does not bring the individual to a normal weight, may improve his or her health, functional ability, and quality of life. An increasing number of children are overweight. Children need to be encouraged to choose from a variety of low-fat foods from the Food Guide Pyramid (described later in this chapter), and they should be provided only rarely with foods high in fats and added sugars.

Individuals with eating disorders attempt to control their weight in unhealthful ways. Frequent binge eating, with or without periods of food restriction, preoccupation with body weight or food, dramatic weight loss, excessive exercise, self-induced vomiting, and laxative abuse are signs of eating disorders.

Be physically active every day

Physical activity reduces the risk of heart disease, colon cancer, and type 2 diabetes (see Chapter 17). In addition, it strengthens muscles, bones, and joints; improves psychological well-being; and helps to control high blood pressure and body weight. Adults need at least 30 minutes of moderate physical activity daily, and children need at least 60 minutes. A regular exercise program is one way to be physically active, but it is also possible to incorporate an adequate amount of physical activity into the daily routine (e.g., climb the stairs rather than taking an elevator or use a bicycle rather than a car to run errands).

Build a Healthy Base

Let the pyramid guide your food choices

No single food provides all of the necessary nutrients in the amounts needed. By using many different foods, a person has the best chance of obtaining the different nutrients needed. Most food choices should be made from the five primary groups in the Food Guide Pyramid (discussed later in this chapter): grains (breads, cereals, rice, pasta); vegetables; fruits; milk (milk, yogurt, and cheese); and meat and beans (meat, poultry, fish, dry beans, eggs, and nuts). Fats and sweets can be used occasionally to add variety to the diet. Although the food guide is currently being revised, choosing a wide variety of foods from different groups will remain a tenet of the new guide. Food choices are determined by many factors, including culture, family background, religion and beliefs, life experiences, food intolerances and allergies, and cost and availability of food. It is possible to obtain a healthful diet with many different eating patterns. For example, milk is a good source of calcium, but adults in many cultures do not drink milk. By making wise food choices (e.g., using cheese, tofu or other soy products fortified with calcium, and fruit juices with added calcium), adequate calcium can be obtained without milk. In general, however, avoiding a whole group places the person at risk for deficiencies of one or more nutrients. For example, people who do not include vegetables and fruits in their diets regularly may not consume enough of the vitamins A and C. Dietary supplements may be needed by some individuals. Women who could become pregnant need a folic acid supplement or regular intake of folic acid–fortified foods. Older adults and people with little sun exposure may need a vitamin D supplement. Individuals who eat no animal products (and many older adults) need a supplement of vitamin B_{12}.

Choose a variety of grains daily, especially whole grains

Whole grains, fruits, and vegetables are an excellent source of fiber. Enriched grains are a good source of folic acid and other B vitamins. Folic acid taken during pregnancy reduces the risk of serious congenital disorders known as neural tube defects and may reduce the risk of coronary artery disease and certain cancers.

Choose a variety of fruits and vegetables daily

Vegetables and fruits are good sources of vitamins, minerals, complex carbohydrates (starch and dietary fiber), and other nutrients and **phytochemicals** (chemical components of a plant, especially those having health-protective effects). Most plant foods are also naturally low in fat. Fiber intake is likely to be low among individuals in many industrialized countries, which can contribute to constipation and an increased risk of cardiovascular disease, diverticulosis, colon cancer, and diabetes. Fiber intake can be increased with a diet that includes whole grains, dry beans, and fiber-rich vegetables and fruits daily (see Appendix B). Dark green leafy and yellow vegetables and yellow fruits such as cantaloupes and mangoes are good sources of β-carotene and other vitamin A precursors and should be chosen frequently.

Phytochemicals include a variety of diverse compounds that act in many ways to prevent or delay chronic illnesses. For example, polyphenols found in tea (especially green tea), cereal grains, and many fruits and vegetables have **antioxidant** properties and may help reduce the risk of both heart disease and cancer. Flavonoids in citrus and other fruits, vegetables, grains, wine, and tea apparently act by several mechanisms to reduce tumor initiation and growth. Genistein from soy inhibits the growth of human breast and prostate cancer cells, and soy also has cholesterol- and triglyceride-lowering effects. In this respect, soy serves as a **nutraceutical** or **functional food** (a foodstuff that provides health benefit beyond its nutritional value). Because the identities of all the beneficial phytochemicals and nutraceuticals, their optimal intakes, and their potential interactions with other phytochemicals and nutrients remain unclear, a varied diet with ample servings of plant foods appears the best way to obtain them.

Keep food safe to eat

Food-borne illness results from eating food that contains harmful bacteria, toxins, parasites, viruses, or chemical contaminants. Appendix K summarizes approaches to maintaining food safety. General rules to follow are to ensure that hands, preparation surfaces, and utensils are clean before preparing food; avoid cross-contamination (e.g., cutting fresh vegetables for salad on a board that has not been cleansed since it was used for trimming raw meat); and keep foods at optimal temperatures (either hot or cold) for reducing bacterial proliferation.

Choose Sensibly

Choose a diet that is low in saturated fat and cholesterol and moderate in total fat

A diet high in saturated fat and cholesterol is linked to elevated blood cholesterol levels and to heart disease. A diet high in total fat is linked to obesity and increased risk of some cancers (e.g., colon, breast). Fat is higher in calories than either protein or carbohydrate, and a high-fat diet (more than 30% of calories from fat) may make it difficult to get the variety of nutrients needed without consuming excessive energy.

The *Dietary Guidelines* recommend that fat supply no more than 30% of calories in the diet, saturated fat account for no more than 10% of calories, and cholesterol intake total no more than 300 mg/day. (These guidelines do not apply to children under the age of 2 years.) Most of the fat in the diet should be **monounsaturated** and **polyunsaturated fatty acids** (Figure 1-1), which are found in olive, canola, sunflower, safflower, soybean, and corn oils; nuts; and high-fat fish. **Trans fatty acids**, found in **hydrogenated fats** (in most shortenings and stick margarines and many processed foods), raise low-density-lipoprotein (LDL) cholesterol levels, and elevated LDL cholesterol is a risk factor for heart disease. A safe level of trans fatty acid intake has not been established, but the best current advice is to avoid trans fats as much as possible. Check the ingredient listings on food products and to consume those products containing hydrogenated fats only occasionally. Trans fat content will appear on food labels by 2006.

Eating fish regularly appears to reduce the risk of heart disease. Many fish from cold waters are rich in *omega-3 fats*, which are used in synthesis of eicosanoids (vital compounds regulating many body processes); omega-3 fatty acids may help to reduce blood pressure and to prevent clumping of platelets, which can block cardiac blood vessels and contribute to myocardial infarction. However, the FDA recommends that pregnant women and women of childbearing age who may become pregnant, as well as nursing mothers and young children, not eat shark, swordfish, king mackerel, and tilefish because these fish often contain relatively high levels of methylmercury. Consumption of up to 12 ounces (360 g) a week of a variety of other types of fish and seafood is believed to be safe.

In order to control the intake of fat and saturated fat, individuals should use fats and oils sparingly. The Nutrition Facts Label (described later in this chapter) helps consumers choose foods lower in fat, saturated fat, and cholesterol. Fruits, vegetables, and grain products (without added fat) are good choices. Other ways to reduce fat intake include using low-fat milk products, lean meats, fish, and poultry and replacing animal proteins with dried beans (navy, pinto, kidney, garbanzo, etc.) and peas often.

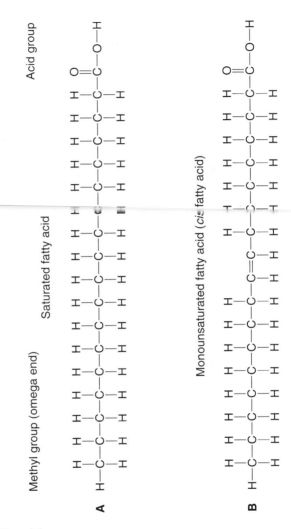

Figure 1-1
Structures of some common fatty acids and triglycerides. Fatty acids containing only single bonds *(A)* are saturated. The *cis* arrangement of double bonds *(B)* is usually found in naturally occurring unsaturated fats.

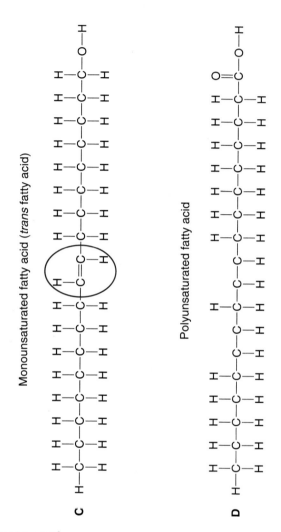

Figure 1-1, cont'd
Trans fatty acids *(C)* are found primarily in partially
hydrogenated vegetable oils, where many of the remaining
unsaturated bonds take on the *trans* arrangement (circled). *D*
and *E* are polyunsaturated fatty acids. Fatty acids are often
described by the number of carbon atoms they contain and by
the number and location of double bonds. One system is to
count the carbon atoms starting at the methyl (or omega) end.

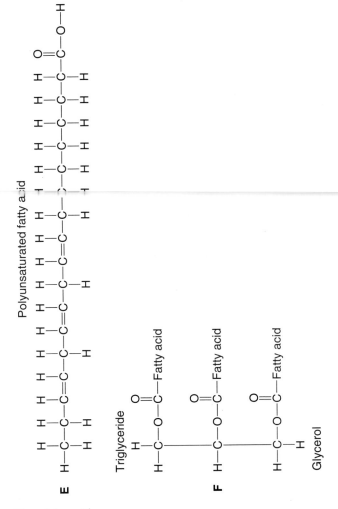

Figure 1-1, cont'd
Using this system, the fatty acid marked *(E)* is an omega-3 fatty
acid (also known as an *n*-3 fatty acid). Most dietary fat is in the
form of triglycerides *(F)*.

Choose beverages and foods to moderate your intake of sugars

Sugars are one form of carbohydrates. During digestion, all carbohydrates except fiber break down into sugars, and many foods are either natural sources of sugars or have sugar added during preparation. Frequent eating of foods high in sugars and starches between meals and failure to brush the teeth after eating carbohydrates increase the risk of tooth decay. Sugar should be used only in moderation and should be used sparingly if energy needs are low. The nutrition label lists the amount of sugars in foods.

Choose and prepare foods with less salt

Most sodium and sodium chloride (salt) in the diet is added during processing and preparation of foods. The suggested **Daily Value (DV)** for sodium on the Nutrition Facts Label is no more than 2400 mg, but most North Americans consume at least 1.5 to 2 times this amount. The DV is a reference value based on the RDA and is used on food labels to provide a guide to the amount of a particular nutrient that the daily diet should contain. Many people at risk for hypertension reduce their chances of developing this condition by reducing their sodium intake. To help reduce sodium intake, choose fresh fruits and vegetables, most of which are naturally low in sodium; read nutrition labels to help identify foods lower in sodium within each group; and flavor foods with herbs and spices rather than salt or seasoning salts.

If you drink alcoholic beverages, do so in moderation

Alcoholic beverages provide energy but few nutrients. Current evidence suggests that moderate drinking is associated with a lower risk for coronary heart disease in some individuals and that red wine, in particular, may be beneficial. Moderate consumption is defined as no more than one drink per day for women or two drinks per day for men. A drink equals 12 oz (360 ml) of regular beer, 1 glass (5 oz or 150 ml) of wine, or 1.5 oz (1 jigger or 45 ml) of distilled spirits. Higher levels of alcohol intake raise the risk for hypertension, stroke, elevated triglyceride levels (a risk factor for heart disease), certain cancers, accidents, violence, suicides, birth defects, and overall mortality. Excessive alcohol intake may cause cirrhosis of the liver, pancreatitis, cardiomyopathy, and damage to the brain. Heavy drinkers also are at risk of malnutrition because of the poor nutrient density of alcoholic beverages and because heavy alcohol intake increases urinary loss of some nutrients (e.g., magnesium and zinc).

Some people should not drink alcoholic beverages at all. These include children and adolescents, individuals of any age who cannot restrict their drinking to moderate levels, women who are trying to conceive or who are pregnant, individuals who plan to drive or take part in activities that require attention or skill, and individuals using many prescription and over-the-counter medications. These individuals can obtain the health benefits of wine by consuming purple grape juice instead.

Food Guide Pyramid

The Food Guide Pyramid (Figure 1-2) is a simple tool for helping individuals to ensure a varied diet. The grain group is at the base and is the largest to demonstrate that it should provide the basis for a healthful diet. The vegetable and fruit groups are next in size to emphasize their importance in nutrition. At the next level are milk products and the group containing meats and plant sources of protein. These groups provide valuable nutrients such as calcium, protein, and iron, but some of the foods in these groups are also rich in fat. Thus, excessive servings from these groups are undesirable. The narrow apex of the pyramid is assigned to fats, oils, and sweets, to illustrate that they should be used in only limited amounts. Many combination foods such as soups, stews, pizza, and casseroles contain servings from more than one food group.

In the proposed revision of the food guide (CNPP, 2003), the major food groupings in the food guide—fruits, vegetables, grains, milk, and meat and beans—are retained. "Meat and beans" reflects a shortening of the current group title, "meat, poultry, fish, dry beans, eggs, and nuts." The suggested changes include expanding the number of food intake patterns (from the three levels in the current guide [1600, 2200, and 2800 kcal daily] to 12, ranging from 1000 to 3200 kcal daily, to meet the public's energy needs more accurately); basing food intake recommendations on a sedentary lifestyle, in recognition that this describes much of the population, while encouraging increased physical activity; using the most up-to-date versions of the *Dietary Guidelines for Americans* (USDA & USDHHS, 2000) and Dietary Reference Intakes (Food and Nutrition Board, 1999, 2000a, 2000b, 2002a, 2002b) as the basis for the food guide; emphasizing low-fat food choices within each food group (e.g., fat-free milk);

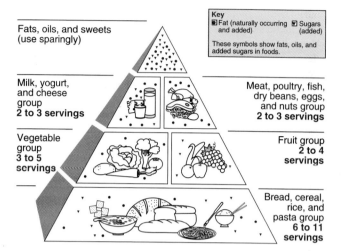

Food group*   Serving size

Grain products   1 slice bread, 1 roll or muffin, 1/2 bagel or
                 hamburger bun
                 1 oz ready-to-eat cereal
                 1/2 cup rice, pasta, cooked cereal

Vegetable   1 cup raw leafy greens
                 1/2 cup of all others, cooked or raw
                 1/4 cup vegetable juice

Fruit   1 medium apple, orange, pear, banana
                 1/2 cup chopped, cooked, or canned fruit
                 1/4 cup juice

Milk   1 cup milk or yogurt
                 1 1/2 oz natural cheese or 2 oz processed
                 cheese

Meat and beans   2 to 3 oz cooked lean meat, poultry, or
                 fish
                 (1/2 cup cooked dried beans or peas or 1
                 egg = 1 oz lean meat; 2 tbsp peanut
                 butter or 1/3 cup nuts = 1 oz meat)

* Some foods fit into more than one group. Dry beans, peas, and lentils can be counted as
servings in either the meat and beans group or vegetable group, but not in both groups.

Figure 1-2
Food Guide Pyramid: a guide to daily food choices.
(From U.S. Department of Agriculture and U.S. Department of Health and Human
Services.)

and creating subgroups within the major groups to emphasize that not all members of the groups are equivalent in nutrition content. The proposed subgroups are "dark-green," "deep-yellow," "legumes," "starchy," and "other" within the vegetable group, as well as "whole grains" and "other grains" within the grains group (with at least half of the grains consumed being whole grains). Specific recommendations may be made for the subgroups—for example, a serving of a dark-green vegetable every other day and a deep-yellow vegetable twice a week. A group of "additional fats" is proposed, to include those fats added in food preparation or at the table and those consumed when higher fat selections are made from the major food groups. It is recommended that 60% of intake from additional fats be derived from oils and soft margarines, which are sources of certain beneficial fats, including monounsaturated, omega-3, and essential long-chain fatty acids. Solid fat such as that from shortening; hard margarines; fat from meat, poultry, and milk products; and butter should be limited to 40% of the intake in this category. An "added sugars" category will include the sugars and syrups added to foods and beverages in processing or preparation, but not the naturally occurring sugars in fruits or milk. There are no recommendations for amounts of added sugars, but instead there is a representation of the amount that can be included without overconsumption of energy.

Dietary Approaches to Stop Hypertension (DASH)

A diet plan that was originally designed to be part of the therapy for hypertension has proven to be a healthful and practical plan for nonhypertensive individuals as well. The DASH plan is consistent with the Food Guide Pyramid, but it provides more emphasis on the importance of fruits and vegetables; beneficial fats and oils; and nuts, seeds, and legumes in the diet and more guidance in limiting intake of saturated fat, cholesterol, salt, and sweets. The DASH plan is summarized briefly in Table 1-2 and described in more detail in Chapter 14.

Nutrition Labeling

Nutrition labeling is required on almost all processed foods, meat, and poultry (Figure 1-3). Similar information also appears near fresh produce in many markets. This labeling is a valuable source of information for the consumer who is trying to choose a healthful diet or modify his or her diet (e.g., reduce fat or sodium intake) and

Table 1-2   The DASH Eating Plan

Food Group	Daily Servings (except as noted)			Serving Sizes
	1600 kcal	2000 kcal	2400 kcal	
Grains and grain products	6	7-8	9-10	1 slice bread; 1 oz dry cereal; ½ c cooked rice, pasta, or cereal
Vegetables	3-4	4-5	5	1 c raw leafy vegetable; ½ c cooked vegetable; 1.5 c vegetable juice
Fruits	4	4-5	5	1.5 c fruit juice; 1 medium fruit; ¼ c dried fruit; ½ c fresh, frozen, or canned fruit
Low-fat or fat-free dairy foods	2-3	2-3	3	1 c fat free or low-fat milk; 1 c low-fat yogurt; 1.5 oz low-fat or fat-free cheese
Meats, poultry, and fish	Less than 2 (total of 5 oz)	2 or less (total of 6 oz)	2 or less (total of 6 oz)	3 oz cooked meats, poultry, or fish

Nuts, seeds, and dry beans	4-5/wk	4-5/wk	6-7/wk	½ c or 1.5 oz nuts; 2 tbsp or ½ oz seeds; ½ c cooked dry beans or peas
Fats and oils	2 or less	2-3	2-3	1 tsp soft margarine; 1 tbsp low-fat mayonnaise; 2 tbsp light salad dressing; 1 tsp vegetable oil
Sweets	Less than 5/wk	5/wk	5/wk	1 tbsp sugar, jelly, or jam; ½ oz jelly beans; 1 c lemonade; 1 frozen fruit ice bar, no sugar added

c, Cup (240 ml); oz, ounce (approx. 30 g); tbsp, tablespoon (15 ml); tsp, teaspoon (5 ml).
The number of daily servings can be modified to suit individuals with different energy needs.
From The DASH eating plan. Available at www.nhlbi.nih.gov/health/public/heart/hbp/dash/, updated May 2003. Accessed November 6, 2003.

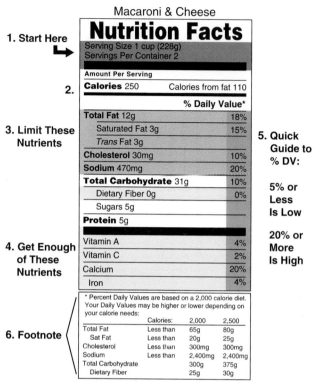

Macaroni & Cheese

Nutrition Facts

1. **Start Here** ➡️

Serving Size 1 cup (228g)
Servings Per Container 2

Amount Per Serving

Calories 250   Calories from fat 110

% Daily Value*

Total Fat 12g	**18%**
Saturated Fat 3g	**15%**
Trans Fat 3g	
Cholesterol 30mg	**10%**
Sodium 470mg	**20%**
Total Carbohydrate 31g	**10%**
Dietary Fiber 0g	**0%**
Sugars 5g	
Protein 5g	
Vitamin A	4%
Vitamin C	2%
Calcium	20%
Iron	4%

2.

3. **Limit These Nutrients**

4. **Get Enough of These Nutrients**

5. **Quick Guide to % DV:**

5% or Less Is Low

20% or More Is High

6. **Footnote**

* Percent Daily Values are based on a 2,000 calorie diet. Your Daily Values may be higher or lower depending on your calorie needs:

	Calories:	2,000	2,500
Total Fat	Less than	65g	80g
Sat Fat	Less than	20g	25g
Cholesterol	Less than	300mg	300mg
Sodium	Less than	2,400mg	2,400mg
Total Carbohydrate		300g	375g
Dietary Fiber		25g	30g

Figure 1-3

Sample nutrition label. To read the label, note the following: (1) the serving size and how it compares with the amount you usually eat or plan to eat; all nutrition information on the label is based on the stated serving size; (2) the total Calories (kcal) and fat kcal per serving; (3) the food components that should be limited in the diet: total fat, saturated fat, *trans* fat, cholesterol, and sodium; (4) nutrients that should be encouraged in the diet; (5) the % Daily Value provided by this serving size, based on a 2000 kcal diet; and (6) daily values for energy intakes in addition to the 2000 kcal diet (optional information).

(From *Guidance on how to understand and use the nutrition label.* Available at www.cfsan.fda.gov/~dms/foodlab.html. Accessed November 30, 2003.)

is a useful tool for health care professionals engaged in educating their patients about nutrition. The total energy (kilocalorie, or kcal) content and kcal from fat must appear on the label to help consumers meet the dietary guidelines recommending no more than

30% of kcal from fat. Also included on the label are the amounts of total fat, saturated fat, cholesterol, sodium, total carbohydrate, fiber, sugars, and protein. Information about most macronutrients is expressed in both units of weight (g or mg) and % Daily Value (DV). Labels must express DV in relation to a 2000 kcal diet, a caloric level that meets the energy needs of many adults. For example, fat should provide no more than 30% of the total kcal intake (600 kcal or approximately 65 g per day for the person consuming 2000 kcal). A food that provides 12 g of fat in one serving (see Figure 1-3) provides nearly 20% of the fat included in a 2000 kcal diet. Food labels may contain information about DVs for other caloric intakes, if there is room. Polyunsaturated and monounsaturated fat and potassium content of foods are optional. Various vitamins and minerals appear on the label, depending on the food's nutritional composition. A shortened form of the food label may be used on small food packages.

The U.S. Food and Drug Administration (FDA) has created guidelines to make food labels more informative for consumers who want to choose a healthful diet. These guidelines include definitions for the use of specific terms, such as *low fat* and *light*, in food labeling (Box 1-1), as well as a description of 10 types of health claims (relationships between diet and specific diseases) that can be included on food labels (Box 1-2).

Cultural Influences on Nutrition

Not all food choices are made because of nutritional considerations, of course. Economic constraints, peer pressure, persuasive advertising, and convenience are just a few of the factors influencing food choices. Cultural practices, including those shaped by national, ethnic, or religious background, can exert strong influences on eating patterns.

Immigrants and their families gradually adopt the typical American diet, especially as new generations are born in North America. This transition occurs both because it may be difficult or expensive to obtain particular foods and because of a desire to fit in with the dominant society. Nevertheless, it is helpful to be aware of some characteristic cultural food practices. Appreciation of distinct cultural food habits helps the health care professional to demonstrate respect for both the individual and the culture and to be aware of food habits that may need modification. It may be possible to use cultural pride to reinforce or promote healthier eating habits.

Box 1-1   Some Terms Used on Food Labels and Their Definitions

Free: Contains none, or an insignificant amount, of a particular component (fat, saturated, cholesterol, sodium, sugars, or calories). Per serving a fat-free food contains <0.5 g fat, a sugar-free food contains <0.5 g sugar, and a sodium-free food contains <5 mg sodium.

Good Source or High: Good source: contains 10%-19% of the Daily Value for a particular nutrient. High (or "rich in" or "excellent source of"): contains 20% or more of the Daily Value for a particular nutrient. Usually applied to fiber or a vitamin or mineral.

Lean or Extra Lean: Lean: contains <10 g fat, <4 g saturated fat, and < 95 mg cholesterol per serving and per 100 g. Extra lean: contains <5 g fat, <2 g saturated fat, and <95 mg cholesterol per serving and 100 g. Used in describing the fat content of meat, poultry, seafood, and game.

Light or Lite: Contains one third fewer calories or one half the fat of the reference food.* A low-calorie, low-fat food can also be referred to as "light in sodium" if it contains 50% or less sodium than that reference food.

Reduced or Less: Contains at least 25% less of a particular (sugar, fat, cholesterol, saturated fat, or sodium) per serving than the reference food.

Low: Contains only a small amount of a particular food component, e.g., per serving (or per 50 g, if the normal serving size is 30 g or 2 tablespoons or less); low calorie means 40 calories or less, low fat means 3 g fat or less, low cholesterol means 20 mg or less, and low sodium means 140 mg or less. "Very low," applies only to sodium, means 35 mg or less per serving.

More or Added Fiber: Contains at least 2.5 g more fiber per serving than the reference food.

Adapted from U.S. FDA CFSAN: *A food labeling guide*, 1994, rev. 1999. Available at www.cfsan.fda.gov/~dms/flg-6a.html. Accessed October 12, 2003.

*A reference food is a non–nutritionally altered version of the same food product; for example, a regular chocolate cake mix would be the reference food for a chocolate cake mix labeled "low-fat," or a dissimilar food that may generally be substituted for the labeled food (e.g., potato chips for pretzels).

Box 1-2   Health Claims Permitted on Food Labels*

Calcium and Reduction in the Risk of Osteoporosis

Foods or supplements must be "high" in bioavailable calcium and must not contain more phosphorus than calcium.

Sodium and Reduction in the Risk of Hypertension (High Blood Pressure)

Foods must meet the criteria for "low sodium."

Dietary Fat and Reduction in Cancer Risk

Foods must meet the definition of "low fat," the claim must refer to total fat rather than any specific type of fat, and the claim must be limited to "some cancers" or "some types of cancers."

Dietary Saturated Fat and Cholesterol and Reduction in Risk of Coronary Heart Disease

Foods must meet the definition of "low saturated fat," "low cholesterol," and "low fat."

Fiber-Containing Grain Products, Fruits, and Vegetables and Reduction of Cancer Risk

Foods must meet the definition for "low fat" and, without fortification, be a "good source" of dietary fiber. The claim must not mention particular types of fiber.

Fruits, Vegetables, and Grain Products that Contain Fiber, Particularly Soluble Fiber, and Reduction in the Risk of Coronary Heart Disease

Food must meet the definition of "low saturated fat," "low cholesterol," and "low fat." It must contain, without fortification, at least 0.6 g soluble fiber per reference amount, and the soluble fiber amount must be listed.

Fruits and Vegetables and Reduction of Cancer Risk

Foods must meet the criteria for "low fat" and, without fortification, be a "good source" of fiber, vitamin A, or vitamin C.

Folate and Reduction in the Risk of Neural Tube Defects

Foods must meet the criteria for "good source" of folate and must not provide more than 100% of the Daily Value for vitamins A and D because of their potential risk to fetuses.

Continued

Box 1-2   Health Claims Permitted on Food Labels*—cont'd

Dietary Sugar Alcohol and Reduction in the Risk of Dental Caries (Cavities)

Foods or sugarless gums must meet the criteria for "sugar-free" and must contain a sugar alcohol that does not promote tooth decay.

Dietary Soluble Fiber, such as that Found in Whole Oats and Psyllium Seed Husk, and Reduction in the Risk of Coronary Heart Disease

Foods must meet the definition of "low saturated fat," "low cholesterol," and "low fat." Foods that contain whole oats or psyllium must provide at least 0.75 or 1.7 g soluble fiber per serving, respectively.

Adapted from U.S. FDA CFSAN: *A food labeling guide*, 1994, rev. 1999 and 2000. Available at www.cfsan.fda.gov/~dms/flg-6a.html. Accessed October 12, 2003.

The claims cannot state that a particular food or nutrient will prevent disease; "may" and "might" are the preferred terms. The claims must state that disease risk depends on factors other than a particular food or nutrient. For example, regular exercise, in addition to calcium intake, reduces the risk of osteoporosis.

Some cultural food practices that are prevalent in the United States are summarized in Table 1-3. Native Americans are not included in the table because the eating patterns of such a diverse group are not easily categorized. Alcoholism is a serious problem among most Native American groups, however, and diabetes is increasingly common among many tribal groups, particularly those in the Southwest.

Two types of vegetarian diets are described in the table, but many others exist, including pescovegetarians, who avoid animal products except fish, and individuals who avoid red meats but eat all other animal products. Thus, the term *vegetarian* tells little about food intake, and the health care provider will need to get more information in order to assess the diet and determine whether intervention and teaching are needed. A new vegetarian food guide pyramid has been developed to aid in diet planning (Messina et al., 2003). The pyramid is similar to the standard Food Guide Pyramid described previously, but it suggests five servings of legumes, nuts,

Text continued on p. 42

Table 1-3 Cultural Food Practices

Characteristic Food Practices	Health Implications
African American*	
Cooking methods: Frying common; vegetables often boiled for prolonged periods and seasoned with salt pork (fat-back); gravy often served.	*Positives:* Many different vegetables consumed.
Foods enjoyed: Chicken, barbecue pork, ham, chitterlings (boiled or fried pig intestines), grits (coarsely ground corn that is boiled and usually served with cheese, butter or margarine), greens (especially collards, mustard), okra (boiled or fried), tomatoes, sweet and white potatoes, cornbread, biscuits, melons, peaches, pecans, and peanuts.	*Concerns:* Fat and sodium intake often high; many adults have little milk intake (lactose intolerance common); pica (eating nonfood items such as soil and clay) occurs especially among women and may inhibit iron absorption.
	Prevalent nutrition-related problems: Obesity, diabetes, hypertension, and heart disease; iron deficiency anemia among women.
Mexican American (also applies to some Central Americans)	
Cooking methods: Boiling, stewing; vegetables often cooked for a long time.	*Positives:* Wide variety of fruits and vegetables liked.

*This diet is often referred to as African American "soul food," but many African Americans have Southern roots. These foods and cooking methods are also typical "home cooking" of Southern whites.

Continued

Table 1-3   Cultural Food Practices—cont'd

Characteristic Food Practices	Health Implications
Foods enjoyed: Dry beans (pinto, garbanzo, black beans; beans often mashed and cooked with lard), beef, pork, chicken, fish, goat, eggs, hot sausage, tripe (beef stomach), rice, corn or flour tortillas, sweet pastries, cookies, candies (often candied fruits), chilies, pumpkin, chayote squash, corn, prickly pear cactus leaves (nopales), avocado, tomatoes, citrus, papaya, cilantro.	*Concerns:* High fat intake; lard used in Mexico and by recent immigrants; margarine, oils, and mayonnaise widely used in the U.S.; little milk used by adults; sugar intake high. *Prevalent nutrition-related problems:* Diabetes and obesity.
Puerto Rican *Cooking methods:* Frying, boiling, or simmering for prolonged periods with lard or salt pork for seasoning. *Foods enjoyed:* Café con leche (coffee with 2 to 5 oz milk), beans (esp. red or white), rice, pork, chicken, eggs, viandas (mixture of plantains, sweet potatoes, and green bananas), breadfruit, mango, avocado, corn, okra, chayote, safrito (relish of tomatoes, green peppers, chilies, onions, spices, and oil or lard).	*Positives:* Many fruits and vegetables used in Puerto Rico. *Concerns:* High fat intake; adults have little milk intake unless coffee intake is also high; foods used in Puerto Rico are often expensive on the North American mainland, so diets there may have little variety.

Food beliefs: Diseases are categorized as hot or cold, and foods are divided into hot, cold, and cool; suitability of a food in sickness or postpartum depends on its category; malt beer believed to be nutritious, often given to children and lactating women.

Prevalent nutrition-related problems: Obesity; megaloblastic anemia among women in the mainland because of poor folate intake.

Southeast Asian (Vietnamese, Cambodian)

Cooking methods: Stir-frying, steaming.
Foods enjoyed: Fish, duck, chicken, eggs, pork, tofu (soybean curd), chicken—rice noodle soup, green leafy vegetables, white rice, "cellophane" (bean starch) noodles, French bread and pastries, tea.

Positives: Low-fat cooking methods; limited intake of high-fat animal products; high complex carbohydrates and low sugar intakes.
Concerns: Little milk product use among adults.
Prevalent nutrition related problems: Osteoporosis among women, anemia, dental caries.

Japanese

Cooking methods: Stir-frying, steaming, broiling, simmering.
Foods enjoyed: Rice, noodles, many vegetables, fish, tofu and other soy products, pickles, green tea.

Positives: Traditional diet low in fat, high in complex carbohydrates, rich in vegetables.
Concerns: Japanese diet ~4 times as high in sodium as American; gastric cancer rate high in Japan, probably related to use of dried, smoked fish high in nitrates; little milk intake among adults; raw fish

Continued

Table 1-3   Cultural Food Practices—cont'd

Characteristic Food Practices	Health Implications
Chinese *Cooking methods:* Broiling, steaming, frying, or simmering. *Foods enjoyed:* Rice, noodles, tofu and other soybean products, pork, chicken, many vegetables, tea.	(sashimi) consumed by Japanese, potential for food poisoning and tapeworms. *Positives:* Vegetables used often. *Concerns:* Sodium intake can be high; lactose intolerance common among adults.
Former Soviet Union *Cooking methods:* Boiling, steaming, stewing, pickling of vegetables. *Foods enjoyed:* Breads, rice, pasta, dumplings, pancakelike breads (blini, oladi), cabbage, potatoes, beets, cucumbers, mushrooms, carrots, berries, pears, cherries, grapes, apples, goose, fresh or smoked salted fish, ground beef, cold cuts, eggs, oil, butter, salad dressings, sour cream or soured milk, whole milk, tea, jams.	*Positives:* Frequent use of grain products (encourage whole-grain breads and flours); use of vegetables in soups, stuffed pastries, salads. *Concerns:* Very high-fat diet; sodium intake can be high (pickled vegetables, salted fish). *Prevalent nutrition-related problems:* Heart disease, a tradition of heavy alcohol use.

Jewish

Cooking methods: Boiling, stewing, many meats salted; "Kashruth," or Jewish food laws, are followed; milk products and meat are not combined in food preparation; utensils used to prepare or serve meat not used for milk products and vice versa; milk consumption must occur at least 3 to 6 hours after meat; "pareve" foods (e.g., fish, eggs, some margarines, and breads) contain neither meat nor dairy products and may be used with either.

Foods enjoyed: Milk, cheese, eggs, fish with scales and fins, wide variety of vegetables, fruits, and breads; beef, lamb, poultry must be slaughtered and prepared in kosher manner; packaged foods are marked with a K, U, or other symbol to indicate that they are kosher.

Foods not used: Pork, horsemeat, or meat of any other 4-footed animal that does not chew a cud and/or have split, hooves; fish without fins and scales; shellfish; insects; reptiles; during Passover (8 days in spring), certain foods (e.g., bread products) must be "kosher for Passover" and no leavenings are used.

Positives: A wide variety of foods from all groups are included in the Kashruth.

Concerns: Meats salted; fasting is practiced several times a year, but pregnant and nursing women and sick individuals are not required to fast; wine is a necessary part of the Passover seder, but grape juice may be substituted or very small amounts of wine consumed.

Continued

Table 1-3   Cultural Food Practices—cont'd

Characteristic Food Practices	Health Implications
Ovolactovegetarian (e.g., Seventh-Day Adventist)	*Positives:* Lower rates of certain cancers than general population; diet tends to be lower fat; provides all known nutrients.
Cooking methods: All.	*Concerns:* Iron and zinc intake must be assessed.
Foods enjoyed: Milk and milk products, eggs, all fruits, vegetables, soy, and grain products; Seventh-Day Adventists use cereal-based beverages (Postum) and meat analogues made from soy or other vegetable proteins.	
Foods not used: Meat, poultry, fish; Seventh-Day Adventists avoid caffeinated beverages.	
Strict Vegetarian (e.g., vegan)	*Positives:* Tends to be low in fat and high in fiber, reducing risk of heart disease, obesity, and some cancers; combining grains, legumes, nuts, and seeds yields adequate protein.
Cooking methods: All, steaming and stir-frying popular.	
Foods enjoyed: Grains (esp. whole grains), fruits, vegetables, soy and fermented soy products, oils, nuts and seeds.	

Foods not used: Any animal products (milk, eggs, cheese, yogurt, meat, fish, poultry); some avoid fortified and processed foods.

Concerns: Vitamin B_2 is found only in foods of animal origin, supplements, and fortified foods; fermented soy products (miso and tempeh) are not reliable sources of vitamin B_{12}; calcium intake often low; absorption of iron and zinc often poor; inadequate energy density for optimal growth in children.

Middle Eastern (Syria, Lebanon, Turkey, Jordan, Iraq, Iran, Greece, Israel, Egypt)

Cooking methods: Meats cooked in a large amount of animal fat (butter or ghee, a clarified butter from sheep, goat, or camel milk) or oil (olive, sesame).

Foods enjoyed: Breads (have almost sacred status), rice, pilaf, beans, lentils, yogurt, cheese, lamb, goat, olives, cucumbers, citrus, onions, tomatoes, eggplant, dates, figs, pomegranates, baklava (layered pastry with honey and nuts), seasonings of cinnamon, mint, and oregano.

Foods not used: Muslims avoid alcohol and pork.

Positives: Fruit served for dessert except on special occasions; breads usually whole-grain and rich in fiber; yogurt used in many foods; avoidance of alcohol-related health problems by Muslims.

Concerns: High-fat cooking methods; females assigned lower status by some Middle Easterners, so may have to eat after males; quantity and variety of available food less for females; fasting during daylight hours required of Muslims for the month of Ramadan; pregnant and lactating women, travelers, or the sick may delay the fast until later in the year.

or other protein sources and eight servings of calcium-rich foods daily. One half cup (120 ml) of cow milk or 21 g (¾ oz) of cheese is one calcium-rich serving. Individuals who do not use dairy products can obtain one calcium serving by consuming alternatives such as 120 ml calcium-fortified juice; 28 g (1 oz) fortified breakfast cereal; 240 ml (1 cup) cooked greens, bok choy, okra, or broccoli (or 480 ml of the uncooked vegetables); or 60 ml (¼ cup) almonds.

Additional information is available online in the series *Cultural Diversity: Eating in America*, at http://ohioline.osu.edu/hyg-fact/5000.

Physiologic Influences on Nutrition: Digestion and Absorption

During digestion, foods are broken down mechanically by chewing and by mixing motions in the stomach and small intestine. Most carbohydrates, proteins, and fats in the diet are too large to be absorbed even after this mechanical breakdown and must be further digested by enzymes (proteins that produce chemical changes in specific nutrients) in the lumen or brush border of the intestine (Figure 1-4).

Energy-Providing Nutrients and the Products of Their Digestion
Carbohydrates

Carbohydrates can be large, small, or intermediate in size. *Polysaccharides* such as the starches are the largest carbohydrates. They are found in grains, legumes, potatoes, and other vegetables. Polysaccharides are formed from many *monosaccharide* (glucose, fructose, mannose, or galactose) units, and they must be broken down into monosaccharides or small oligosaccharides so that they can be absorbed. *Dextrins* and *oligosaccharides* are compounds made up of chains of glucose molecules (usually 3 to 20 glucose units). They are formed during digestion of starch, and they are used commercially in the manufacturing of medical foods for enteral tube feedings and nutritional supplements. *Disaccharides* are sugars composed of two monosaccharides. Sucrose is a disaccharide composed of glucose and fructose. It is found in table sugar, brown sugar, maple syrup, and molasses. Lactose is a disaccharide found in milk and consisting of glucose and galactose. Maltose is a

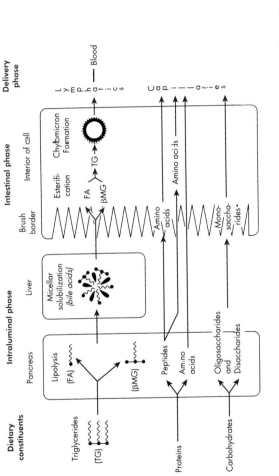

Figure 1-4

Digestion and absorption of triglycerides (fat), proteins, and carbohydrates. *FA*, Fatty acid; *MG*, monoglyceride; *TG*, triglyceride.

(From Silverman A, Roy CC: *Pediatric clinical gastroenterology*, ed 3, St Louis, 1983, Mosby.)

disaccharide consisting of two glucose molecules; maltose is not common in the diet, but it is produced during digestion of starch. In addition to being building blocks for larger carbohydrates, the monosaccharides glucose and fructose are found by themselves in foods such as honey and fruits. Monosaccharides and disaccharides are often called *simple sugars.*

Proteins

Dietary *proteins* are compounds made up of hundreds of *amino acids,* or nitrogen-containing molecules. During the digestion of a protein, *polypeptides* (or compounds containing fewer than 100 amino acids) and *peptides* (shorter chains of amino acids) are formed from the protein. These intermediate products must be further digested into amino acids or dipeptides and tripeptides (compounds containing two or three amino acids) to be absorbed. After absorption, the dipeptides and tripeptides are further digested to amino acids, which can be used for synthesis of body proteins.

Fats or lipids

Most dietary fat, and most fat stored in the body, is in the form of *triglycerides* (see Figure 1-1). A triglyceride is a molecule formed from glycerol, a three-carbon alcohol, bonded (esterified) to three fatty acids. A *fatty acid* is a chain of carbon atoms (usually two to 22 atoms long) with hydrogen attached; the chain contains a methyl group (CH_3) on one end and an acid group (COOH) on the other end. Fatty acids can be saturated (with no carbon-carbon double bonds) or unsaturated (with one or more carbon-carbon double bonds). Triglycerides must be digested into smaller forms to be absorbed. A *diglyceride* is a molecule composed of glycerol bound to two fatty acids; it is produced during triglyceride digestion. A diglyceride is broken down further, into a *monoglyceride* (a molecule composed of glycerol bound to one fatty acid) or to glycerol and fatty acids, and these products can be absorbed.

Process of Digestion and Absorption

Table 1-4 summarizes the major enzymes involved in digestion, the sites where they are released, and the products of their action. Most nutrients are absorbed in the duodenum, jejunum, and ileum (Figure 1-5); therefore, damage to or surgical removal of a significant portion of the small intestine often leads to malabsorption of a nutrient or nutrients. Fat malabsorption is especially likely because

Table 1-4   Summary of the Major Digestive Enzymes

Enzyme	Site of Production	Process of Digestion
Carbohydrate Digestion		
Salivary amylase	Mouth	Starch → Oligosaccharides, dextrins, and maltose
Pancreatic amylase	Pancreas (released into intestine)	Starch → Oligosaccharides, dextrins, and maltose
"Brush border" enzymes	Small intestine (inside mucosal cell)	
Isomaltase and Glucoamylase		Oligosaccharides and dextrins → Maltose and glucose
Lactase		Lactose → Glucose and galactose
Maltase		Maltose → Glucose
Sucrase		Sucrose → Glucose and fructose
Protein Digestion		
Pepsin	Stomach	Proteins → Polypeptides
Trypsin, chymotrypsin	Pancreas (released into small intestine)	Proteins, polypeptides → Small polypeptides
Carboxypeptidase	Pancreas (released into small intestine)	Polypeptides → Small peptides, amino acids

Continued

Table 1-4   Summary of the Major Digestive Enzymes—cont'd

Enzyme	Site of Production	Process of Digestion
Aminopeptidase	Intestine	Polypeptides, small peptides → Smaller peptides, amino acids
Dipeptidase	Intestine	Dipeptides → Amino acids
Fat Digestion		
Lingual lipase (significant only in infants); gastric lipase	Mouth; stomach	Triglycerides → Diglycerides (glycerol linked to 2 fatty acids), monoglycerides (glycerol linked to 1 fatty acid), glycerol, fatty acids
Lipase	Pancreas (released into small intestine)	Fat → Diglycerides, monoglycerides, glycerol, fatty acids

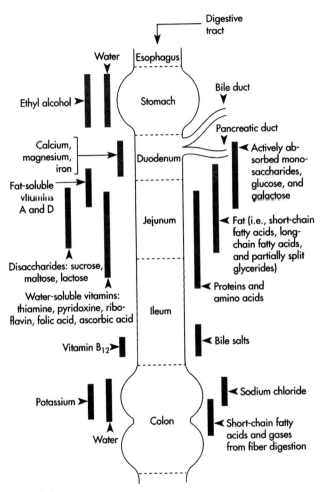

Figure 1-5
Sites of nutrient absorption.
(From Heimburger DC, Weinsier RL: *Handbook of clinical nutrition*, ed 3, St Louis, 1997, Mosby.)

fat and fat-soluble vitamin absorption is a complicated process requiring adequate production of bile salts and adequate bowel surface area for absorption (see Chapter 8). Bile salts are reabsorbed in the ileum and reused, and therefore an intact ileum is needed for normal fat absorption.

REFERENCES

Center for Nutrition Policy and Promotion (CNPP), US Department of Agriculture: *The food guide pyramid update.* Available at www.cnpp.usda.gov/pyramid-update. Accessed December 10, 2003.

Dietary Guidelines Advisory Committee: *Meeting summary*, Washington, DC, September 23, 2003. Available at www.cnpp.usda.gov/dietary_guidelines. Accessed December 10, 2003.

Food and Nutrition Board, National Academy of Sciences, Institute of Medicine: *Dietary reference intakes: calcium, phosphorus, magnesium, vitamin D, and fluoride*, Washington, DC, 1999, National Academy Press.

Food and Nutrition Board, National Academy of Sciences, Institute of Medicine: *Dietary reference intakes for thiamin, riboflavin, niacin, vitamin B_6, folate, vitamin B_{12}, pantothenic acid, biotin, and choline*, Washington, DC, 2000a, National Academy Press.

Food and Nutrition Board, National Academy of Sciences, Institute of Medicine: *Dietary reference intakes for vitamin C, vitamin E, selenium, and carotenoids,* Washington, DC, 2000b, National Academy Press.

Food and Nutrition Board, National Academy of Sciences, Institute of Medicine: *Dietary reference intakes for vitamin A, vitamin K, arsenic, boron, chromium, copper, iodine, iron, manganese, molybdenum, nickel, silicon, vanadium, and zinc,* Washington, DC, 2002a, National Academy Press.

Food and Nutrition Board, National Academy of Sciences, Institute of Medicine: *Dietary reference intakes for energy, carbohydrate, fiber, fat, fatty acids, cholesterol, protein, and amino acids (macronutrients),* Washington, DC, 2002b, National Academy Press.

US Department of Health and Human Services: *Healthy people 2010,* Washington, DC, 2000, USDHHS.

Messina V, Melina V, Mangels AR: A new food guide for North American vegetarians, *J Am Dietet Assoc* 103:771, 2003.

US Department of Agriculture, US Department of Health and Human Services: *Nutrition and your health: dietary guidelines for Americans,* ed 5, Washington, DC, 2000, USDA and USDHHS.

SELECTED BIBLIOGRAPHY

Gans KM et al: Baseline fat-related dietary behaviors of white, Hispanic, and black participants in a cholesterol screening and education project in New England, *J Am Diet Assoc* 103:699, 2003.

Graves DE, Suitor CW: *Celebrating diversity—approaching families through their food,* Arlington, VA, 1998, National Center for Education in Maternal and Child Health.

Milner JA: Functional foods and health: a US perspective, *Br J Nutr* 88(suppl 2):S151, 2002.

Position of the American Dietetic Association and Dietitians of Canada: Vegetarian diets, *J Am Dietet Assoc* 103:748, 2003.

Schneeman BO: Gastrointestinal physiology and functions, *Br J Nutr* 88(suppl 2):S159, 2002.

Thomas J: Nutrition intervention in ethnic minority groups, *Proc Nutr Soc* 61:559, 2002.

Xie B et al: Effects of ethnicity, family income, and education on dietary intake among adolescents, *Prev Med* 36:30, 2003.

Nutrition Assessment

2

An individual's nutritional status affects performance, well-being, growth and development, and resistance to illness. **Nutrition assessment** is the process used to evaluate nutritional status, identify disorders of nutrition, and determine which individuals need nutritional instruction and/or nutrition support.

Types of Malnutrition

Malnutrition includes both undernutrition and overnutrition. It can result from inadequate intake; disorders of digestion, absorption, or assimilation; or excessive intake of nutrients.

Undernutrition

Protein-energy malnutrition

Protein-energy malnutrition (PEM) or **protein-calorie malnutrition (PCM)** is defined as undernutrition resulting from inadequate intake, digestion, or absorption of protein and/or energy. Weight loss, fat loss, muscle wasting and weakness, impaired immune function, poor wound healing, and reduction of protein synthesis are characteristics of PEM. Two forms of PEM are termed *marasmus* and *kwashiorkor*. Marasmus describes a condition in which weight loss and wasting of muscle and fat are the predominant signs. It occurs when intake of energy nutrients are inadequate to meet the person's needs, such as under conditions of famine. Kwashiorkor, on the other hand, refers to a condition in which the most evident symptoms are related to impaired protein synthesis. Levels of serum proteins such as albumin, prealbumin or transthyretin (a protein participating in thyroxine transport), and retinol binding protein are reduced. These proteins are termed *visceral proteins*, since they are produced by the liver. Serum oncotic pressure (a function of serum protein concentrations) falls in kwashiorkor, allowing edema and sometimes ascites to develop. In severe kwashiorkor, skin lesions, changes in hair color (including flag sign, in which individual strands of hair demonstrate banding of different color), and hepatomegaly (largely due to fatty infiltration of the liver resulting from impaired ability to synthesize the lipoproteins that transport lipid from the liver to other tissues) are evident. Classically, kwashiorkor has been viewed as a disease occurring when energy intake is adequate or near-adequate but protein intake is very low; it was first described in African infants weaned from human milk to a diet consisting almost entirely of cereal. It can occur in developed countries among children and adults with inadequate vegetarian or alternative diet patterns (Carvalho et al., 2001; Liu et al., 2001).

PEM occurs not only in developing countries but among ill individuals in all nations when their intakes are inadequate to meet their needs for energy and tissue synthesis. It has been suggested that kwashiorkor among sick patients results at least partly from the presence of inflammation and that the signs and symptoms of kwashiorkor are brought about by elevated levels of the inflammatory **cytokines** (immunoregulatory proteins such as the interleukins, tumor necrosis factor, and interferon that are secreted by cells, especially those of the immune system). In any case, inflammation and trauma can alter serum protein levels so that they are not reliable indicators of PEM (see the later section Biochemical or Laboratory Analyses).

Vitamin and mineral deficiencies

Vitamin and mineral deficiencies develop in a progressive manner, with depletion of tissue stores occurring first, followed by biochemical abnormalities (e.g., decrease in activity of enzymes requiring a particular vitamin or mineral), and finally the development of overt clinical signs and symptoms. The clinical signs and symptoms may be subtle and nonspecific (e.g., cracking skin may be a sign of deficiency of riboflavin or biotin or a sign of excess vitamin A intake). The most common nutritional disease in this category is iron deficiency anemia. Suboptimal intakes of vitamins and minerals may result in adverse outcomes even if overt deficiency is not present. For example, inadequate folate intake among women in the childbearing years contributes to births of infants with neural tube defects, even though macrocytic anemia (which can be a nutritional deficiency disease resulting from folate deficiency) is not prevalent.

It is common for multiple vitamin and mineral deficits to be present or for these deficits to occur in conjunction with PEM. For example, the individual who consumes no animal products is at risk of deficiency of vitamin B_{12}, calcium, iron, and zinc; additionally, protein and energy intake may be suboptimal unless the diet is carefully planned.

Overnutrition

The most common forms of overnutrition, present in more than half of American adults, are overweight and obesity. Overweight and obesity refer to an excess of body fat, but for simplicity they are often defined as being 10% and 20%, respectively, greater than the ideal body weight. These conditions are associated with numerous health risks, including hypertension, heart disease, type 2 diabetes, stroke, gallbladder disease, osteoarthritis, sleep apnea and other respiratory disorders, and certain cancers.

Overnutrition can also occur with excessive intakes of fat-soluble vitamins and some minerals. For instance, excessive intake of vitamin A, especially an intake of 10 mg or more daily over a period of several months, can cause increased intracranial pressure, liver damage, bone and joint pain, and scaly skin. Water-soluble vitamins are usually excreted in the urine without ill effects, but very large amounts of these vitamins may also result in side effects. Megadoses of vitamin C (usually more than 1 g/day), for example, can cause diarrhea, false-negative results on tests for occult blood in the stool, and interference with anticoagulant therapy.

Assessment Procedures

Assessment of nutritional status has four components:

A, anthropometric measurements
B, biochemical or laboratory analyses
C, clinical (physical) assessment
D, diet or nutritional history

Anthropometric Measurements

Anthropometric measurements are measurements of the human body. Essential measurements include height (or length for children less than 2 to 3 years) and weight. Head circumference is included for children less than 2 years of age. Anthropometric measurements are sometimes compared with standard measurements. Appendix C lists healthy weight for height for adults. An estimate of the ideal body weight (IBW) for adults may also be obtained with these rules of thumb:

Women: IBW = 100 lb for the first 5 ft of height + 5 lb for every inch over 5 ft

Men: IBW = 106 lb for the first 5 ft of height + 6 lb for every inch over 5 ft

Using these equations, the desirable body weight is within 10% of the estimated IBW. These simple equations yield only rough estimates of IBW. Because of variations in body build and other factors, the values determined by these equations may not be very accurate for a particular individual.

The **body mass index (BMI)** is a simple tool for evaluating the appropriateness of weight for height (Box 2-1). It does not involve measurement of body composition, and thus it is not an accurate method for assessing the percentage of lean body mass or fat. However, the BMI correlates well with many measures of body fat content, as well as with risk of morbidity. In addition, it is quickly and easily performed in virtually any setting. A chart for determining BMI without making any calculations can be found inside the back cover of this book, and an automatic BMI calculator can be found on the World Wide Web at http://www.nhlbisupport.com/bmi/.

Appendix D contains the standardized growth charts for children, showing percentile rankings of height and weight for age and weight for height, as well as BMI for age. In long-term undernutrition, children exhibit growth retardation, with height low in relation to expected height for age. (Length or height will be below the 5th percentile). Short stature is also found in endocrine and other disorders unrelated to nutrition in children. When short-term undernutrition has occurred, height may be normal for age but weight will be low for height. (Weight for height below the 5th percentile indicates undernutrition; see Appendix D.) Overweight children have a weight for height or BMI that is above the 95th percentile. Those with a BMI between the 85th and 95th percentile are at risk for overweight.

Adjustments to ideal or desirable body weights

Certain physical body changes require adjustments to the ideal or desirable body weights. For amputees, reduce IBW by the

---

Box 2-1   Body Mass Index (BMI)*

Calculating BMI

$$BMI = \frac{Weight\ (kg)}{Height^2\ (m)} \quad OR \quad BMI = \frac{Weight\ (lb)}{Height^2\ (in)} \times 704.5$$

Example: An individual weighs 65 kg (143 lb), and is 1.7 m (5′7″) tall.

BMI = $65/(1.7)^2 = 22.5$ kg/m^2

Classification of BMI

Underweight: <18.5

Normal: 18.5-24.9

Overweight: 25.0-29.9

Obese: ≥30.0

Extreme obesity ≥40.0

Classification is from the *Clinical guidelines on the identification, evaluation, and treatment of overweight and obesity in adults*, Washington, DC, 1998, NHLBI and NIDDK.

*A nomogram for determining BMI without making any calculations can be found inside the back cover.

following percentages, depending on the extremity lost: hand and forearm, 2.3%; total arm, 5%; foot and lower leg, 6%; and total leg, 16%. These percentages are derived largely from white individuals and may require some adjustment for other racial and ethnic groups. Blacks have proportionally longer lower extremities, and Chinese have shorter extremities than whites. The calculations are based on height, so preamputation values must be used for individuals with loss of both lower extremities. For paraplegic individuals, IBW is approximately 5% to 10% less than the calculated value, and for quadriplegic individuals, IBW is 10% to 15% less than calculated.

For bed-ridden individuals and those with severe spinal curvature, total height may be estimated from knee height. To measure knee height, bend the knee 90 degrees and measure from the heel to the anterior surface of the thigh:

Men: height in cm = $71.85 + (1.88 \times K)$

Women: height in cm = $70.25 - (0.06 \times A) + (1.87 \times K)$

A = age in years, K = knee height in cm

Body composition

The body composition—particularly the relative proportions of body fat and lean body mass (or fat-free mass) and the distribution of body fat—is much more relevant to health and fitness than the simple determination of the appropriateness of weight for body weight. Numerous methods are available for measuring body composition (Box 2-2).

Not only total body fat but also regional distribution of fat is important in relation to long-term health. Abdominal fat is a predictor of cardiovascular risk, and abdominal fat exists in more than depot, including the deep fat associated with the visceral organs **(visceral fat)** and the more superficial subcutaneous abdominal fat. Visceral fat is especially closely related to health risk. Only a limited number of the available methods (i.e., computerized tomography [CT] and magnetic resonance imaging) assess visceral fat. CT and dual energy x-ray absorptiometry (DEXA) involve radiation exposure, albeit a very small amount with DEXA. This is a consideration in vulnerable populations such as pregnant women and children, as well in performing repeated measurements in the same subject.

Biochemical or Laboratory Analyses

Good clinical judgment must be used in selecting laboratory analyses to be performed and interpreting test results. A thorough physical assessment and nutritional history can be as effective in identifying many cases of malnutrition as a battery of laboratory analyses.

Laboratory assessment of protein nutritional status is especially difficult (Table 2-1). Circulating proteins provide the simplest index of protein nutrition, but their serum or plasma concentrations rise and fall in sick or injured individuals for many reasons that have little to do with nutrition. The liver increases synthesis and release of **acute-phase reactants**, such as C-reactive protein, fibrinogen, serum amyloid A, and α_1-acid glycoprotein, in response to injury, trauma, inflammation, and infection. The same conditions can suppress circulating levels of albumin, transferrin, and prealbumin (*reverse acute-phase reactants),* as hepatic protein synthesis priorities are directed toward the acute-phase reaction. Fluid loss and fluid resuscitation also alter serum protein concentrations. A thorough physical assessment and diet/nutritional history provides

---

Box 2-2   Methods of Assessing Body Composition

Anthropometric Measurements

- Height and weight

  Description: Weight is measured with a calibrated scale and height with a stadiometer.

  Advantages: Inexpensive; easy to perform; readily obtained; can be used for calculation of BMI, which correlates well with other measures of body fatness.

  Disadvantages: No direct information about total body fat* or regional fat distribution.

- Skinfold measurements

  Description: Skinfold(s) are measured with calipers at one or more sites, e.g., triceps (Figure 2-1), subscapular, suprailiac, and midthigh.

  Advantages: Inexpensive, easy to perform, correlate well with size of subcutaneous fat deposits.

  Disadvantages: Substantial intra- and interobserver variation in measurements; skinfolds may be too large to measure with calipers in obese individuals; inaccurate when edema is present in the area measured; subcutaneous fat distribution may vary among races.

- Waist circumference

  Description: The circumference is measured in a standing subject at the level of the iliac crest, at the end of normal expiration. The measuring tape must be parallel to the floor and snug, without compressing the skin.

  Advantages: Inexpensive; easy to perform; highly correlated with visceral fat, with waist circumferences of 102 cm (40 in) in men and 88 cm (35 in) in women indicating risk for the metabolic syndrome (see Chapter 5); may be more predictive of cardiovascular risk in some groups, such as Asian Americans, than BMI measurement.

  Disadvantages: Visceral adiposity may vary among racial and ethnic groups.

Tissue Conductivity Techniques

- Bioimpedance analysis (BIA)

  Description: BIA requires passage of small electrical current, undetectable to the individual, between two electrodes placed on the body. Tissues rich in water (muscle and other lean tissues) are good electrical conductors,

Box 2-2   Methods of Assessing Body Composition—cont'd

whereas fat is a poor conductor. BIA measures body water and from that estimates fat content.

Advantages: Relatively inexpensive, portable equipment; easy and fast to perform; reproducible; can measure intra- and extracellular water compartments; segmental analysis allows estimation of muscle and fluid in segments of the body, e.g., trunk or extremity.

Disadvantages: Accuracy is affected by numerous factors that may be hard to control: changes in hydration, electrolyte concentrations, hematocrit, and skin temperature (fever or cold exposure), as well as recent eating, drinking, exercise, and position changes; inaccurate in cases of limb amputation or regional alterations of skeletal muscle, e.g., muscular dystrophy.

Comments: To decrease error, measurements should be taken after at least 4 h of fasting and sedentary activity and 10 min after assuming a supine position. Do not use in individuals with a cardiac pacemaker or implantable defibrillator.

■ Total body electrical conductivity (TOBEC)

Description: The subject is surrounded by a low-level electromagnetic field in a detection chamber; the conductivity of hydrated tissues allows estimation of fat vs. FFM.

Advantages: Easy and fast to perform; reproducible; accurate.

Disadvantages: Expensive equipment; not widely available; little information about regional fat distribution.

■ Near-infrared interactance

Description: A wand emitting near-infrared wavelengths of light is applied to the midpoint of the biceps in the dominant arm (midway between the antecubital fossa and axilla), and FFM and fat mass are differentiated by the relative amounts of light reflected and absorbed (FFM reflects and fat absorbs the light).

Advantages: Relatively inexpensive, portable equipment; easy and fast to perform; reproducible.

Disadvantages: Accuracy is not as high as some of the other methods requiring instrumentation, and error may

Continued

Box 2-2   Methods of Assessing Body Composition—cont'd

be greatest with very lean and very obese; no data for
children under 5 years; little information about regional
fat distribution.

Density Measurements
- Hydrodensitometry or underwater weighing
  Description: The subject exhales maximally and is
  weighed while submerged in water, and pulmonary
  residual volume is measured and deducted from the volume of water displaced. Fat mass and fat-free mass
  (FFM) are estimated from standard density measurements for fat and FFM derived from cadavers.
  Advantages: Reproducible; easy to perform.
  Disadvantages: Not suited to subjects that are unable or
  unwilling to be totally submerged in water; depends on
  accurate measurement of pulmonary reserve volume;
  provides no information about regional fat distribution.
- Air displacement plethysmography (Bod Pod)
  Description: Displacement of air is measured while the
  person sits inside a small chamber; calculation is similar
  to that for hydrodensitometry.
  Advantages: Reproducible, easy to perform, suited to individuals up to 227 kg (500 lb).
  Disadvantages: Depends on accurate measurement of pulmonary reserve volume; subject must remain very still,
  with no change in breathing during test; provides no
  information about fat distribution.

Imaging Techniques
- Dual energy x-ray absorptiometry (DEXA) or dual x-ray
  absorptiometry (DXA)
  Description: Two x-ray beams with differing energies are
  passed through the body; their attenuation is used to
  estimate bone mineral density, fat mass, and lean body
  mass.
  Advantages: Reproducible; easy to perform; provides a
  "multicompartment model," i.e., is able to separate the
  mass of bone from other FFM.

Box 2-2   Methods of Assessing Body Composition—cont'd

Disadvantages: Radiation exposure (very low); expensive equipment, requires trained radiology personnel to administer and interpret the scan; most current equipment is limited to use in individuals weighing 136 kg (300 lb) or less.

- Computerized tomography (CT)

  Description: Radiographic and computer analysis are used to determine the structure of internal organs.

  Advantages: Provides a very accurate indication of regional body composition, e.g., visceral and subcutaneous abdominal fat.

  Disadvantages: Radiation exposure (significant); expensive equipment, requires trained radiology personnel to administer and interpret the scan; infants and small children usually need sedation to remain still.

- Magnetic resonance imaging (MRI)

  Description: A powerful magnet is used to alter motion of atoms within the body; from these changes, computerized images of internal body tissues are produced.

  Advantages: Provides an indication of regional body composition; enhanced technology has made it possible to measure fat stores within the muscle and the liver; no radiation exposure.

  Disadvantages: Expensive equipment, requires trained personnel to administer and interpret the scan; subject must be completely still (infants and small children usually need sedation).

- Ultrasonography

  Description: A two-dimensional image of internal body structures is formed via use of ultrasonic frequencies.

  Advantages: Equipment relatively widely available; no radiation exposure.

  Disadvantages: Moderately expensive, requires skilled technicians to perform the tests.

Isotopic Techniques

- Isotope dilution

  Description: Two fluid samples (blood, saliva, or urine) are collected: one just before administration of a radioactive

Continued

Box 2-2   Methods of Assessing Body Composition—cont'd

or stable (nonradioactive) isotope, to determine the natural background levels, and the second sample after waiting a sufficient amount of time for the isotope to equilibrate within the body. Typically the subject drinks water labeled with deuterium (^{2}H), tritium (^{3}H), or ^{18}O to label the body water pool; urine samples are collected for isotope analysis. Total body water is calculated, and from this fat mass and FFM are estimated.

Advantages: No radiation exposure if stable isotopes such as deuterium or ^{18}O are used; with the "double-labeled water" technique, water can be labeled with both deuterium and ^{18}O, allowing simultaneous measurement of body composition and energy expenditure in free-living individuals going about their daily activities.

Disadvantages: Moderately expensive; requires skilled technicians to analyze the samples; no measurement of regional body composition.

■ Total body potassium

Description: The body is scanned for the presence of gamma emissions from trace amounts of naturally occurring radioactive potassium, which is concentrated in the FFM.

Advantages: No radiation exposure; accurate and reproducible.

Disadvantages: Very expensive; equipment not widely available; no measure of regional fat distribution.

FFM, Fat-free mass.

*Formulas have been developed for estimation of % total body fat from BMI in U.S. adults. For females, % body fat is estimated as follows: European Americans = 79.145 − 1105.59 × 1/BMI; African Americans = 76.955 − 1072.573 × 1/BMI; Hispanic Americans = 73.175 − 915.644 × 1/BMI. For males, % body fat is estimated as: European Americans = 64.813 − 1084.43 × 1/BMI; African Americans = 65.832 − 1146.108 × 1/BMI; Hispanic Americans = 69.622 − 1210.938 × 1/BMI. (From Fernandez JM et al: Is percentage body fat differentially related to body mass index in Hispanic Americans, African Americans, and European Americans? *Am J Clin Nutr* 77:71, 2003.)

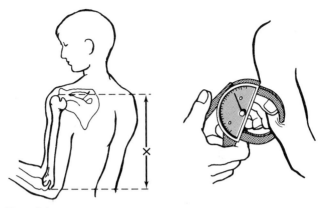

Figure 2-1
TSF measurements are performed at the midpoint of the upper arm.
(From Heimburger DC, Weinsier RL: *Handbook of clinical nutrition*, ed 3, St Louis, 1997, Mosby.)

more information about the presence of nutritional risk in acutely sick or injured individuals than measurement of circulating proteins does. However, serum protein measurements do have a role in monitoring the response of stable patients to nutritional therapy, and they can provide an objective measure of the redirection of liver protein synthesis away from the acute phase and toward visceral proteins. Prealbumin's short half-life and small body pool make it one of the most sensitive visceral proteins for assessment of nutritional status. (*Sensitivity* is the probability that a test indicates a nutrient deficiency, given that the person actually does have a deficiency. *Specificity* is the probability that a test indicates no nutrient deficiency, given that the person does not have a deficiency.)

Table 2-2 lists representative tests used in nutritional assessment of selected minerals and vitamins. Reference values for nutrition-related laboratory tests are provided in Appendix F. Blood, plasma, or serum concentrations are among the easiest values to obtain and the most commonly used tests for most vitamins and minerals. Nevertheless, with the exception of selenium, the circulating nutrient concentrations are unlikely to be sensitive or specific indicators of nutritional status. For many vitamins and minerals, homeostatic mechanisms maintain normal or near-normal circulating

Text continued on p. 67

Table 2-1 Laboratory Assessment of Protein Status

Protein Compartment and Test	Comments
Visceral proteins (serum or plasma proteins)	Synthesized in liver, decreased in liver disease; fall during the acute-phase response
Albumin	Long half-life (14-20 days) and thus relatively insensitive to nutritional change; lost in urine in nephrotic syndrome; "capillary leak" can cause loss from circulation in critical illness
Transferrin	Half-life 7-8 days; elevated in iron deficiency
Prealbumin (transthyretin)	Half-life 2-3 days
Retinol binding protein	Half-life 12-14 hours; elevated in renal failure
Somatic (muscle) proteins	Urinary excretion is an indicator of muscle mass
Creatinine excretion Expected 24-hr urinary excretion: 20 mg/kg body weight for children, 17 mg/kg for women, and 23 mg/kg for men	Requires accurate 24-hr urine collection; altered by renal failure; not a valid nutritional indicator in the presence of diseases affecting muscle
3-Methylhistidine (urine)	Specific indicator found only in muscle

Nitrogen balance Balance = [24-hour protein intake (g) × 0.16] − [24-hr urine urea nitrogen (g) + 4 g]*	Negative values occur when more nitrogen is lost than consumed (inadequate intake or catabolism), positive values are observed when more nitrogen is consumed than lost (e.g., nutritional repletion, growth, pregnancy) Requires accurate 24-hr urine collection and food intake records; altered by liver and renal failure

*Protein intake is multiplied by 0.16 because protein is approximately 16% nitrogen.
4 g represents an estimate of daily fecal and skin losses, but severe diarrhea, fistula drainage, exudative losses, and so forth can increase this value.

Table 2-2   Laboratory Assessment of Selected Minerals and Vitamins

Nutrient	Tissue Concentrations	Indicators of Body Stores	Functional Indices Associated with Deficiency
Iron	Serum iron	Plasma or serum ferritin concentration* Serum transferrin saturation† Plasma-soluble serum transferrin receptor concentration (sTfR; specific and sensitive but not yet universally available)	↓ Hgb, Hct, MCV (deficiency must be well advanced to be detected) ↑ Red cell distribution width (RDW) ↑ Erythrocyte protoporphyrin concentration
Calcium		Bone mineral density	
Zinc	Plasma zinc†	Red or white blood cell zinc Hair zinc Metallothionein monocyte messenger RNA (experimental, but promising results)	↓ Activity of zinc-dependent enzymes such as alkaline phosphatase, copper-zinc superoxide dismutase, lymphocyte 5′-nucleotidase
Iodine	Urine iodine		↑ Thyroid-stimulating hormone ↓ Thyroxine (T4) Thyroid gland enlargement (may also indicate tumor)

Selenium	Plasma selenium	↓ Plasma glutathione peroxidase activity
Copper	Plasma copper and ceruloplasmin (copper transport protein)	Hair and nail selenium	↓ Activity of copper-dependent enzymes such as cytochrome c oxidase in platelets and white blood cells
Folate	Serum or plasma folate	Red cell folate	↑ Urinary excretion of FIGLU following an oral dose of histidine (may also be ↑ in vitamin B_{12} deficiency) Macrocytic anemia (↓ Hct, ↓ Hgb, ↑ MCV; also a sign of B_{12} deficiency)
Vitamin A	Serum retinol	Minimal dose response (measure baseline serum retinol and repeat measurement after small dose of vitamin A)	
Vitamin C (ascorbic acid)	Serum ascorbate	Leukocyte ascorbate	
Vitamin K	Serum vitamin K		↑ Prothrombin time

Continued

Table 2-2 Laboratory Assessment of Selected Minerals and Vitamins—cont'd

Nutrient	Tissue Concentrations	Indicators of Body Stores	Functional Indices Associated with Deficiency
Vitamin B_{12}	Serum vitamin B_{12}		Macrocytic anemia ($\downarrow$ Hct, $\downarrow$ Hgb, $\uparrow$ MCV; also seen in folate deficiency)
Vitamin E	Serum tocopherol		$\uparrow$ Hemolysis (red cell peroxidation test)

FIGLU, Formiminoglutamate; *Hct,* hematocrit; *Hgb,* hemoglobin; *MCV,* mean (red blood) cell volume.

*Increased by acute-phase reaction, ethanol intake, and hyperglycemia. Directly correlated with BMI.

†Decreased during acute-phase reaction.

concentrations of the nutrient even though intake is inadequate and tissue stores are decreasing. However, alternative analyses are not always readily available. In many instances, measurements of tissue stores are poorly standardized (as in the case of hair and nail analyses) or difficult to apply on a wide basis. Functional tests (e.g., reduction in activity of an enzyme requiring a particular nutrient) are of great practical benefit, because they provide an indicator of a change in normal physiology and metabolism related to a nutritional deficit. To be most beneficial, functional indices must be specific for a deficiency of only one nutrient, a difficult criterion to meet. The most definitive indication of deficiency of many vitamins and minerals is the response to supplementation; for example, an increase in hemoglobin concentration within a month of initiating iron supplementation is consistent with the presence of iron deficiency.

Nutritional anemias

Nutritional anemias, resulting from deficiencies of iron, folate, vitamin B_{12}, and other nutrients, are characterized by low hematocrit and hemoglobin concentrations. In order to distinguish between the types of anemia, judicious use of laboratory tests is essential (Figure 2-2). However, caution must be used in interpreting the tests. For example, the mean cell volume (MCV), a measure of the red blood cell size, is useful in differentiating the types of anemia, but it may be misleading for a number of reasons: (1) the MCV is normal in the early stages of virtually all anemias; (2) the reticulocyte, an immature form of the red blood cell, is larger than the mature cell, so that a marked increase in reticulocytes (e.g., following an acute hemorrhage) can elevate the MCV; and (3) combined deficiencies, as of iron and folate, may result in a normal MCV. Ferritin is an acute-phase reactant, and this can complicate the diagnosis of iron deficiency when inflammation is present. Although not yet widely available, the serum transferrin receptor (sTfR) assay may prove to be a more sensitive indicator of iron deficiency. Bone marrow aspiration may be necessary to determine whether marrow iron is depleted (i.e., in iron deficiency) or normal to high (as it may be in anemia of chronic disease) and to differentiate nutritional and nonnutritional (e.g., hemolytic anemias, leukemia) causes of macrocytic anemia.

Anemia of chronic disease is a complex disorder that occurs in a variety of conditions, including infection, inflammation, renal

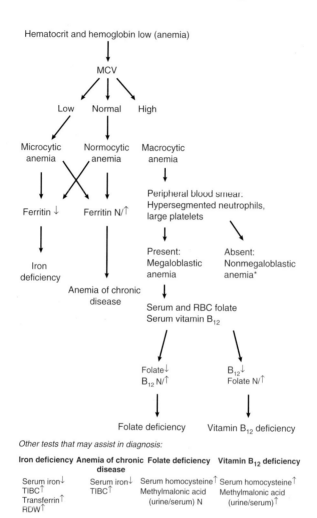

Figure 2-2

Decision tree for laboratory tests differentiating among nutritional anemias. Anemia of chronic disease is not a nutritional anemia but is among the most common disorders in hospitalized and chronically ill patients and may coexist with nutritional anemias. *MCV,* Mean cell volume; ↓, decreased; ↑, elevated; *N,* normal; *TIBC,* total iron binding capacity; *RBC,* red blood cell; *RDW,* red blood cell distribution width. *Nonnutritional anemia; requires further evaluation.

disease, and cancer. Contributing factors include suppression of bone marrow function by inflammatory cytokines, accelerated red blood cell breakdown with sequestration of iron in the reticuloendothelial system, and abnormalities in iron mobilization and delivery. Because of its prevalence among sick individuals, it is important to distinguish it from the nutritional anemias and recognize that it can occur concurrently with nutritional anemias.

If vitamin B_{12} deficiency is present, the cause (e.g., inadequate intake as in strict vegetarianism or inadequate absorption following ileal resection) must be determined. A subset of deficient individuals are lacking in intrinsic factor and are said to have pernicious anemia. Intrinsic factor, secreted in the stomach, is required for vitamin B_{12} absorption. The presence of anti–intrinsic factor antibodies in the serum or an abnormal result on the Schilling test (an indicator of B_{12} absorption in the presence and absence of intrinsic factor) is indicative of intrinsic factor deficiency. Lifetime parenteral or intranasal vitamin B_{12} therapy is required in intrinsic factor deficiency, while low-dose oral therapy (2 to 3 μg/day) will correct dietary inadequacy and large oral doses (1000 μg/day) may be sufficient to correct a deficiency caused by impaired absorption. Vitamin B_{12} deficiency is associated with nerve damage that results in numerous neuropsychiatric symptoms including abnormal gait, paresthesias, memory loss, disorientation, psychosis, spasticity, and visual loss (optic nerve atrophy). These symptoms may improve but are unlikely to be fully reversed with correction of the deficiency. Thus it is essential that B_{12} deficiency be diagnosed as early as possible and treated appropriately. High doses of folic acid can correct the anemia of vitamin B_{12} deficiency without correcting the nerve damage. Intake of folic acid from supplements and foods should be limited to 1 mg daily to reduce the risk of masking vitamin B_{12} deficiency. (Most over-the-counter folic acid supplements contain 0.4 mg in a daily dose, fortified cereals contain 0.1 mg folic acid per serving, and fortified flour and cornmeal provide 0.43 to 1.4 mg folic acid per pound [454 g].)

Clinical or Physical Assessment

Many nutrient deficiencies and excesses become apparent during careful physical assessment of the individual. Table 2-3 describes findings that may indicate malnutrition.

Table 2-3   Signs That Suggest Nutrient Imbalance

Area of Concern	Possible Deficiency	Possible Excess
Hair		
Dull, dry, brittle	Pro	
Easily plucked (with no pain)	Pro	
Hair loss	Pro, Zn, biotin	Vit A
Flag sign (loss of hair pigment in strips around head)	Pro, Cu	
Head and Neck		
Bulging fontanel (infants)		Vit A
Headache		Vit A, D
Epistaxis (nosebleed)	Vit K	
Thyroid enlargement	Iodine	
Eyes		
Conjunctival and corneal xerosis (dryness)	Vit A	
Pale conjunctiva	Fe	
Blue sclerae	Fe	
Corneal vascularization	Vit B$_2$	
Mouth		
Cheilosis or angular stomatitis (lesions at corners of mouth)	Vit B$_2$	

Finding	Nutrient	
Glossitis (red, sore tongue)	Niacin, folate, vit B_{12}, other B vit	
Gingivitis (inflamed gums)	Vit C	
Hypogeusia, dysgeusia (poor sense of taste, distorted taste)	Zn	
Dental caries	Fluoride	
Mottling of teeth		Fluoride
Atrophy of papillae on tongue	Fe, B vit	
Skin		
Dry, scaly	Vit A, Zn, EFA	
Follicular hyperkeratosis (resembles gooseflesh)	Vit A, EFA, B vit	Vit A
Eczematous lesions	Zn	
Petechiae, ecchymoses	Vit C, K	
Nasolabial seborrhea (greasy, scaly areas between nose and lip)	Niacin, vit B_{12}, B_6	
Darkening and peeling of skin in areas exposed to sun	Niacin	
Poor wound healing	Pro, Zn, vit C	
Nails		
Spoon-shaped nails	Fe	
Brittle, fragile	Pro	
Heart		
Enlargement, tachycardia, failure	Vit B_1	

Continued

Table 2-3   Signs That Suggest Nutrient Imbalance—cont'd

Area of Concern	Possible Deficiency	Possible Excess
Small heart	Energy	
Sudden failure, death	Se	
Arrhythmia	Mg, K, Se	
Hypertension	Ca, K	
Abdomen		
Hepatomegaly	Pro	Vit A
Ascites	Pro	
Musculoskeletal Extremities		
Muscle wasting (especially temporal area)	Energy	
Edema	Pro, vit B₁	
Calf tenderness	Vit B₁ or C, biotin, Se	
Beading of ribs, or "rachitic rosary" (child)	Vit C, D	
Bone and joint tenderness	Vit C, D, Ca, P	
Knock-knee, bowed legs, fragile bones	Vit D, Ca, P, Cu	

Neurologic	
Paresthesias (pain and tingling or altered sensation in the extremities)	Vit B_1, B_6, B_{12}, biotin
Weakness	Vit C, B_1, B_6, B_{12}, energy
Ataxia, decreased position and vibratory senses	Vit B_1, B_{12}
Tremor	Mg
Decreased tendon reflexes	Vit B_1
Confabulation, disorientation	Vit B_1, B_{12}
Drowsiness, lethargy	Vit B_1
Depression	Vit B_1, biotin, B_{12}
	Vit A, D

Pro, Protein; *vit*, vitamin(s); *Cu*, copper; *Fe*, iron; *K*, potassium; *Zn*, zinc; *EFA*, essential fatty acids; *Ca*, calcium; *Mg*, magnesium; *Na*, sodium; *Se*, selenium; *P*, phosphorus.

Diet or Nutritional History

Several methods can be used to obtain information about nutrient intake, depending upon the depth and type of information needed.

24-hour recall

The individual is asked to recall everything he or she consumed the previous day. If the previous day's intake was atypical for the person, a recent, more typical day may be substituted. A sample tool for collection of a 24-hour recall is shown in Box 2-3. The advantage of this method is that it is easily and quickly done; however, the person being interviewed may not be able to recall his or her intake accurately, and snacks, beverages, and supplements tend to be omitted. The interviewer must be trained in prompting and questioning the individual to obtain complete and accurate information. Serving sizes, in particular, may be reported incorrectly. Having available measuring cups, spoons, and dishes of different sizes may help the interviewee to describe serving sizes more accurately.

Food frequency questionnaire

The health professional collects information regarding the number of times per day, week, or month the individual eats particular foods. A sample tool, focusing on cholesterol and saturated fat intake, is shown in Box 2-4. When used with a 24-hour recall, the questionnaire can help validate the accuracy of the recall and provide a more complete picture of the individual's intake. If the goal of the nutritional history is to find out about intake of particular food components or nutrients (e.g., cholesterol and saturated fat), then the questionnaire can be designed to focus on those items. The food frequency method is economical in terms of time but provides limited information in comparison to some of the other methods that reveal time and circumstances of food intake, which may be of help in identifying and changing poor eating habits (e.g., nighttime snacking during television viewing).

Food record

In keeping a food record, the individual records all the foods he or she consumes, with portions weighed, measured, or estimated. Usually this is done for 3 days—a weekend day and 2 weekdays. The food record provides more information than the 24-hour recall, particularly in quantifying the amounts eaten. Nevertheless, a food

---

Box 2-3   24-Hour Recall

The following questions may be used to elicit a 24-hour recall:

1. What time did you get up yesterday? _____
2. When was the first time you had anything to eat or drink? _____ (Avoid mentioning specific meals, e.g., "What did you have for breakfast?")
   What did you have? How much? _____ (For each food, ask for details if type or preparation method is unclear, e.g., was chicken fried or baked?; was milk whole, low-fat, or skim?)
3. When did you eat or drink something again? _____
   What did you have and how much? _____
   (Repeat question 3 until the individual has described the entire day.)
4. Did you eat or drink anything else? _____ (Review the day with the individual to see if any snacks have been omitted.)
5. Did you put anything else in your mouth and swallow it? _____ (Ask specifically about supplements: vitamin/mineral, health foods, herbal medications, etc.) Do you usually take any supplements or herbal medications that you did not take yesterday? _____
6. Was this day's intake different from usual? If so, in what way? _____
7. Do you eat differently on weekends than on weekdays? If so, in what way? _____

---

record relies heavily on the individual's cooperation. Also, food intake may be atypical during the recording period. In some cases, the act of recording one's intake results in a change in eating patterns.

Food records are a valuable part of a program of weight control. Keeping food records on a regular basis increases the likelihood of success in weight loss and maintenance of weight loss.

Diet history

The individual is extensively interviewed to elicit detailed information about nutritional status, as well as general health, socioeconomic status, and cultural impact on nutrition. The diet history

Box 2-4   Food Frequency List for Cholesterol and Fat Intake

Mark the box showing how often you eat or drink each of the following:

	Daily	Several times a week	Once a week	Once or twice a month or less	Never
Whole milk	☐	☐	☐	☐	☐
Butter	☐	☐	☐	☐	☐
Cheese (regular)	☐	☐	☐	☐	☐
Cheese (low-fat)	☐	☐	☐	☐	☐
Cream	☐	☐	☐	☐	☐
Cream cheese	☐	☐	☐	☐	☐
Ice cream	☐	☐	☐	☐	☐
Eggs	☐	☐	☐	☐	☐
Liver	☐	☐	☐	☐	☐
Beef, pork, goat, or mutton/lamb	☐	☐	☐	☐	☐
Poultry	☐	☐	☐	☐	☐
Shellfish	☐	☐	☐	☐	☐
Salmon, tuna, sardines, or mackerel	☐	☐	☐	☐	☐
Other fish	☐	☐	☐	☐	☐

Lard	☐	☐	☐	☐	☐
Hydrogenated shortening	☐	☐	☐	☐	☐
Stick margarine	☐	☐	☐	☐	☐
Soft (tub or squeeze) margarine	☐	☐	☐	☐	☐
Corn, sunflower, or safflower oils	☐	☐	☐	☐	☐
Olive, peanut, or canola oils	☐	☐	☐	☐	☐
Pastries	☐	☐	☐	☐	☐
Gravies	☐	☐	☐	☐	☐
Walnuts or flax seed	☐	☐	☐	☐	☐
Cashews or macadamias	☐	☐	☐	☐	☐
Peanuts, mixed nuts, or peanut butter	☐	☐	☐	☐	☐

usually includes information similar to that collected by the 24-hour recall and food frequency questionnaire, as well as other information listed in Box 2-5. An accurate diet history requires an experienced interviewer, and it can be very time consuming. This method provides more information than either the 24-hour recall or the 3-day food record, however, and it can give an indication of food habits over several months or years. Table 2-4 illustrates diet history findings that may indicate nutritional deficits.

Evaluating nutrient intake

Tables of food composition or computer databases can be used to calculate the amount of each nutrient in the diet. There are numerous commercial databases available. A free downloadable database can be found at http://www.nal.usda.gov/fnic/foodcomp. The same website provides links to databases for foods from African, East Asian, Middle Eastern, Latin American, and various European countries, and it also includes data about food components (e.g., **isoflavones** and flavenols) that can be difficult to find elsewhere.

Once nutrient intake is calculated, it is then compared with some standard, usually the Dietary Reference Intakes (DRIs) (see Chapter 1). The DRIs are set so that they cover the needs of practically all of the healthy people in the U.S., and thus an individual's intake may be adequate even though lower than the DRI. Comparison of the individual's intake with the Estimated Average Requirement (EAR) for his/her life stage and gender group reveals the likelihood that the individual has an inadequate diet. Half of all healthy individuals consuming the EAR will have an inadequate intake. For nutrients with an Adequate Intake (AI), rather than an EAR, healthy individuals that consume as much as the AI for the nutrient are unlikely to have an inadequate intake, but intakes below the AI cannot be assessed.

The food composition method can provide specific information about a wide group of nutrients and food components, and computer databases make the process rapid and easy. Some caveats should be noted, however, in the use of any nutrient database. Diet analysis is limited by the accuracy of the food intake records, which depends on the skill and motivation of the record keeper. In addition, foods consumed may not have exactly the same nutrient composition as those in the database because of variations in growing and storage conditions, food processing, cooking procedures, and changes in fortification or formulation. Moreover, gaps exist in

Box 2-5   Diet History

I. Socioeconomic data
- A. Income
  1. Adequate for food purchasing
  2. Eligibility for food stamps or other public assistance
- B. Ethnic or cultural background
  1. Influence of culture or religion on eating habits
  2. Educational level

II. Food preparation
- A. Problems in shopping for or preparing food
  1. Skill of person who shops and cooks
  2. Availability of market(s)
  3. Adequacy of facilities for cooking, food storage, and refrigeration
- B. Use of convenience foods

III. Physical activity
- A. Occupation—type, number of hours per week, activity level
- B. Exercise—type and frequency
- C. Handicaps

IV. Appetite and perception of taste and smell—quality, any changes over the last 12 months

V. Allergies, intolerances, food avoidances, and special diets
- A. Foods avoided and reason
- B. Special diet—what kind, why followed, and who recommended it

VI. Oral health/swallowing
- A. Dentures; completeness of dentition
- B. Problems with chewing, swallowing, and salivation

VII. Gastrointestinal problems
- A. Heartburn, bloating, gas, diarrhea, vomiting, constipation—frequency of problems, any association with food intake or other occurrences
- B. Remedies used—laxatives, antacids

VIII. Medical or psychiatric illnesses
- A. Type of disease
- B. Type and duration of treatment

Continued

Box 2-5   Diet History—cont'd

IX. Medications
  A. Vitamins, minerals, or other nutritional supplements—frequency, type, amount, and recommended or prescribed by whom
  B. Other medications, including over-the-counter and herbal—frequency, type, amount, and duration of use
X. Recent weight change
  A. Amount of loss or gain and over what period of time (most significant if during past year)
  B. Intentional or unintentional; if intentional, what method was used
XI. Usual food intake—description of a "typical" day's intake, or 24-hour recall with use of food frequency questionnaire

---

the food composition data in published tables and databases. Many foods have not been analyzed for all trace elements, for example. Despite these caveats, the databases are among the most useful and widespread methods for nutrition analysis. An interactive "healthy eating index" program for consumers is available at the website of the U.S. Department of Agriculture Center for Nutrition Policy and Promotion (http://www.usda.gov/cnpp/). Individuals enter their own food intake data and receive a nutritional analysis of their diet, with a comparison to the appropriate Dietary Reference Intakes, as well as a score based on the comparison of their intake with the Food Guide Pyramid and the Dietary Guidelines for Americans.

Nutrition Screening

Health care providers rarely have the time to perform a complete nutrition assessment on every patient. It is most important that individuals who are nutritionally at risk or those who are malnourished be identified quickly; thorough assessment can then be performed on these individuals and intervention can be planned as necessary. Nutrition screening of individuals consists of gathering some readily available subjective and objective information. Any of the

Table 2-4   Evaluation of Nutritional History

Area of Concern	History	Possible Deficiency
Inadequate intake	Alcohol abuse	Energy, pro, vit B_1, niacin, folate
	Avoidance of food groups:	
	Fruits and vegetables	Vit A, C
	Breads and cereals	Vit B_1 and B_2, fiber
	Meat, eggs, dairy products	Vit B_{12}, pro, Fe, Zn
	Dairy products	Ca, vit B_2
	Constipation, hemorrhoids, diverticulosis	Fiber
	Poverty, disadvantaged environment	Various nutrients, especially pro and Fe
	Multiple food allergies	Depends on specific allergies
	Weight loss	Energy, other nutrients
Inadequate absorption	Drugs (especially antacids, cimetidine, anticonvulsants, cholestyramine, neomycin, antineoplastics, laxatives)	Various nutrients (see Appendix H)
	Malabsorbtion (diarrhea, weight loss, steatorrhea)	Energy, vit A, D, E, K; pro; Ca; Mg; Zn
	Parasites	Fe
	Surgery	
	Gastrectomy	Vit B_{12}, Fe, folate
	Intestinal resection	Energy; vit A, D, E, K; Ca; Mg; Zn; vit B_{12} if distal ileum

Continued

Table 2-4 Evaluation of Nutritional History—cont'd

Area of Concern	History	Possible Deficiency
Impaired utilization	Drugs (especially antineoplastics, oral contraceptives, isoniazid, colchicines, corticosteroids)	Various nutrients (see Appendix H)
	Inborn errors of metabolism (by family history)	Depends on disorder
Increased losses	Diabetes	Zn, Cr
	Alcohol abuse, cirrhosis of the liver	Mg, Zn
	Blood loss	Fe
	Diarrhea, fistula	Pro, Zn, fluid, electrolytes
	Draining abscesses or wounds	Pro, Zn
	Nephrotic syndrome	Pro, Zn
	Peritoneal dialysis or hemodialysis	Pro, water-soluble vit, Zn
Increased requirements	Fever	Energy, vit B_1
	Hyperthyroidism	Energy
	Physiologic demands (infancy, adolescence, pregnancy, lactation)	Fe, Ca, energy; other nutrients
	Surgery, trauma, burns, infection	Energy, pro, vit C, Zn
	Neoplasms (some types)	Energy, pro, other nutrients

Modified from Heimburger DC, Weinsier RL: *Handbook of clinical nutrition*, ed 3, St Louis, 1997, Mosby.

Pro, Protein; *vit*, vitamin(s); *Fe*, iron; *Ca*, calcium; *Mg*, magnesium; *Zn*, zinc; *Cr*, chromium.

following findings may indicate the presence of malnutrition or nutritional risk:

- Unplanned loss of ≥10% of usual body weight within 6 months or ≥5% of usual body weight in 1 month; in infants (after the first week of life) and children, any weight loss (or failure to gain adequate weight) that causes deviation from the child's usual percentile on standardized growth charts (see Appendix D)
- Body mass index (see Box 2-1) >25 or <18.5, or weight 10% greater than or less than ideal body weight; in infants and children, weight, length, or BMI less than the 10th percentile or greater than the 85th percentile (see Appendix D)
- Presence of chronic disease
- Increased metabolic requirements (e.g., trauma, burns, systemic infection)
- Altered diet or diet schedules (e.g., recent surgery, serious illness, receiving total parenteral nutrition or tube feedings)
- Inadequate food intake (for adults, risk is greater if inadequate intake continues or is expected to continue for 7 days or more; infants and children are considered at risk with a shorter period of inadequate intake)

Estimating Nutrient Needs
Energy Needs

Energy expenditure can be divided into three components: (1) **basal energy expenditure,** or energy required for basic life processes such as respiration, cardiac function, and maintenance of body temperature; (2) the thermic effect of food, or the energy required for ingestion, digestion, absorption, and metabolism of nutrients from food (generally a rather small contribution to energy expenditure); and (3) physical activity. Basal (or resting) energy expenditure (BEE) is determined largely by the amount of lean body mass (also known as the fat-free mass). It can be measured by indirect calorimetry. This technique, which requires a metabolic cart, is not available in all settings, and therefore a variety of formulas are used in estimation of energy needs.

Table 2-5 provides rough estimates of energy needs that are sometimes used for a quick assessment of the adequacy of energy intake and for teaching lay individuals. These estimates may not reflect accurately the energy expenditure of a particular person.

Table 2-5   Estimates of Daily Energy Needs for Adults

Status/Activity Level	kcal/kg	kcal/lb
Obese	21	9.5
Sedentary or hospitalized	25-30	11-13.5
Moderately active (regular aerobic exercise plus routine activities)	30-35	13.5-16
Very active (manual laborer, athlete) or patient with major burns or trauma	40	18

A number of more detailed formulas are used in clinical practice in an effort to derive more individualized estimates of energy expenditure. Some of the common formulas are shown in Table 2-6. These formulas yield basal or resting energy expenditure. Generally they are multiplied by an activity factor to obtain an estimate of total energy expenditure (Box 2-6). Alternative methods have been proposed for calculation of total energy expenditure in ill patients (see Box 2-6).

The lean body mass (LBM, or fat-free mass) is responsible for most of the energy expenditure. Obese people contain more of both fat and LBM than do normal-weight individuals, but LBM accounts for only about 25% of the excess weight in the obese. Elderly people have less LBM and a higher fat content, on average, than their younger counterparts. LBM decreases approximately 10% between the ages of 25 and 60 years, another 10% between 60 and 75, and then declines more rapidly (as much as 20% to 25% more by age 90). For this reason, estimates of energy needs for elderly persons should usually fall at the bottom end of the suggested range. Rather than drastically limiting their energy intake to maintain a desirable body weight, elderly people should be encouraged to exercise at a moderate intensity on a regular basis (e.g., walk as briskly as can be tolerated for 30 to 60 minutes almost every day). Regular exercise has two advantages: maintenance of LBM and increase in energy expenditure. With increased energy expenditure, and thus an increase in energy needs, it is easier for the elderly to obtain a diet adequate in vitamins, minerals, and other nutrients.

Protein Needs

Protein needs vary with the physiologic demands, degree of malnutrition (if present), and stressors. Estimated needs for growth in

Table 2-6 Selected Equations Used in Estimating Resting Energy Expenditure (kcal/day)

Age Group	Males	Females
Harris-Benedict Equations		
Adults	$66 + 13.7(W)$ $+ 5(H) - 6.8(A)$	$655 + 9.6(W)$ $+ 1.7(H) - 4.7(A)$
Owen Equations		
Adults	$879 + (10.2 \times W)$	$795 + (7.18 \times W)$
World Health Organization		
0-3 yr	$(60.9 \times W) + 54$	$(61.0 \times W) + 51$
3-10 yr	$(22.7 \times W) + 495$	$(22.5 \times W) + 499$
10-18 yr	$(17.5 \times W) + 651$	$(12.2 \times W) + 746$
18-30 yr	$(15.3 \times W) + 679$	$(14.7 \times W) + 996$
30-60 yr	$(11.2 \times W) + 879$	$(8.7 \times W) + 829$
>60 yr	$(13.5 \times W) + 987$	$(10.5 \times W) + 596$

W, Weight in kg (1 lb = 0.45 kg); H, height in cm (1 in = 2.54 cm); A, age in years.
Modified from Harris JA, Benedict FG: Standard basal metabolism constants for physiologists and clinicians. In The Carnegie Institute of Washington: *A biometric study of basal metabolism in man,* Publication 279, Philadelphia, 1919, JB Lippincott, p 223; Owen OE: Resting metabolic requirements of men and women, *Mayo Clinic Proc* 63:503, 1988; World Health Organization: *Energy and protein requirements. Report of a Joint FAO/WHO/UNU Expert Consultation,* Technical Report Series 724, Geneva, 1985, World Health Organization.

healthy children can be found in Table 1-1. For healthy adults or those undergoing elective surgery, 0.8 to 1 g/kg body weight is usually adequate. Athletes and individuals in catabolic states (sepsis, major trauma, and burns) may need as much as 1.2 to 2.0 g/kg daily. Individuals with liver or kidney failure may require lower protein intakes (see Chapters 11 and 16).

Assessing State of Hydration

The state of hydration is an important part of nutritional assessment. On one hand, fluid overload is a hazardous state that may compromise cardiorespiratory function. It is usually reflected in rapid weight gain (more than approximately 0.1 to 0.2 kg [¼ to ½ lb]/day in an adult over a period of several days). On the other hand, fluid

Box 2-6   Selected Equations Used in Estimation of Total Energy Expenditure

Equations Based on Basal or Resting Energy Expenditure
Used for both well and sick individuals

Multiply the basal or resting expenditure (see Table 2-6) by an activity factor to obtain an estimate of total energy expenditure.

Sedentary, obese, or hospitalized individual: 1.2 to 1.3

Active nonhospitalized normal weight individual: 1.4 to 1.6

Example: A woman who has a sedentary job is 26 years old, 162.5 cm (5′4″) tall, and 84 kg (185 lb).

$$BEE = 655 + 9.6(84) + 1.7(162.5) - 4.7(26) = 1615 \text{ kcal/day}$$

Estimated total energy expenditure = $1615 \times 1.2 = 1938$ kcal/day

Ireton-Jones Equations*
Developed in and used for sick hospitalized patients†

$$EEE(v) = 1784 - 11(A) + 5(W) + 244(S) + 239(T) + 804(B)$$

$$EEE(s) = 629 - 11(A) + 25(W) - 609(O)$$

EEE = estimated total energy expenditure in kcal/day, v = ventilator-dependent, s = spontaneously breathing, A = age in years, W = actual weight in kg, S = sex (m = 1, f = 0). Diagnosis: T = trauma, B = burn, O = obesity (if present = 1, absent = 0).

Example: If the woman in the example above suffered respiratory failure and needed ventilatory support following a near-drowning incident, her EEE would be as follows:

$$\begin{aligned} EEE(v) &= 1784 - 11(26) + 5(84) + 244(0) + 239(0) + 804(0) \\ &= 1918 \text{ kcal/day} \end{aligned}$$

*Both of the Ireton-Jones equations can be applied to obese individuals, although obesity appears as a factor only in the equation for spontaneously breathing patients.

†Ireton-Jones C, Jones JD: Improved equations predicting energy expenditure in patients, the Ireton-Jones equations. *Nutr Clin Pract* 17:29, 2002.

deficits (**dehydration**) can become severe enough to cause shock and coma.

There are three types of dehydration, which can be distinguished by the serum sodium level:

1. *Hypertonic or hypernatremic:* Serum sodium >150 mEq/L. This occurs because loss of water is greater than loss of sodium. Causes include inadequate water intake (e.g., hospitalized elderly individuals who may not feel or be able to express thirst, infants given improperly diluted powdered or concentrated formula, individuals with diarrhea and inadequate fluid intake) and osmotic diuresis (e.g., excessive urination in hyperglycemia).

2. *Isotonic:* Serum sodium 130 to 150 mEq/L. This is the most common form of dehydration; it occurs because of loss of balanced amounts of sodium and water. Causes include diarrhea, vomiting, and nasogastric suction with inadequate replacement of fluid and electrolytes.

Table 2-7   Judging Severity of Fluid Deficit

	Mild, 3%-5%	Moderate, 6%-9%	Severe, ≥10%
Blood pressure	N	N	N to ↓
Pulses	N	N to ↓	↓↓
Heart rate	N	↑	↑*
Skin turgor	N	↓ to ↓↓	↓↓ to ↓↓↓
Fontanelle (infants)	N	Sunken	Sunken
Mucous membranes	Slightly dry	Dry	Dry
Eyes	N	Sunken	Deeply sunken
Capillary refill	N	Delayed	Delayed†
Mental status	N	N to ↓	N to ↓↓↓
Urine output	↓	↓↓‡	↓↓↓‡
Thirst	↑	↑↑	↑↑↑

N, Normal; ↓, slightly decreased; ↓↓, moderately decreased; ↓↓↓, severely decreased; ↑, slightly increased; ↑↑, moderately increased; ↑↑↑, severely increased.
*May become bradycardic in very severe dehydration.
†Skin cool and mottled.
‡<1 ml/kg/hr.

3. *Hypotonic or hyponatremic:* Serum sodium <130 mEq/L. Sodium is lost in excess of water. Causes include viral gastroenteritis with rehydration with plain water, tea, or other low-sodium fluids; excessive sweating without fluid and electrolyte replacement; cystic fibrosis; diuretic therapy.

Dehydration can be graded as mild, moderate, or severe. The amount of weight loss, along with clinical signs (Table 2-7), can be used to determine the severity of the fluid deficit.

REFERENCES

Carvalho NF et al: Severe nutritional deficiencies in toddlers resulting from health food milk alternatives, *Pediatrics* 107:e46, 2001.

Liu T et al: Kwashiorkor in the United States, *Arch Dermatol* 137:630, 2001.

SELECTED BIBLIOGRAPHY

Battezzatti A et al: Body composition assessment: an indispensable tool for disease management, *Acta Diabetol* 40:S151, 2003.

Brugler L et al: The role of visceral protein markers in protein calorie malnutrition, *Clin Chem Lab Med* 40:1360, 2002.

Brugnara C: Iron deficiency and erythropoiesis: new diagnostic approaches, *Clin Chem* 49:1573, 2003.

Ellis KJ: Human body composition: in vivo methods, *Physiol Rev* 80:649, 2000.

Hambidge M: Biomarkers of trace mineral intake and status, *J Nutr* 133: 948S, 2003.

Ireton-Jones C, Jones JD: Improved equations for predicting energy expenditure in patients: the Ireton-Jones equations, *Nutr Clin Prac* 17:29, 2002.

Lopez-Hellin J et al: Usefulness of short-lived proteins as nutritional indicators in surgical patients, *Clin Nutr* 21:119, 2002.

Mathieu J: NSI: providing simple tools for our nation's health, *J Am Diet Assoc* 102:1394, 2002.

National Institutes of Health, National Heart, Lung, and Blood Institute, and North American Association for the Study of Obesity: *The practical guide: identification, evaluation, and treatment of overweight and obesity in adults,* Washington, DC, 2000, NIH, NHLBI, and NAASO.

Niggemann B, Grüber C: Side-effects of complementary and alternative medicine, *Allergy* 58:707, 2003.

Raguso C, Dupertuis YM, Pichard C: The role of visceral proteins in the nutritional assessment of intensive care unit patients, *Curr Opin Clin Nutr Metab Care* 6:211, 2003.

Treuth MS et al: Body composition in prepubertal girls: comparison of six methods, *Int J Obesity* 25:1352, 2001.

US Department of Agriculture, Agricultural Research Service. *USDA nutrient database for standard reference, release 15*, Washington, DC, 2002, USDA. Available at www.nal.usda.gov/fnic/foodcomp. Accessed June 11, 2004.

Pregnancy and Lactation

3

Pregnancy

There is a growing recognition that nutrition during pregnancy is important not only because it contributes to the health of the mother and her newborn but also because it establishes the nutritional foundations for a healthy adult life. Poor growth in utero, for example, increases the risk of cardiovascular disease and diabetes in later life.

Needs for most nutrients increase at least modestly during pregnancy (see Table 1-1). Nutritional deficiencies during pregnancy can have adverse effects on both the mother and her infant. Maternal diets are most likely to be low in iron, zinc, calcium, and folic acid. Requirements for some important nutrients are described later in this chapter. Food sources of these nutrients are listed in Appendix A.

Objectives of nutritional care during pregnancy are for the woman to do the following: (1) recognize and alter any practices or findings that could interfere with optimal nutritional status and pregnancy outcome, (2) establish with the health care provider a goal for weight gain within the recommended range and achieve this goal with an appropriate rate of gain, and (3) cope with physiologic changes during pregnancy that interfere with optimal nutritional intake or comfort.

Assessment

Nutrition assessment, summarized in Table 3-1, should be carried out even before conception if possible. If any maternal nutritional problems (e.g., poor eating habits; inappropriate weight for height; inadequate folate intake; and poor control of chronic maternal diseases such as hypertension, diabetes, or phenylketonuria), they should be addressed before pregnancy or as soon after conception as possible. Nutritional status should be reevaluated at each prenatal visit. Pregnancy alters the normal ranges for many laboratory tests commonly used in nutrition assessment (Box 3-1).

Box 3-1   Changes in Laboratory Values during Pregnancy

↓ Hematocrit
↓ Hemoglobin
↑ Lymphocyte count
↓ Serum albumin
↓ Serum ferritin
↑ Serum cholesterol
↓ Blood urea nitrogen
↓ Serum creatinine

Nutrition Needs

Preconceptual weight, weight gain, and energy needs

Enlargement of maternal breasts, uterine tissue, blood volume, and energy (fat) stores, as well as development of the placenta, amniotic fluid, and fetus, contribute to maternal weight gain during pregnancy (Table 3-2). Appropriate weight gain does not necessarily equal good nutritional status, of course, but the amount of weight gain during pregnancy is closely related to pregnancy outcome. The mother's weight before pregnancy is another factor involved in pregnancy outcome. Maternal and fetal risks are increased in the following cases:

1. *Underweight:* Women who are underweight before pregnancy are more likely to experience preterm labor and to deliver **low-birth-weight (LBW;** less than 2500 g or 5.5 lb) infants. LBW is the single greatest risk factor for the survival of the newborn.
2. *Overweight:* Women who are overweight before pregnancy are more likely to have hypertension and diabetes. Fetal death rates are highest in pregnancies where the mother weighs more than 77.3 kg (170 lb).
3. *Inadequate weight gain:* For normal-weight and underweight women, maternal weight gain is directly related to infant birth weight, and the risk of delivering an LBW infant is increased by inadequate gain.
4. *Excessive weight gain:* Overeating, multiple gestation, edema, and pregnancy-induced hypertension are some of the causes of greater-than-expected weight gain. There is increased risk of

Text continued on p. 97

Table 3-1 Assessment of Nutrition in Pregnancy and Lactation

Areas of Concern	Significant Findings
Inadequate Energy, Intake, and Weight Gain	*History* Limited income; body image concerns; nausea and vomiting; lack of knowledge about optimal gain during pregnancy, nutritional needs during pregnancy and lactation; stress or fatigue; prepregnant BMI <19.8; poor obstetric history during previous pregnancies (e.g., spontaneous abortion, delivery of an LBW infant); heavy smoking; illicit drug use; adolescent pregnancy *Physical Examination* Pregnancy: failure to demonstrate adequate weight gain; lactation: poor milk production, inadequate gain by infant
Excessive Energy Intake	*History* Emotional stress, indulgence, and boredom from interruption of job routine; decrease in activity because of awkwardness during pregnancy or interruption of job routine; prepregnant BMI >25 *Physical Examination* Pregnancy: weight gain > recommended range; lactation: weight gain or maintenance of BMI >25
Inadequate Protein Intake	*History* Limited income; strict vegetarianism*: nausea and vomiting during pregnancy; lack of knowledge about needs; fatigue (especially during lactation); frequent pregnancies (>3 within 2 years) or high parity; poor obstetric history during

previous pregnancies (e.g., spontaneous abortion, delivery of an LBW infant); alcohol or illicit drug use; multiple gestation

Physical Examination

Edema (some lower-extremity edema is normal during pregnancy; look for edema in hands and periorbital area); changes in hair color and texture; hair loss

Laboratory Analysis

Serum albumin <3.2 g/dl; prealbumin <10 mg/dl

Inadequate Vitamin Intake

Vitamin C

History

Failure to consume vitamin C–containing food daily because of poverty, alcohol or drug abuse, or dislike of these foods; increased needs because of smoking, long-term oral contraceptive or salicylate use; multiple gestation

Physical Examination

Bruising, petechiae, bleeding gums

Laboratory Analysis

↓ Serum or leukocyte vitamin C

Folate

History

Failure to use a daily folic acid supplement or foods rich in folate; delivery of a previous infant with a neural tube defect; increased needs because of alcohol or drug abuse, smoking, or multiple gestation

Physical Examination

Pallor; glossitis

Continued

Table 3-1   Assessment of Nutrition in Pregnancy and Lactation—cont'd

Areas of Concern	Significant Findings
Vitamin B_{12}	*Laboratory Analysis* Hct <33%; ↑ MCV; ↓ serum and RBC folate *History* Strict vegetarian with failure to use a supplement or foods fortified with vitamin B_{12}; ileal resection or disease *Physical Examination* Maternal findings: glossitis, pallor, ataxia; infant breastfed by strict vegetarian: delayed growth, pallor, glossitis, developmental delay *Laboratory Analysis* ↓ Hct; ↑ MCV (in mother or infant); ↓ serum vitamin B_{12} (in mother or infant
Vitamin D	*History* Failure to consume vitamin D–fortified milk because of strict vegetarianism, lactose intolerance, dislike of milk, or cultural practices; little exposure of skin to sunlight because of residence in northern latitudes in winter or cultural prohibitions against exposing the body
Inadequate Mineral Intake Iron (Fe)	*History* Failure to consume a daily supplement and foods rich in Fe because of vegetarianism, limited income, or dislike of these foods; frequent pregnancies or high parity with depletion of stores; adolescent with increased needs for her

growth as well as that of the fetus; anemia during a previous pregnancy; pica; menorrhagia; multiple gestation

Physical Examination

Pallor, especially of conjunctiva; blue sclerae; spoon-shaped nails

Laboratory Analysis

Hct <33%; Hgb <11 g/dl; ↓ MCV, serum ferritin, serum Fe; ↑ free erythrocyte protoporphyrin (FEP)

Zinc (Zn)

History

Use of supplement containing >30 mg Fe (competition between Zn and Fe for absorption); use of folate or calcium supplement; avoidance of animal protein foods; frequent pregnancies or high parity with depletion of stores; adolescent with increased needs for her growth as well as that of the fetus; pica; alcoholism with increased excretion

Physical Examination

Seborrheic dermatitis; alopecia; diarrhea; poor sense of taste; distorted taste

Laboratory Analysis

↓ Serum Zn

Calcium (Ca)

History

Lactose intolerance; dislike of milk products; strict vegetarianism or cultural food patterns that avoid milk (e.g., Asian); frequent pregnancies or high parity with depletion of stores; adolescent with increased needs for her growth as well as fetus

Continued

Table 3-1   Assessment of Nutrition in Pregnancy and Lactation—cont'd

Areas of Concern	Significant Findings
Potentially Harmful Substances (during Pregnancy)	
Caffeine	*History*
	Daily consumption of coffee, tea, and soft drinks (other than caffeine-free), especially if more than the equivalent of 2 cups coffee/day; use of over-the-counter cold or analgesic medications (not usually recommended during pregnancy; the woman should consult her physician before using)
Alcohol	*History*
	Use of alcoholic beverages, especially if >1 oz/day or more than 3 or 4 times/wk during pregnancy
Cocaine/other illicit drugs	*History*
	Use of drugs, especially on a regular basis, during pregnancy
	Laboratory Analysis
	Positive urinary drug screen

*Strict vegetarians consume no milk products, eggs, meat, poultry, or fish. Lactovegetarians use milk products, and ovolactovegetarians use both milk products and eggs.

RBC, Red blood cell.

Table 3-2   Components of Maternal Weight Gain at Term Gestation

Tissue	Pounds	Kilograms
Fetus	7.9	3.6
Placenta	1.1	0.5
Amniotic fluid	2.5	1.1
Increased uterus and breast tissue	4.0	1.8
Increased blood volume	4.4	2.0
Increased fat and other tissues	5.5	2.5
TOTAL	25.4	11.5

fetopelvic disproportion, operative delivery, birth trauma, and infant mortality with very high total weight gain, especially in short women (less than 157 cm or 62 in). Moreover, excessive fat stores tend to be retained after pregnancy, increasing the woman's likelihood of being overweight or obese.

Intervention and teaching

Optimal energy intake and weight gain. The optimum amount of weight gain during pregnancy is determined largely by the mother's weight before pregnancy. Recommendations have been developed for desirable ranges for total weight gain and rate of weight gain based on body mass index (BMI), an indicator of the appropriateness of weight for height. See Chapter 2 for the method of calculating BMI, or consult the chart inside the back cover of this book.

Recommended total weight gain during pregnancy is as follows: underweight women (BMI <19.8), 12.5 to 18 kg (28 to 40 lb); normal-weight women (BMI 19.8 to 26), 11.5 to 16 kg (25 to 35 lb); overweight women (BMI 26 to 29), 7 to 11.5 kg (15 to 25 lb); and obese women (BMI >29), ≥6.8 kg (15 lb) (National Academy of Sciences, 1992). Young adolescents (less than 2 years past menarche) should be encouraged to make their weight gain goal the upper end of the recommended range for their BMI because their infants are smaller than those of adult women for any given amount of maternal gain. Outcome of a twin pregnancy appears to be best if weight gain is approximately 16 to 20.5 kg (35 to 45 lb). Although there are insufficient data to make a conclusive recommendation, the National Academy of Sciences (2002) has suggested that a gain of at least 22.7 kg (50 lb) be the goal for triplet gestations.

Women may be surprised to learn how large the desirable weight gain in pregnancy is, and women who have always worked to keep their weight under control may be resistant to achieving the recommended weight gain. Explanation of the components of that weight gain (see Table 3-2) may help them to understand the importance of weight gain. On the other hand, excessive weight gain is associated with the development of diabetes and hypertension, and women who gain more than the recommended amount during pregnancy are more likely to remain overweight afterward.

The pattern of weight gain is important in evaluating weight changes during pregnancy. Most women gain approximately 1.5 to 2 kg (3 to 5 lb) during the first trimester of pregnancy, when the fetus and the changes in maternal tissues are relatively small. Current data indicate that fetal outcome in multiple gestation is better if the mother has some weight gain during the first trimester of pregnancy. Recommended weekly weight gains during the second and third trimesters are 0.5 kg (1.1 lb) for underweight women, 0.4 kg (1 lb) for normal-weight women, and 0.3 kg (0.66 lb) for overweight women. Gain of 1 kg (2.2 lb) or less per month in the second or third trimester by normal-weight women and 0.5 kg or less (1 lb) by obese women should be investigated, as should a gain of 3 kg (6.6 lb) or more per month. In twin gestations, the goal is a gain of approximately 0.75 kg (1.65 lb) a week during the second and third trimesters.

The Dietary Reference Intakes (DRIs) (National Academy of Sciences, 2002) suggest that during the second and third trimesters the woman should consume 340 and 452 kcal/day (respectively) more than her nonpregnant intake to promote an adequate gain. (See Chapter 1 for discussion of DRIs.) The extra energy (kcal) needed daily is easily obtained by increasing intake of milk products by 1 or 2 servings per day and making small increases in intake of protein foods, fruits, and vegetables. There is little room in the diet for high-energy foods that are low in nutrients. Problems occur when women restrain their intake too much or, alternatively, eat excessively during pregnancy. Therefore it is especially important that pregnant women know their weight gain goal and understand how to follow a food plan to achieve it.

Healthful food plan. Nutritional needs for healthy pregnant women, except perhaps those for iron, can be met through a varied diet of

Table 3-3   Composition of a Representative Prenatal Multivitamin-Multimineral Supplement

Nutrient	Amount
Vitamin A	800 µg
Vitamin D_3	10 µg
Vitamin E	20 mg
Vitamin C (ascorbic acid)	120 mg
Folic acid	1 mg
Vitamin B_1 (thiamin)	3 mg
Vitamin B_2 (riboflavin)	3.4 mg
Vitamin B_6 (pyridoxine)	10 mg
Niacinamide	20 mg
Vitamin B_{12} (cyanocobalamin)	12 µg
Biotin	30 µg
Pantothenic acid	10 mg
Calcium	250 mg
Iodine	150 µg
Iron	27 mg
Magnesium	25 mg
Copper	2 mg
Zinc	25 mg
Chromium	25 µg
Molybdenum	25 µg
Manganese	5 mg

normal foods (e.g., the DASH diet described in Chapters 1 and 14). Adequate calcium is contained in 3 or 4 servings of milk, yogurt, cheese, or calcium-fortified juices or soy milk daily. A minimum of 5 to 6 servings of fruits and vegetables, 2 to 3 servings of meat or protein-rich substitutes (e.g., nuts or cooked dry beans), and 6 to 11 servings of whole and enriched grain products supply the remainder of the needed nutrients. Vitamin-mineral supplements (Table 3-3) are commonly prescribed during pregnancy to ensure that intake of these nutrients is adequate.

Physical activity during pregnancy. Moderate physical activity is recommended in healthy women without obstetrical conditions that would contraindicate such activity. No pregnant woman should participate in such activity without the guidance of her health care provider. Activities such as cycling, swimming, and walking are recommended, and those such as skiing, water skiing, surfing, scuba diving, and mountaineering at high altitudes are discouraged. A moderate level of physical activity is one that would result in a heart rate (beats per minute) of approximately 140 to 155 in women less than 20 years of age, 135 to 150 in women 20 to 29 years of age, 130 to 145 in women 30 to 39, and 125 to 140 in women older than 40 years.

Protein

An intake of 1.1g/kg body weight/day, or a total of approximately 71 g of protein per day (25 g more than the nonpregnant recommendation) is recommended. This amount, which is easily provided by the average diet in the United States and Canada, is necessary for normal growth of the fetus, enlargement of the uterus and breasts, formation of blood cells and proteins as the blood volume expands, and production of amniotic fluid.

Intervention and teaching

The extra protein needed in addition to the prepregnant intake can be provided by approximately 1 cup (240 ml) of milk or soy milk and 2 oz (60 g) of meat or an equivalent meat substitute per day. There is no benefit in consuming protein in excess of the recommendations, and doing so increases the cost of the diet.

For low-income women who may have difficulty affording the additional protein foods and other nutrient-rich foods that are needed during pregnancy, the Special Supplemental Food Program for Women, Infants, and Children (WIC) provides vouchers for purchase of selected food items rich in protein, iron, and vitamin C. Low-income women may also be eligible for the Food Stamp program. When the woman's diet is found to be poor and there is little likelihood of its improving, or when other risk factors (adolescent pregnancy, maternal smoking, use of illicit drugs or alcohol, or multiple gestation) exist, vitamin-mineral supplementation is especially important (see the discussion that follows).

Vitamins and minerals

Folate (folic acid)

The recommended daily intake of folate increases from 400 μg for all women who have the potential to become pregnant to 600 μg in pregnancy. It is needed for both maternal red blood cell production and the DNA synthesis entailed in fetal and placental growth. Data indicate that women with folate deficiency are more likely to give birth to infants with neural tube defects.

Intervention and teaching. Folate seems to be especially important during the periconceptual period, before pregnancy may even be suspected, and therefore good nutrition education is needed to ensure adequate intakes by nonpregnant teens and women in their childbearing years.

- Folic acid (from supplements) is better absorbed than folate (from food), and a supplement may be the best way to ensure that intake is adequate. Most over-the-counter multivitamins contain 400 μg folic acid in a daily dose, and prenatal vitamins contain increased amounts (see Table 3-3).
- Fruit, juices, green vegetables, whole grains and enriched flour, and fortified cereals are reliable dietary sources.

Other vitamins

An increase in intake of vitamin C is recommended during pregnancy because of its many roles in metabolism, including its involvement in development of connective tissue. In addition, vitamin C improves iron absorption and facilitates activation of folate. Vitamin D plays an important role in calcium metabolism, and vitamin B_{12} is required for synthesis of nucleic acids, needed for the increased production of maternal red blood cells and growth of fetal tissue.

Intervention and teaching
- *Vitamin C:* An extra 10 mg in addition to the DRI of 75 mg is recommended for adult women during pregnancy, and a total of 80 mg is recommended for pregnant teens. Although vitamin C is contained in prenatal vitamins, the recommended amounts can easily be achieved from a diet rich in foods such as citrus fruits, broccoli, green peppers, strawberries, and melons.
- *Vitamin D:* Regular exposure of the skin to sunlight or consumption of vitamin D–fortified milk and cereals generally provides sufficient amounts. A supplement of 10 μg or 400 IU is suggested for strict vegetarians or other women with little intake of vitamin D–fortified milk, especially for women with little exposure of the

skin to sunlight and those with very dark skin in northern latitudes.

▪ *Vitamin B_{12}:* This vitamin is found only in animal products, and therefore strict vegetarians need a supplement of approximately 2 to 3 μg daily unless they are consuming vitamin B_{12}–fortified food products. Women with pernicious anemia require parenteral or intranasal vitamin B_{12} for life, and those with disease or previous resection of the ileum usually require similar therapy or very-high-dose oral supplements (1000 μg daily).

Iron

The red blood cell mass expands by about 15% during pregnancy, which requires a substantial increase in the maternal content of iron. Iron is also needed for deposition of fetal stores, and inadequate maternal iron intake is linked with delivery of LBW infants (those less than 2500 g). The DRIs include a 50% increase in iron intake during pregnancy, from 18 to 27 mg daily. **Pica,** the consumption of substances usually considered nonfoods, can interfere with iron nutriture in two ways: (1) displacing nutritious foods in the diet (both calcium and iron intakes have been found to be lower in women with pica than those without pica by some investigators), and (2) interfering with absorption of iron and other nutrients from foods and nutritional supplements. Women who practice pica have been found to have significantly lower levels of hemoglobin, mean cell hemoglobin, and ferritin (a storage form of iron) than women who do not practice pica. Risk factors for pica during pregnancy include race (African American), living in a rural area, practicing pica during childhood, and having family members who practice pica. As many as 20% of pregnant women in some of the high-risk groups practice pica. Ice or freezer frost, soil or clay, chalk, glue, cornstarch, and laundry starch are common substances consumed. The substances preferred by a particular woman are usually items that her family members have consumed or that she herself consumed before pregnancy.

Intervention and teaching. A supplement of 30 mg of iron is recommended during the second and third trimesters of pregnancy. Ferrous sulfate, 150 mg, provides 30 mg of elemental iron and is often prescribed because it is inexpensive and relatively well absorbed. Teaching points in relation to iron supplementation and iron nutrition include the following:

- Take the supplement between meals or at bedtime because certain food components interfere with iron absorption. These include phytates (in whole grains), oxalates (in deep green leafy vegetables), and tannins in tea and coffee.
- Take the supplement with liquids other than milk, coffee, and tea, which inhibit iron absorption.
- Take the supplement at bedtime if it causes GI distress.
- Even with supplementation, include in the daily diet good sources of iron, such as meats and legumes, and vitamin C sources, which enhance iron absorption. Cooking foods in cast-iron cookware increases their iron content.
- Keep the supplement out of the reach of children.

Zinc

Zinc is needed for formation of new tissue. The DRI for zinc increases from 8 to 11 mg daily during pregnancy in women over age 18 and from 9 to 12 mg for pregnant adolescents.

Intervention and teaching

- Women need to consume reliable sources of zinc (e.g., shellfish, meats, and tofu and other products made from soybeans) daily. Whole grains, milk, cheese, and eggs contain smaller but important amounts of zinc.
- Vegetarians are especially apt to have marginal zinc status, both because meats and shellfish are some of the richest sources of zinc and because phytates and oxalates found in whole grains and green leafy vegetables inhibit zinc absorption. For this reason, they may need a zinc supplement (15 mg elemental zinc daily).
- Absorption of zinc is inhibited by large intakes of iron and folic acid. Supplements of zinc (15 mg daily) and copper (2 mg daily) are recommended for women who require therapeutic doses of iron (more than 30 mg daily) to treat anemia.

Calcium

Pregnant women are encouraged to consume at least 1000 mg of calcium per day, and pregnant adolescents are advised to consume 1300 mg. This can be achieved with a daily intake of 3 cups of milk or yogurt plus additional foods such as green leafy vegetables or bread products made with milk or the use of calcium-supplemented juices, cereals, or other food products. The requirement for calcium in the fetal skeleton is a major reason for the increase in maternal needs.

Intervention and teaching. Women are encouraged to consume several good dietary sources of calcium daily:

- Dairy products, particularly milk, buttermilk, yogurt, and cheese, are among the richest calcium sources available (Figure 3-1). Three to 4 daily servings meet most of the needs of pregnant women.
- Sardines and other canned fish are excellent calcium sources if the bones are eaten.
- Foods made with milk, such as pancakes, waffles, puddings, and cream soups, provide moderate amounts of calcium.
- Most deep green leafy vegetables contain calcium; however, some of these vegetables, such as Swiss chard and spinach, are poor calcium sources because they contain oxalates that prevent absorption of the calcium.
- A commercial lactase enzyme preparation can be used when consuming milk if the woman has lactose intolerance (cramping, bloating, and diarrhea following milk consumption, resulting from lack of lactase, the enzyme that digests lactose). Lactose-intolerant individuals usually tolerate yogurt and hard cheeses, which contain little lactose. Many individuals with lactose intolerance can tolerate milk as long as they drink only 0.5 to 1 cup at a time.
- Calcium-fortified juices and cereal products are good calcium sources.
- A supplement of 600 mg daily is recommended for women under 25 years of age who consume less than 600 mg of calcium (two 8-oz glasses of milk) a day, because the bones of these women may still be increasing in density. To maximize absorption of the supplement, it should be taken 1 to 2 hours before or after the iron supplement, and it should not be taken with bran or whole-grain cereals.

Harmful and Potentially Harmful Practices
Alcohol

Fetal alcohol syndrome (FAS) results from maternal alcohol intake during pregnancy. This disorder is characterized by some or all of the following features in the infant: microcephaly, prenatal

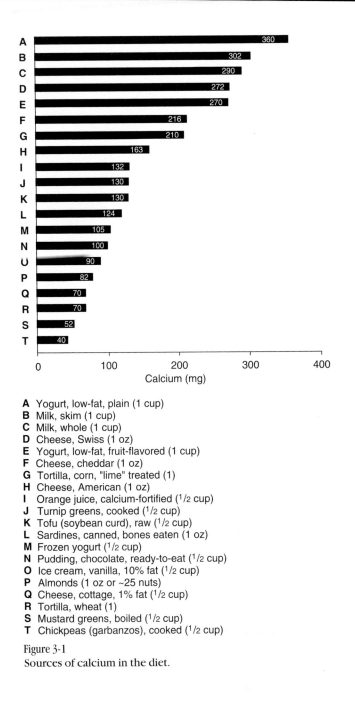

Figure 3-1

Sources of calcium in the diet.

A Yogurt, low-fat, plain (1 cup)
B Milk, skim (1 cup)
C Milk, whole (1 cup)
D Cheese, Swiss (1 oz)
E Yogurt, low-fat, fruit-flavored (1 cup)
F Cheese, cheddar (1 oz)
G Tortilla, corn, "lime" treated (1)
H Cheese, American (1 oz)
I Orange juice, calcium-fortified ($1/2$ cup)
J Turnip greens, cooked ($1/2$ cup)
K Tofu (soybean curd), raw ($1/2$ cup)
L Sardines, canned, bones eaten (1 oz)
M Frozen yogurt ($1/2$ cup)
N Pudding, chocolate, ready-to-eat ($1/2$ cup)
O Ice cream, vanilla, 10% fat ($1/2$ cup)
P Almonds (1 oz or ~25 nuts)
Q Cheese, cottage, 1% fat ($1/2$ cup)
R Tortilla, wheat (1)
S Mustard greens, boiled ($1/2$ cup)
T Chickpeas (garbanzos), cooked ($1/2$ cup)

and postnatal growth failure, mental retardation, facial abnormalities (Figure 3-2), cleft palate, skeletal-joint abnormalities, abnormal palmar creases, cardiac defects, and behavioral abnormalities. There is no known safe level of alcohol intake during pregnancy, and no safe time during pregnancy when alcohol can be consumed. Regular (seven or more drinks a week), heavy (two or more drinks/day), or binge (five or more drinks at a time) drinking are especially to be discouraged. Some children who do not develop all of the characteristics of FAS are said to have alcohol-related birth defects (ARBDs) or alcohol-related neurodevelopmental disorder (ARND), depending on the disorders they display. ARBDs, such as facial anomalies, skeletal abnormalities, and damage to organ systems, most commonly occur because of drinking during the first trimester. Since the brain is forming throughout pregnancy, ARND may be caused by drinking at any time. Growth failure is commonly related to drinking during the last trimester. Hyperactive behavior, learning disabilities, developmental disabilities such as speech and language delays, and poor judgment and reasoning skills are signs of ARND. Difficulty in school and in maintaining employment, inappropriate sexual behavior, and violations of the law are problems likely to be exhibited by individuals with ARND.

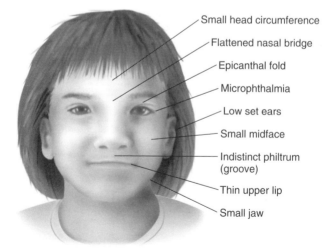

- Small head circumference
- Flattened nasal bridge
- Epicanthal fold
- Microphthalmia
- Low set ears
- Small midface
- Indistinct philtrum (groove)
- Thin upper lip
- Small jaw

Figure 3-2
Abnormal findings of the head in fetal alcohol syndrome.

Intervention and teaching

Avoiding alcohol altogether during pregnancy is the only known way to prevent FAS, ARBDs, and ARND. If the mother does not find this possible, she should be urged to limit her intake to no more than one drink at a time and not to drink every day. Every effort should be made to achieve abstinence from alcohol.

Cigarette smoking

Infants of women who smoke during pregnancy have lower birth weights than infants of nonsmoking mothers. In addition, women who smoke have an increased risk of preterm delivery, perinatal mortality, placenta previa, and possibly spontaneous abortion. The mechanism by which smoking affects the fetus is not completely understood, but it is likely that it causes intrauterine hypoxia, perhaps through reduced placental blood flow. Also, smoking increases the metabolic rate and thus caloric needs. Weight gain and prepregnant weight tend to be lower in smokers than in nonsmokers, and the diets of smokers are reported to be poorer than those of nonsmokers. Women who smoke have decreased levels or increased needs for several nutrients, including vitamin C, folate, zinc, and iron. Women who stop smoking during pregnancy have been successful in increasing the birth weights of their infants.

Intervention and teaching

Vitamin and mineral supplementation of the woman who continues to smoke is advisable, but supplementation does not counteract the detrimental effects of smoking on the fetus. Smoking cessation should be the goal for all women who smoke.

Illicit drugs

Increased risk of intrauterine growth retardation (IUGR) and preterm labor is associated with both marijuana and cocaine abuse. The risk of abruptio placentae is also increased by cocaine. Moreover, infants of mothers who abuse crack cocaine often display persistent learning and behavioral abnormalities. It is difficult to determine exactly what impact illicit drugs have on the nutritional status of the pregnant woman because drug abuse is often accompanied by abuse of other substances, such as alcohol or cigarettes, poverty, and poor education, all of which have detrimental influences on nutritional status.

Intervention and teaching

Vitamin and mineral supplements are recommended for women who abuse drugs, but supplements cannot be expected to correct the problems associated with drug use during pregnancy. Every effort should be made to convince the pregnant woman to stop using drugs.

Methylmercury

Methylmercury is a naturally occurring element and also an industrial pollutant that accumulates in some of the larger, long-lived fish and fish that eat other fish.

Intervention and teaching

- The U.S. Food and Drug Administration (2003a) advises pregnant women, those likely to become pregnant, and lactating women to avoid shark, swordfish, king mackerel, and tilefish, but to eat as much as 12 oz (360 g) of other ocean fish and farm-raised fish per week, as long as they eat a variety of types of fish.
  - Fresh tuna (sashimi) and canned albacore (white) tuna have significant amounts of mercury and should not be used regularly.
  - Croaker, farm raised trout, sardines, and whitefish are among the lowest in mercury content (U.S. Food and Drug Administration, 2003b).
- Check local and state advisories about locally caught fish. If no advisory exists, up to 6 oz (180 g) of locally caught fish can be consumed weekly, as long as no other fish is consumed during the week.

Listeria infection

The food-borne illness known as listeriosis can cause spontaneous abortion, stillbirth, and fetal infection. Pregnant women are about 20 times more likely than normal adults to contract listeriosis.

Intervention and teaching

To avoid listeriosis, pregnant women should not consume any of the following:

- Unpasteurized milk or items made with unpasteurized milk (e.g., cheeses) unless thoroughly cooked.

- Undercooked or raw animal products such as fish, shellfish, eggs, or meat.
- Refrigerated smoked seafood, refrigerated pâtés or meat spreads, deli meats, cold cuts, or hot dogs (which can easily become contaminated after processing) unless they are thoroughly cooked.
- Soft cheeses. Hard cheeses can be consumed.
- Fresh fruits and vegetables before they are thoroughly washed.

Caffeine and artificial sweeteners

The effect of caffeine intake on the fetus is not fully known. Some investigators have found coffee drinking during pregnancy to be associated with spontaneous abortions and a decrease in birth weight, with no ill effects found among drinkers of decaffeinated coffee. The risk seems to be greater in women who consume 600 mg caffeine a day (equivalent to approximately 1 liter or four 8-oz cups of regular coffee) or more, with few side effects evident when women consume 300 mg caffeine (500 ml, or two 8-oz cups) or less daily.

Intervention and teaching

- *Caffeine:* Insufficient data are available to make a recommendation regarding caffeine use during pregnancy; however, until such data are available, it seems prudent to abstain from caffeine use or to limit daily intake to no more than 300 mg (approximately two 8-oz cups or 500 ml of coffee). In addition to coffee, tea, colas, and many over-the-counter medications (which should not be used without the approval of the health care provider) contain caffeine (see Appendix G).
- *Artificial sweeteners:* Four artificial sweeteners—saccharin, aspartame, acesulfame potassium, and sucralose—are approved by the Food and Drug Administration for use in the United States, including consumption during pregnancy. Aspartame (NutraSweet) has not been found to have adverse effects on the normal mother or fetus, but its use should be avoided by pregnant women homozygous for phenylketonuria (PKU).

Pregnancy Complications with Nutritional Implications

Nausea and vomiting

Nausea and vomiting, or "morning sickness," are common during the first trimester of pregnancy. "Morning sickness" is a misnomer because the symptoms can occur at any time of the day. Although annoying, nausea and vomiting are rarely severe and prolonged enough to impair nutritional status. Severe nausea and vomiting that may continue throughout pregnancy occurs in about 3.5/1000 births. Known as **hyperemesis gravidarum,** this condition is associated with electrolyte imbalance, dehydration, weight loss, and ketonemia.

Intervention and teaching

Suggestions for coping with morning sickness are as follows:

- Eat small, frequent meals; hunger can worsen nausea.
- Avoid fluids for 1 to 2 hours before and after meals.
- Consume plain, starchy foods (crackers, dry toast, melba toast, rice, pasta or noodles, plain boiled or baked potatoes, unsweetened cooked or ready-to-eat cereals) during times of nausea because they are easily digested and unlikely to cause nausea. Spicy foods can worsen nausea.
- Decrease intake of fats and fried foods. Fat delays gastric emptying and can increase nausea.
- Minimize exposure to strong food odors. Avoid cooking foods with strong odors during times of nausea, maintain adequate ventilation in the kitchen, and use lids on pots during cooking.
- Avoid brushing teeth immediately after eating because this causes some individuals to gag.
- Try salty foods (e.g., potato chips) or tart foods (e.g., lemonade), which are tolerated well by some women with nausea.

The woman suffering from hyperemesis gravidarum may require hospitalization to receive intravenous fluids for rehydration. Parenteral nutrition (containing glucose, amino acids, vitamins, and electrolytes) or an enteral tube feeding may be used initially to restore fluid and electrolyte balance and maintain an adequate nutrient supply for the mother and fetus. When vomiting has diminished, small amounts of low-fat, easily digested starches, skinless poultry, and lean meats are reintroduced orally, with the diet gradually advanced as tolerated. Occasionally, nausea and vomiting will be so severe and prolonged that the woman requires prolonged enteral tube feeding or parenteral nutrition (see Chapters 7 and 8).

Constipation

Constipation is most common during the last half of pregnancy. Contributing factors include decreased gastrointestinal (GI) motility resulting from increased progesterone levels, increased pressure on the GI tract by the bulky uterus, effects of iron supplementation, and decreased physical activity.

Intervention and teaching

- Maintain a dietary fiber intake of at least 28 g/day (see Appendix B).
- Consume approximately 50 ml fluid/kg body weight daily to ensure that adequate fluid is available to form soft, bulky stools.
- Obtain aerobic exercise (e.g., walk briskly) regularly to improve muscle tone and stimulate bowel motility.

Preeclampsia

Preeclampsia is a form of hypertension that occurs only in pregnancy. Also termed **pregnancy-induced hypertension (PIH),** preeclampsia is characterized by not only hypertension but also proteinuria, and usually by excessive edema. It generally occurs in the third trimester. The cause is unknown, but diets adequate in protein, energy, calcium, magnesium, zinc, and sodium are associated with the lowest incidence of preeclampsia. Obesity increases the risk of preeclampsia. Bed rest and antihypertensive medications are used in the treatment of PIH. A severe sodium restriction (1 to 1.5 g daily) was previously used in treatment of hypertension associated with pregnancy, but recognition that adequate sodium is necessary for normal expansion of blood volume during pregnancy has reduced the use of severe sodium restriction.

Intervention and teaching

A moderate restriction of sodium to 2 to 3 g/day may be prescribed to help control pregnancy-induced hypertension. To achieve this level of restriction, omit the following foods and seasonings from the diet: salt, seasoning salts, and obviously salty foods, such as potato chips and pretzels; smoked or canned meats, fish, and poultry; condiments and seasonings, such as prepared mustard, catsup, and Worcestershire or soy sauce; canned soups and vegetables (unless they are low-sodium); bouillon; prepared mixes for cakes, casseroles, breads and muffins, gravies or sauces, and puddings (especially instant); frozen entrees; commercially prepared pies and pastries; and salted butter, margarine, peanut butter, and cheese.

Good choices for a low-sodium diet include fresh, canned, or frozen fruits; fresh vegetables and those canned or frozen without salt (check label); and unprocessed meats, poultry, and fish. Use of herbs and spices (except those containing salt, such as garlic salt) and seasonings such as lemon juice improve food flavors without increasing the sodium content. The Dietary Approaches to Stop Hypertension (DASH) diet described in Chapters 1 and 14, which emphasizes intake of fruits and vegetables, low-fat dairy products, and whole and enriched grain products, is a useful diet pattern for control of pregnancy-induced hypertension.

Diabetes

For the diabetic woman who becomes pregnant or the woman who develops **gestational diabetes mellitus** (GDM; diabetes that is first evident during pregnancy), the goal is to maintain normoglycemia during pregnancy. Women with a high risk of GDM (marked obesity, history of GDM during a previous pregnancy, glucose in the urine, or a strong family history of diabetes) should undergo glucose testing as soon as they enter prenatal care. If they are found not to have GDM initially, they should be retested between 24 and 28 weeks of gestation. Women of average risk should have testing undertaken at 24 to 28 weeks of gestation. Women of low risk of GDM (those meeting all of the following criteria: less than 25 years, normal weight before pregnancy, member of an ethnic group with low prevalence of GDM, no known diabetes in first-degree relatives, no history of abnormal glucose tolerance, and no history of poor obstetric outcome) require no glucose testing. The diagnosis of GDM is made by abnormal results on an oral glucose tolerance test (American Diabetes Association, 2004). GDM in some women can be controlled by dietary measures (medical nutritional therapy) alone; for those who cannot, insulin is the pharmacologic agent most commonly used.

For women with insulin-dependent diabetes before pregnancy, insulin requirements usually decline during early pregnancy but increase during the second trimester and remain high until delivery. Poor control of blood glucose levels during pregnancy is associated with an increased number of congenital malformations and fetal deaths. In fact, it is important for diabetic women to achieve good control before conception; an increased risk of preeclampsia and of producing infants with malformations is present for those who do not.

Intervention and teaching

The diet for diabetes in pregnancy is discussed in Chapter 17.

- Tight control of blood glucose reduces the risk of congenital deformities of the fetus. Insulin-dependent women receive several daily injections or continuous infusions with an insulin pump.
- Self-monitoring of blood glucose, usually several times daily, is associated with better control than periodic monitoring by the health care provider.
- Moderate physical activity is recommended as a part of treatment for women without physical or obstetric contraindications to exercise.
- For obese women, a moderate energy restriction (~25 kcal/kg per day) has been shown to reduce hyperglycemia and hypertriglyceridemia without increasing urine ketone excretion. Restriction of carbohydrate to about 35% to 40% of total energy improves maternal and fetal outcomes (American Diabetes Association, 2004).

Maternal phenylketonuria (PKU)

Individuals with PKU, an inborn error in the metabolism of the amino acid phenylalanine to tyrosine, appear to have better neurologic and mental function if they maintain a low phenylalanine diet for life. However, those women who have relaxed their dietary control need counseling to return to the diet and achieve target blood phenylalanine concentrations before conception. If conception occurs before control is achieved, every effort should be made to achieve good control by 8 weeks of gestation. Pregnant women with PKU in poor control are at risk of delivering infants with defects that include low birth weight, microcephaly, and congenital heart disease. Although maternal blood phenylalanine concentrations of 120 to 360 μmol/l are desirable, it is difficult to achieve such stringent control. Adequate protein intake and weight gain reduce the incidence of delivering infants with microcephaly and congenital heart defects (Matalon et al., 2003), but the diet must be carefully planned. Special low protein foods are included, and much of the protein comes from a low phenylalanine formula (medical food). Education and follow-up by a dietitian skilled in working with individuals with PKU is essential.

Lactation

Human milk is an ideal food for the infant, and any mother who is interested in breastfeeding should be encouraged to do so. The advantages of breastfeeding are summarized in Box 3-2.

The objectives of nutritional care in lactation are for the woman to do the following: (1) maintain an adequate diet to replenish stores that were diminished during pregnancy and produce sufficient milk for growth of the infant, (2) lose the weight gained during pregnancy, (3) avoid nutritional practices that could harm the infant, and (4) establish a successful breastfeeding relationship with her infant.

Assessment

Assessment is summarized in Table 3-1.

Nutritional Requirements
Energy

The DRI for energy intake during the first 6 months of lactation is set at 330 kcal per day more than nonpregnant needs, and during the second 6 months it is 400 kcal a day more than nonpregnant needs. During the first 6 months of lactation, the DRI is calculated to be approximately 170 kcal/day less than needed to meet the mother's needs. Therefore consuming the DRI would result in continuing weight loss, helping the woman to return to her prepregnant weight more rapidly than women who do not breastfeed. During the second 6 months, the mother's weight is assumed to be stable, but the DRI is increased only slightly because milk intake by the older infant is reduced as more and more foods are added to the infant's diet.

Intervention and teaching

The increased energy needs should be met by use of additional milk products and small increases in meat and meat substitutes, fruits and vegetables, and whole-grain or enriched breads and cereals. Fatigue and the demands of the infant on the woman's time may interfere with food preparation. Commercially prepared foods such as low-salt and low-fat frozen meals may be helpful during the early postpartum period.

The Dietary Approaches to Stop Hypertension plan (see Chapters 1 and 14), with inclusion of approximately 3 to 4 servings of milk, yogurt, or cheese, is appropriate during lactation. A variety of foods from all food groups should be consumed.

Box 3-2   Advantages of Breastfeeding

Infant Benefits

- Reduced risk of diarrheal diseases, respiratory diseases, bacterial meningitis, and otitis media. Human milk contains a variety of antiinfective factors and immune cells—such as IgA, IgM, IgG, B and T lymphocytes, neutrophils, macrophages, complement, and lactoferrin—that are not found in infant formula. In addition, human milk appears to contain immunomodulation factors that stimulate the infant to produce interferon and other agents of immunity.
- Reduced risk of overfeeding.
- Ease of digestion. Lactalbumin protein in human milk forms a soft, easily digested curd in the infant's stomach. Lipase enzyme in human milk improves the digestion of milk fat.
- Improved absorption of zinc and iron, compared with absorption from formula.
- Potential for enhanced cognitive development. Infants fed human milk have been found to have higher scores on intelligence tests at school age than those fed formula. These findings may be related to the fact that human milk is rich in certain long-chain polyunsaturated fatty acids believed to be needed for neurologic development. These fatty acids are especially important for preterm infants, who are more immature neurologically than term infants.

Maternal Benefits

- Less postpartum bleeding and more rapid uterine involution. Oxytocin levels are increased in the breastfeeding mother.
- Convenience (once lactation is established).
- Economy.
- More rapid postpartum weight loss.
- Increased child spacing because of delayed resumption of ovulation. Note that this does not mean that breastfeeding is a reliable method of contraception.
- Reduced risk of ovarian and premenopausal breast cancer.
- Improved bone mineralization in the postpartum period, with a reduced risk of postmenopausal hip fractures.

Mutual Benefits

Promotion of mother-infant bonding.

It is important to exercise regularly after the birth of the baby to promote weight control, reshape the figure, and foster a feeling of health and well-being. The lactating woman can participate in any activity she enjoys. It is essential that she have adequate fluid intake during and after exercise to replace losses in perspiration and to avoid interfering with milk production. After very heavy exercise, lactic acid may accumulate in the milk and cause the infant to reject the following feeding. This condition is usually temporary, with the infant nursing well at the next feeding.

Protein

Recommendations for protein during lactation are the same as during pregnancy (1.1 g/kg/day, or approximately 71 g per day). This amount is easily obtained in the U.S. diet; women often consume this much protein or more even before becoming pregnant.

Intervention and teaching

Most of the extra protein needed is provided by the consumption of 1 to 2 extra servings of milk or equivalent products per day, along with an additional 2 oz (60 g) of meat or meat substitutes.

Vitamins, minerals, and fluid

Vitamin B_{12}, calcium, and fluid are of special concern during lactation. Most normal adults have long-lasting stores of vitamin B_{12}, but approximately two thirds of lactating women who have followed strict vegetarian diets for several years are lacking in reserves of this vitamin, and their milk contains little or no vitamin B_{12}. Megaloblastic (macrocytic) anemia, poor growth, and neurologic abnormalities have occurred in infants breastfed by such mothers (Centers for Disease Control, 2003). The DRI for calcium during lactation remains the same as during pregnancy (1000 mg/day for adult women, and 1300 mg/day for teens).

Intervention and teaching

- *Vitamin B_{12}:* Strict vegetarian (vegan) mothers need a supplement (at least 2 to 3 µg of vitamin B_{12}) or daily consumption of sufficient food sources fortified with vitamin B_{12} (e.g., at least 2 to 3 servings of vitamin B_{12}–fortified soy milk).
- *Calcium:* For women who do not drink milk, other good sources of calcium are listed in Figure 3-1 or Appendix A. The use of milk in cooking (e.g., in mashed potatoes, grain products, and soups)

can greatly increase milk intake. If the woman's diet appears likely to be inadequate, a daily calcium supplement is advisable.

- *Fluid:* To produce adequate milk, women need 35 to 50 ml of fluid/kg of body weight per day (16 to 23 ml/lb/day) plus an additional 500 to 1000 ml.
  - Water, milk, tea, decaffeinated coffee, soft drinks, fruit juices, and ices can be used to meet fluid needs.
  - If energy intake is likely to be excessive, then emphasis should be placed on skim milk and calorie-free beverages. Women may perceive 100% fruit juices as healthful drinks, but these contain about 60 kcal in 120 ml and are a significant source of energy if used to quench thirst.

Diabetes

Breastfeeding may have a positive effect on blood glucose control in women with type 1 diabetes. Successful breastfeeding is associated with a kcal prescription of at least 31 kcal/kg of maternal weight (14 kcal/lb). Women with diabetes should be carefully monitored for mastitis because it is more common in diabetic than in nondiabetic women.

Potentially Harmful Practices

In a few circumstances, mothers should not be encouraged to breastfeed. These include the following:

- Galactosemia (congenital inability to metabolize galactose, a component of lactose) in the newborn.
- Serious maternal infections that pose a threat to the infant, such as sputum-positive tuberculosis. Human T-lymphotrophic virus infection and active herpes simplex on the breast may also be contraindications to breastfeeding. In the United States and other industrialized nations, women positive for the human immunodeficiency virus (HIV) are advised not to breastfeed because the virus is present in milk. In developing countries, however, the issue is more complicated. The antiinfective properties of human milk, which protect the infant from many diarrheal and respiratory infections associated with high mortality, may outweigh the risk of transmission of HIV posed by breastfeeding.
- Maternal need for certain drugs secreted in milk that may have deleterious effects on the infant (for an extensive listing of specific drugs, see Lawrence & Lawrence, 1999).
- Maternal disinclination to breastfeed.

Certain medical conditions are compatible with breastfeeding as long as there is careful supervision by the health care provider:

- *Phenylketonuria (PKU) in the infant:* Human milk is relatively low in phenylalanine, and many PKU infants can be totally or partially breastfed if their phenylalanine levels are closely monitored.
- *Severe "breast milk jaundice"* (serum bilirubin concentration approaching 20 mg/dl): Human milk contains an inhibitor of bilirubin conjugation and excretion, and therefore in some cases of severe hyperbilirubinemia, pediatricians may recommend temporary interruption of breastfeeding. After 12 to 24 hours of formula feeding, bilirubin usually declines, and breastfeeding can continue. The mother should be reassured that her milk is not bad for the infant and assisted in pumping her breasts if necessary during the interruption of breastfeeding.
- *Hepatitis B:* Carriers of hepatitis B may breastfeed as long as their infants have received hepatitis B immune globulin at birth and hepatitis B vaccine before hospital discharge.

Some specific foods and lifestyle practices may have negative effects on the success of lactation or the health of the infant.

- *Alcohol and drugs of abuse:* Maternal alcohol intake during lactation can impair the mother's milk ejection reflex. In addition, alcohol and other drugs appear in breast milk. Controversy exists regarding whether or not maternal alcohol intake has a detrimental effect on infant motor development. If a woman chooses to drink alcohol during lactation, it would be best for her to limit her intake to no more than one drink per day, and preferably she should not drink alcohol on a daily basis. Drugs of abuse, including amphetamines, cocaine, heroin, marijuana, and phencyclidine hydrochloride (angel dust), should be avoided during lactation.
- *Coffee and caffeine:* The iron content of milk from mothers drinking three or more cups of coffee per day has been found to be approximately one third lower than in mothers drinking less than three cups. Only 1% of the caffeine consumed by the mother is passed into her milk, but infants are unable to metabolize and excrete caffeine as effectively as adults. Some infants of mothers who consume caffeine have been noted to have irritability and insomnia, and mothers who note these symptoms would be well

advised to limit to 300 mg daily their intake of caffeine from coffee, tea, chocolate, soft drinks, and over-the-counter drugs.

- *Smoking:* Smoking should be avoided. Nicotine appears in milk, but the major risk to the infant is from "passive smoking"—exposure to tobacco pollutants within the home environment. This increases the risk of asthma and other respiratory diseases.

- *Antigens in foods:* Where there is a family history of atopic disease (an allergy, probably hereditary, characterized by symptoms such as asthma, hay fever, or hives produced upon exposure to a particular antigen), evidence suggests that lactating mothers who avoid antigenic foods reduce the risk of atopy in their infants (Kramer and Kakuma, 2003). Some common antigenic foods include peanuts, tree nuts, cow milk, eggs, and shellfish.

- *Spicy and "gas-forming" foods:* Lactating women are sometimes told to avoid "gas-forming" foods such as onions, cabbage, legumes, chocolate, and spicy foods. There is little basis for these prohibitions. Very rarely a mother will note that some food she consumes causes a rash, diarrhea, or irritability in her infant on a consistent basis. Elimination of this food from her diet readily corrects this problem.

- *Methylmercury in fish:* See advice under pregnancy, previously discussed.

Establishing Successful Breastfeeding

Many actions by health care providers can enhance the likelihood of successful breastfeeding. Early and sustained contact between the infant and mother (e.g., the opportunity to breastfeed within the first hour of life and to room in with the infant in the hospital) is an important measure. The infant should not be supplemented with water, glucose solutions, or formula unless the infant's medical condition makes supplementation necessary. A supportive layperson that has breastfed successfully can be a valuable resource for new breastfeeding mothers. In general, supplements and pacifiers should be used only after lactation is established, if at all. When juices, formula, and solid foods are introduced, the mother's milk production declines, and these foods and fluids are generally unnecessary until at least 6 months of age. Growth spurts occur during infancy, and the infant may seem continually hungry at these times. The mother can be reassured that this is normal and that her milk is sufficient; more frequent feedings will increase her milk supply so that the infant's needs are met.

For the infant, some signs of successful breastfeeding include a moist tongue and good hydration, weight gain of 15 to 30 g/day after the milk comes in, at least three to four bowel movements and four to six urinations daily after the third day of life, and rhythmic sucking with audible swallowing during breastfeeding. Signs of success in the mother include milk "coming in" by 72 hours after delivery (the breasts feel full and warm, and milk may leak), comfortable feedings, and letdown of milk, evidenced by the infant's swallows, leaking of milk, and softening of the breasts after feeding.

REFERENCES

American Diabetes Association: Gestational diabetes mellitus, *Diabetes Care* 27(suppl 1):S88, 2004.

Centers for Disease Control and Prevention: Neurologic impairment in children associated with maternal dietary deficiency of cobalamin—Georgia, 2001, *JAMA* 289:979-980, 2003.

Kramer M, Kakuma R: Maternal dietary antigen avoidance during pregnancy and/or lactation for preventing or treating atopic disease in the child, *Cochrane Database Syst Rev* 4:CD000133, 2003.

Lawrence RA, Lawrence RM: *Breastfeeding: a guide for the medical profession,* ed 5, St Louis, 1999, Mosby.

Matalon KM, Acosta PB, Azen C: Role of nutrition in pregnancy with phenylketonuria and birth defects, *Pediatrics* 112:1534, 2003.

National Academy of Sciences, Institute of Medicine: *Nutrition during pregnancy and lactation*, Washington, DC, 1992, National Academy Press.

National Academy of Sciences, Institute of Medicine: *Dietary reference intakes for energy, carbohydrates, fiber, fat, protein and amino acids (macronutrients)*, Washington, DC, 2002, National Academy Press.

U.S. Food and Drug Administration: Advice for women who are pregnant, or who might become pregnant, and nursing mothers, about avoiding harm to your baby or young child from mercury in fish and shellfish, 2003a. Available at http://www.fda.gov/oc/opacom/mehgadvisory1208.html. Accessed December 30, 2003.

U.S. Food and Drug Administration: Mercury levels in various fish, 2003b. Available at http://www.fda.gov/ohrms/dockets/ac/03/briefing/4010b1-11-fish-data.pdf. Accessed December 30, 2003.

SELECTED BIBLIOGRAPHY

American College of Obstetricians and Gynecologists: Breastfeeding: maternal and infant aspects, *Int J Gynaecol Obstet* 74:217, 2001.

Dennis CL: Breastfeeding initiation and duration: a 1990-2000 literature review, *J Obstet Gynecol Neonatal Nurs* 31:12, 2002.

Gabbe SG, Graves CR: Management of diabetes mellitus complicating pregnancy, *Obstet Gynecol* 203:857, 2003.

Hamaoui E, Hamaoui M: Nutritional assessment and support during pregnancy, *Gastroenterol Clin North Am* 32:59, 2003.

Hasenau SM, Covington C: Neural tube defects, *MCN Am J Matern Child Nurs* 27:87, 2002.

Kaiser LL, Allen L: Position of the American Dietetic Association: nutrition and lifestyle for a healthy pregnancy outcome, *J Am Diet Assoc* 102:1479, 2002.

Kuscu NK, Koyuncu F: Hyperemesis gravidarum: current concepts and management, *Postgrad Med J* 78:76, 2002.

Luke B et al: Specialized prenatal care and maternal and infant outcomes in twin pregnancy, *Am J Obstet Gynecol* 189:934, 2003.

Olson CM et al: Gestational weight gain and postpartum behaviors associated with weight change from early pregnancy to 1 y postpartum, *Int J Obes Relat Metab Disord* 27:117, 2003.

Ong KK, Dunger DB: Perinatal growth failure: the road to obesity, insulin resistance and cardiovascular disease in adults, *Best Pract Res Clin Endocrinol Metab* 16:191, 2002.

Oumachigui A: Prepregnancy and pregnancy nutrition and its impact on women's health, *Nutr Rev* 60:S64, 2002.

Picciano MF: Nutrient composition of human milk, *Pediatr Clin North Am* 48:53, 2001.

Ramakrishnan U: Nutrition and low birth weight: from research to practice, *Am J Clin Nutr* 79:17, 2004.

Rasch V: Cigarette, alcohol, and caffeine consumption: risk factors for spontaneous abortion, *Acta Obstet Gynecol Scand* 82:182, 2003.

Thackray H, Tifft C: Fetal alcohol syndrome, *Pediatr Rev* 22:47, 2001.

Infancy, Childhood, and Adolescence

4

During infancy, childhood, and adolescence, adequate nutrition is essential for the promotion of growth and the establishment of a framework for lasting health. Growth is the simplest and most basic parameter for evaluation of nutritional status in children.

Evaluating Growth

Adequate nutrition is reflected in a child's progress on standardized growth charts depicting height/length for age, weight for age, weight for stature, head circumference for age (up to 36 months of age), and body mass index for age. Sex- and age-specific charts are available for children from birth through 20 years (see Appendix D).

Each child establishes an individual growth pattern and should follow this pattern consistently. Children should be evaluated for nutritional or medical disorders when one of the following occurs:

- They are consistently below the 5th or above the 95th percentile for any growth parameter. Some normal children fall outside the boundaries of the 5th and 95th percentile markings, but all children outside these boundaries should be evaluated to be sure that their growth patterns are reasonable for them (e.g., consistent with the size of their parents and other family members).
- They fail to stay within one percentile marking of their previous growth parameter (e.g., weight has been at 75th percentile marking and it then declines below the 50th percentile).
- Weight and height (or length) are inconsistent with each other (e.g., weight is at the 90th percentile but height is at the 25th percentile).

Infancy

Goals of nutritional care are to assist the infant to consume an adequate diet for optimal growth and development; to avoid practices that may contribute to obesity, poor dentition, or other health problems; and to begin to develop good food habits.

Assessment

Assessment is summarized in Table 4-1.

Nutrition for Normal Growth and Development

Either human milk or iron-fortified infant formula meets the nutritional needs of term infants for the first 4 to 6 months of life. The formula-fed infant may grow more rapidly than the breastfed one, but more rapid growth has not been shown to be an advantage for a healthy term infant.

Infants vary considerably in their feeding patterns, but after the first few weeks of life many breastfed infants feed at approximately 3-hour intervals and formula-fed infants feed at 4-hour intervals. Overfeeding is more likely than underfeeding, but parents frequently worry about whether they are feeding their infants enough, especially if the infants are breastfed. Infants who are gaining weight steadily and are wetting at least six to eight diapers per day are usually taking in enough milk or formula.

The American Academy of Pediatrics (AAP) Committee on Nutrition (2003a) recommends that infants receive human milk or iron-fortified formula for the first year of life. Infants given cow's milk before 12 months of age are likely to develop iron deficiency anemia. Cow's milk, whether whole, low-fat (1% or 2% fat), or skim, can cause gastrointestinal blood loss in infants. Also, cow's milk is extremely low in iron and has excessive amounts of protein, calcium, phosphorus, and sodium for infants; excreting the unneeded nitrogen and minerals can place stress on the kidneys by increasing the renal solute load. It is especially important that skim milk not be used. Skim milk lacks essential fatty acids, which are needed for optimal growth and maintenance of skin integrity.

Recommended supplements

The AAP Committee on Nutrition (2003a) has made the following recommendations:

Text continued on p. 127

Table 4-1   Assessment in Growth and Development

Areas of Concern	Significant Findings
Inadequate Energy or Protein Intake	*History* Poverty; chronic illness or frequent acute illnesses; altered parent-infant relationship manifested by failure to feed infant adequately; fear of becoming obese; obsession with thinness (older children and adolescents); poorly planned vegetarian diet *Physical Examination* Length, height, or weight <5th percentile, or >10% decrease in these parameters; edema, ascites; hair changes: alopecia, loss of pigmentation (flag sign), altered texture; muscle wasting; TSF <5th percentile for age; tooth erosion, gastric bleeding, weak and flabby muscles, poor skin turgor (signs of self-induced vomiting) *Laboratory Analysis* ↓ Serum albumin, transferrin and prealbumin, serum K^+ (self-induced vomiting)
Excessive Energy Intake	*History* Overfeeding; sedentary lifestyle: frequent and prolonged television viewing, lack of regular physical activity; one or both parents overweight or obese *Physical Examination* BMI >85th percentile; TSF >85th percentile for age

Table 4-1   Assessment in Growth and Development—cont'd

Areas of Concern	Significant Findings
Inadequate Mineral Intake	
Iron (Fe)	*History* Poverty; dislike of iron containing foods; vegetarianism; increased needs (especially adolescent females); excessive milk consumption by toddlers; infant receiving cow's milk before 12 months of age *Physical Examination* Pallor; blue sclerae; spoon-shaped nails; short attention span; diminished learning ability *Laboratory Analysis* ↓ Hgb, Hct, MCV, serum Fe, serum ferritin; ↑ free erythrocyte protoporphyrin (FEP)
Zinc (Zn)	*History* Poverty; dislike of zinc-containing foods; vegetarianism (large intake of grains and vegetables containing phytates and oxalates that impede absorption); abnormal losses (severe or prolonged diarrhea) *Physical Examination* Seborrheic dermatitis; anorexia; diarrhea; alopecia; poor growth *Laboratory Analysis* ↓ Serum Zn
Calcium (Ca)	*History* Failure to consume milk products, calcium-fortified soy milk or formula, or a calcium supplement daily because of

Continued

Table 4-1   Assessment in Growth and Development—cont'd

Areas of Concern	Significant Findings
	food preferences, vegetarianism, dieting, or frequent reliance on fast foods
Inadequate Vitamin Intake	
A	*History*
	Failure to consume vitamin A (liver; deep green, leafy, or deep yellow vegetables) at least every other day; frequent reliance on fast foods
	Physical Examination
	Dry skin, mucous membranes, or cornea; follicular hyperkeratosis (resembles gooseflesh); poor growth, susceptibility to infection
	Laboratory Analysis
	↓ Serum retinol
B_{12}	*History*
	Child or adolescent following strict vegetarian diet without a supplement or use of fortified soy milk[*]; ileal resection or disease; infant breastfed by strict vegetarian mother
	Physical Examination
	Pallor; glossitis; neurologic abnormalities (altered sensation, altered sense of balance); confusion, depression
	Laboratory Analysis
	↓ Serum vitamin B_{12}, Hct; ↑ MCV

[*]Young children should not follow strict vegetarian regimes because of the difficulty of ensuring that the diet contains adequate energy and protein for growth. Lactovegetarian diets and ovtolactovegetarian diets can be adequate for children.

- *Vitamin D:* all infants, whether breastfed or formula fed, should receive 5 µg (200 IU) daily.
- *Vitamin B_{12}:* approximately 0.3 to 0.5 µg daily is needed for breastfed infants of strict vegetarian mothers.
- *Iron:* 10 mg daily is recommended for breastfed infants older than 6 months if they do not consume food sources of dietary iron (such as iron-fortified infant cereal) daily.
- *Fluoride:* 0.25 mg fluoride daily is needed for infants over 6 months of age who are fed human milk, ready-to-feed formula, or formula reconstituted with water containing less than 0.3 parts per million (ppm) fluoride. No fluoride supplementation is recommended before 6 months of age.

Human milk feedings

Human milk is ideally suited to meet the needs of the term infant (see Box 3-2). The composition of human milk changes over the first few weeks of lactation. **Colostrum,** the milk produced for about the first 3 to 5 days, is yellowish, rich in immunoglobulins and lymphocytes, and higher in protein than mature human milk. Mature human milk is produced after about 10 to 14 days. It appears watery and may be bluish; it has more lactose and lipid than does colostrum. Transitional milk, produced in the period between colostrum and mature milk production, has some features of each type of milk.

Intervention and teaching

The following information should be included when instructing the breastfeeding mother:

- Make sure that the infant "latches on" well. The infant's mouth should cover as much of the areola (the dark area around the nipple) as possible and never cover just the nipple (Figure 4-1). If the infant is grasping only the nipple or nursing is painful to the mother, then she should insert her finger between the breast and the infant's mouth to break the seal and then reposition the infant's mouth before beginning again. Improper grasp of the nipple makes nipples sore and may lead to cracking.
- Feed the infant from both breasts at each feeding. Begin each feeding with the breast the infant ended with at the last feeding, to ensure that the breast is drained at least every other feeding. Emptying the breasts encourages milk production. If twins are being breastfed,

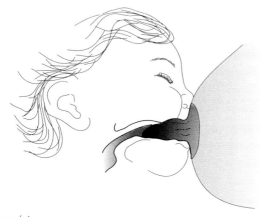

Figure 4-1
Infant properly latched on at the breast. Note that most of the areola is in the infant's mouth.

feed each baby on alternate breasts every other feeding. One baby is likely to be a more vigorous feeder than the other.

■ Exposing the nipple to the air helps to heal it if it becomes sore or cracked (e.g., leave flaps of nursing bra down for 20 minutes after feedings). Massaging a drop of colostrum or milk into the nipple is also helpful. Begin with brief feedings (< 5 minutes per breast) to avoid nipple soreness, but progress to 15 to 20 minutes per breast. Milk fat is usually released only after 10 to 20 minutes of suckling, and the infant needs the fat to grow properly and to be satisfied between feedings.

■ Avoid offering bottle feedings (expressed human milk or formula) until the mother's milk supply is established, usually 4 to 6 weeks after birth. The artificial nipple is different and may confuse the infant, causing him or her to refuse the breast. After that time, it may be possible to give a bottle so that the mother can be away from the infant. Many mothers who return to work outside the home continue to breastfeed for months, either by pumping their breasts during breaks at work or by adjusting to partial breastfeeding (e.g., only two to three feedings per day).

■ Use different infant positions (e.g., cradle hold across the mother's body; lying beside the mother; and football hold with the infant's head in the mother's hand, nursing from the breast on the same side of the body as that hand) to drain different portions of the breast and decrease the risk of clogging the milk ducts. Clogging causes discomfort and may lead to mastitis or breast infection. If signs of clogging or mastitis (redness, enlargement, and pain in a portion of the breast) occur, then the mother should nurse more frequently, beginning on the affected side. The baby is hungrier at the beginning of the feeding and will nurse more effectively, helping to relieve the clogging.

Formula feeding

Commercial formulas closely resemble human milk. Standard formulas and human milk contain about 20 kcal/oz (66 kcal/100 ml). Commercial formulas contain higher levels of protein and most minerals than human milk to compensate for less complete absorption and utilization. The formulas are manufactured with or without added iron. The low-iron formulas are virtually iron free, as is cow's milk. Anemia is common in infants receiving low-iron formulas. For infants who are not breastfed, use of iron-fortified formulas for the first year of life provides a reliable source of dietary iron. Commercial formulas are available in three forms: ready-to-feed, concentrate (to be diluted with an equal volume of water), and powder. The three forms are the same in nutritional value (except for fluoride), and the concentrate or powdered forms are almost always less expensive than ready-to-feed.

Intervention and teaching

When teaching the parents of a formula-fed infant, include the following information:

- Hold the infant closely during feedings. Never prop a bottle or leave an infant unattended during feeding, both for safety reasons and because feedings are an important time for nurturing.
- Be attuned to the infant's degree of hunger. Never encourage him or her to take more at a feeding than he or she seems to want. Table 4-2 gives general guidelines as to the amount of formula to feed, but the individual infant may have different needs.
- Burp the infant regularly during feeding, every 0.5 to 1 oz initially and less often as the infant grows.

Solid foods

There is no need to introduce solid foods before 4 to 6 months of age. Reasons for delaying consumption of solid food include the following:

- The tongue extrusion reflex, which tends to push solid foods out of the mouth, does not fade until the infant is about 4 months of age.
- Production of pancreatic amylase, an important enzyme for digestion of starches in infant foods, is low before 4 months.
- Infants can maintain good head control at 4 months of age and can sit fairly well by 6 months of age. Thus, they are better prepared than younger infants to participate in the feeding process; for example, an infant can turn his or her head away from the spoon to indicate that he or she is full.
- Eczema, other atopic diseases, and diabetes are more common in infants who have undergone early introduction of solid foods; the greater the diversity of foods introduced, the greater the risk.
- Early introduction of solid food has no effect on sleep patterns. Many parents introduce solid foods early, erroneously believing that this will cause the infant to sleep through the night.
- Solid foods can inhibit absorption of iron and other nutrients from human milk.
- Introduction of solid foods before 4 to 6 months of age is associated with a shorter duration of lactation.

Intervention and teaching

When introducing solid foods, the parents should follow these guidelines:

- Begin with foods that provide needed nutrients. For breastfed infants, this means good sources of iron, zinc, protein, and energy. Iron-fortified infant cereals and pureed meats, vegetables, and fruits are usually among the first foods. If foods are

Table 4-2   Approximate Daily Amount of 20 kcal/oz Formula Needed by Infants Younger than 6 Months

| Infant Weight | | Caloric Need | Ounces (ml) of Formula Needed |
kg	lb		
3	6.6	324	16.2 (486)
4	8.8	432	21.6 (648)
5	11.0	540	27.0 (810)
6	13.2	648	32.4 (972)

not introduced until at least 4 to 6 months of age, the order of food introduction is not of major importance.

- Introduce only one new food every 3 to 5 days, and observe the infant for hypersensitivity reactions after each food. If a reaction is thought to have occurred, then stop that food for several weeks and try again later. If the same thing occurs after the second or third trial, then the infant is probably sensitive to this food. Use single-grain cereals until it is clear that the infant tolerates all grains contained in mixed cereals.

- Wait until late in infancy or after infancy to introduce egg white and shellfish, which are among the foods most likely to cause allergy. Avoid nuts and nut butters in infancy because of their potential for allergenicity, as well as the choking hazard they pose.

- Begin with about 1 tsp at a time, and advance the amount as the infant seems ready.

- Offer solid foods at the beginning of feedings while the infant is hungry.

- Thin foods with formula or expressed breast milk initially (e.g., 1 spoon of cereal to 6 spoons of formula or milk) to help the infant make the transition from human milk or formula to foods with thicker consistencies.

- Feed the infant with a spoon. Adding foods to formula in a bottle deprives the infant of a chance to learn feeding skills. Infants with certain medical disorders are exceptions to this rule. Thickening the formula with infant cereal may help to control gastroesophageal reflux, for example.

- Never feed the infant from the jar. If any food is left over, amylase enzyme in the saliva will digest starches in the food, making it watery. Also, bacteria from the mouth contaminate the food and might cause spoilage.

- Avoid serving desserts regularly; these are usually low in nutrients and establish a desire for sweets.

- Consider the developmental state of the infant in choosing foods. For instance, between 7 and 9 months of age the infant's purposeful grasp improves and he or she picks objects up and moves them to his or her mouth. This is an ideal time to offer finger foods such as toast, zwieback, dry cereals, and cheese slices.

Some parents may wish to prepare food at home for the infant. When preparing infant foods at home:

- Use fresh or frozen fruits, vegetables, and meats. Canned foods may contain lead, and canned vegetables and meats contain salt unless they are "no salt added" products.
- Cook foods in as little water as possible, and do not overcook; this preparation preserves the vitamin content.
- Add no sugar or salt. Infants have a well-developed sense of taste and do not require flavor enhancers. The infant receives enough sodium from unsalted foods, and routine use of sugar and salt causes the infant to develop a taste for these unnecessary food additives.
- Puree foods in a blender or food grinder initially; chop or mash foods once the infant has more teeth and can chew lumpier foods.
- Freeze prepared foods in ice trays for later use; the appropriate number of cubes can be used each time for an infant-sized serving.

Minimizing the risk of obesity

To minimize the risk of obesity, parents can do the following:

- Reduce formula and milk intake as infants consume more solids.
- Recognize and respond to cues that the infant has reached satiety. Satiety cues from a younger infant include withdrawing from the nipple, falling asleep, closing the lips tightly, and turning the head away. Cues from an older infant include closing the lips tightly, shaking the head "no," playing with or throwing utensils or food, and handing the cup or bottle back to the parent.
- Never insist that the infant finish a bottle, dish, or jar of food. Before 6 months, an average serving size is about 2 to 5 tablespoons, and after 6 months, it is approximately $\frac{1}{2}$ to 1 jar of baby food. Infants' needs vary widely, however, and an individual infant may not need an average serving.

Promoting dental health

Nursing bottle caries is a form of tooth decay resulting from prolonged contact of sugar-containing fluids (milk, juice, fruit drinks) with developing teeth. Although it usually occurs in bottle-fed infants, it can also occur in breastfed infants. To reduce the risk of caries, these guidelines should be followed:

- If infants are put to bed with a bottle, then it should contain only water so that exposure of the teeth to sweet fluids is minimized. When infants are put to bed with a bottle, they suck on it periodically and keep the mouth full of fluid.

- Avoid giving the infant a bottle or breastfeeding whenever he or she cries. Learn to distinguish cries of hunger from cries for other needs, and feed only in response to hunger.
- Infants less than 6 months of age should not be introduced to fruit juice, since it is not required to meet their nutritional needs (AAP, 2001). Infants over 6 months of age should not receive juice in a bottle or any other easily transported container so that they can easily consume juice throughout the day.
- Fruit drinks, even those that contain some fruit juice, are not equivalent to fruit juice and should not be included in the infant diet.

Feeding safety

Infants are at special risk for certain types of food-borne infections and for choking. Infant food safety practices include the following:

- Infants less than 1 year of age should not consume honey. Clostridium botulinum spores in honey can cause infant botulism. Symptoms range from constipation through progressive weakness and diminished reflexes to sudden death. In contrast, botulism in older persons is almost always caused by consuming the toxin released by the bacteria in spoiled food, not by consuming spores.
- When infants are given fruit juice, it should be pasteurized.
- Infants should not receive hot dogs, grapes, hard foods such as raw carrot, or any other food that is likely to cause choking and block the airway.

Nutritional Problems in Infancy

Acute gastroenteritis

Acute episodes of diarrhea and vomiting, usually associated with viral illness, are common during infancy and early childhood. These illnesses damage the intestinal mucosa and diminish the absorptive surface. Lactase, the enzyme required for digestion of the milk sugar *lactose,* is found in the brush border of the intestinal mucosa, and the activity of this enzyme is reduced during acute episodes of gastroenteritis and the recovery period. In addition, the increased motility of the GI tract during gastroenteritis may not allow sufficient time for fat absorption. Fatty foods often worsen diarrhea and delay gastric emptying, which may increase vomiting. Therefore, it is best to choose foods low in fat and high in glucose oligosaccharides or starch during and immediately after a bout of gastroenteritis.

Intervention and teaching

The Centers for Disease Control and Prevention (King et al., 2003) have made specific recommendations regarding management of acute gastroenteritis in children in the United States, based on the presence and degree of dehydration, and these are summarized below. The degree of dehydration can be determined using the criteria in Table 2-7. Treatment takes place in two stages. In the rehydration stage, fluid deficits are replaced over a period of approximately 3 to 4 hours and a state of adequate hydration is achieved. This is followed by the maintenance stage, where maintenance fluid and energy are provided. Nutrition should not be restricted. Breastfeeding should continue throughout therapy, even during rehydration, and bottle-feeding should resume as soon as the rehydration stage is over. The majority of bottle-fed infants tolerate lactose-containing full-strength formulas, although infants with severe malnutrition, diarrhea, or enteropathy (disease of the gastrointestinal tract) may benefit from a lactose-free formula.

Children receiving semisolid or solid foods should continue to receive their usual diet during episodes of diarrhea. Carbonated soft drinks, fruit juice, fruit drinks, gelatin desserts, and other liquids and foods high in simple sugars should be avoided because they may cause osmotic diarrhea. It is often recommended that fat be restricted, but there does not appear to be much clinical evidence that this reduces diarrhea. Very limited diets such as the BRAT (bananas, rice, applesauce, and toast) diet have been commonly recommended. These regimens are unnecessarily restricted and may result in nutritional deficits, especially if the infant or child suffers repeated episodes of gastroenteritis.

Children with diarrhea but minimal or no dehydration. These children should continue to receive an age-appropriate diet with increased fluids to replace losses. A commercial oral rehydration solution (ORS) is preferred for fluid replacement (Table 4-3). Most children with little or no dehydration can be treated at home.

- If the child is hospitalized, soiled diapers can be weighed, with the estimated weight of the dry diaper deducted, and 1 ml fluid administered for every gram of stool output.

Table 4-3   Appropriate and Inappropriate Solutions for Oral Rehydration

Composition	Rehydration Solutions*	Solutions Inappropriate for Oral Rehydration			
		Cola	Apple Juice	Chicken Broth	Sports Drink
CHO	70-140	700	690	0	255
Na	45-90	2	3	250	20
K	20-25	0	32	8	3
Base	30-48	13	0	0	3
Osm	250-310	750	730	500	330

*Carbohydrate–electrolyte solutions that are commercially available (e.g., Pedialyte [Ross], Infalyte [Mead Johnson], Rehydralyte [Ross], WHO/UNICEF oral rehydration salts).

CHO, Carbohydrate; Na, sodium; K, potassium; Osm, osmolality.

All concentrations are mmol/l, except osmolality, which is mOsm/kg water.

- To replace ongoing losses in children at home, parents can be instructed to give 10 ml of ORS per kilogram body weight for each watery stool or 2 ml/kg body weight for each episode of emesis. As an alternative, children weighing <10 kg can be given 60 to 120 ml ORS for each episode of vomiting or diarrheal stool, and those weighing >10 kg can be given 120 to 240 ml.
- Some children object to the salty taste of ORS. The solutions may be better accepted if frozen into ice pops. Some of the commercial solutions are flavored to improve their acceptance.

Children with more severe dehydration

- *Mild to moderate dehydration:* Fluid deficits should be replaced quickly, over 2 to 4 hours, using 50 to 100 ml fluid per kilogram of usual body weight plus additional fluid as needed to replace ongoing losses. Ongoing losses are replaced as described for children with minimal or no dehydration. A commercial ORS (see Table 4-3) is the preferred fluid. Use of an ORS is less expensive than intravenous treatment and is associated with fewer complications. Very small amounts of ORS (e.g., 5 ml every 10 to 15 minutes) should be administered initially, with the volume increased as tolerated. If vomiting prevents oral rehydration, or the infant/child is unable or unwilling to consume sufficient fluid, the ORS can be administered continuously via a nasogastric (NG) tube. NG rehydration has been successful even in the presence of vomiting. After rehydration, many children can undergo maintenance ORS therapy at home, if the parents are carefully instructed in administration of ORS, signs of dehydration, and findings to report to the health care provider and if they have the ability to return to the health care facility if needed.
- *Severe dehydration:* Severe dehydration is a medical emergency requiring immediate rehydration. Lactated Ringer's (LR) solution, normal saline, or a similar isotonic solution should be given intravenously (20 ml/kg body weight for previously healthy infants and small children; 10 ml/kg in frail or malnourished infants, where sepsis might be confused with dehydration) until pulse, perfusion, and mental status return to normal. Monitor the patient closely for edema of the eyelids and extremities, signs of overhydration. Once the mental status has returned to normal, maintenance fluid therapy can be given as described for infants with minimal or no dehydration, using ORS or IV fluids.

Other treatment measures. No medication is required for treatment of most acute diarrheal illnesses, but may be warranted in cases where the disease does not respond to supportive therapy. Nonspecific antidiarrheal agents such as the adsorbents (e.g., kaolin-pectin) and antimotility drugs (e.g., loperamide) have been used, but their efficacy is unproven. The underlying problem in most cases is increased secretion of fluid and electrolytes by intestinal crypt cells. Racecadotril is an antisecretory agent that has shown promise in reducing secretory diarrhea in early studies.

There is some evidence that **prebiotics** (food ingredients that stimulate the growth or activity of nonpathogenic bacteria such as bifidobacteria and lactobacilli in the colon, e.g., oligofructose) and **probiotics** (live microorganisms such as lactobacilli, bifidobacteria, or the nonpathogenic yeast *Saccharomyces boulardii*) can be used to alter intestinal microflora in a beneficial manner, thus reducing the duration of diarrheal diseases. No specific recommendations for the therapeutic use of these agents can be made at this time. The oligosaccharides found in human milk are potent prebiotics, however, and acute diarrhea is less prevalent among breastfed infants, providing an excellent reason for promotion of breastfeeding.

Diarrhea can result from malabsorption of sorbitol and fructose in fruit juices. If diarrhea is chronic, rather than acute, then the child's intake of fruit juices should be evaluated.

Food hypersensitivity

In infants and small children, symptoms of **food hypersensitivity** or allergy (an immunologic reaction to ingestion of a food or food additive) can include anaphylaxis, failure to thrive, vomiting, abdominal pain, diarrhea, rhinitis, sinusitis, otitis media, cough, wheezing, rash, urticaria, and atopic dermatitis. Egg white, cow's milk, peanuts, nuts from trees, and shellfish are among the most allergenic foods for children.

Intervention and teaching

If a mother is breastfeeding an infant that is at high risk for food hypersenstivity (e.g., an infant with a family history of allergies), it may be necessary for her to avoid these foods with high allergenic potential during lactation. There is no need for a mother breastfeeding an infant at low risk of allergy to avoid any specific foods, unless it becomes evident that her infant is displaying allergic symptoms. A significant proportion of infants allergic to cow's milk are also allergic to soy and thus cannot tolerate soy formulas. Protein hydrolysate formulas (in which the protein is broken down so that no large protein molecules are present to stimulate an allergic response) such as Nutramigen are often used for infants with allergic symptoms. About 85% of children with milk allergy outgrow it by their third year of life. Reintroduction of milk or any other suspected allergen into the diet should be done in a setting where epinephrine, intravenous fluids, and respiratory support are available (Mofidi, 2003; Zeiger, 2003).

Failure to thrive

Failure to thrive describes the infant who does not regain his or her birth weight by 3 weeks of age or the infant who exhibits continuous weight loss or failure to gain weight at the appropriate rate (see Appendix D). This condition results from an inadequate food supply or illness in the infant. *Organic* failure to thrive is a condition in which a physiologic reason for the infant's failure to thrive is apparent. Insufficient milk production by the breastfeeding mother and cystic fibrosis in the infant are two examples of this condition. When no physical cause is apparent, the infant has *inorganic* failure to thrive. Impairments in the parent-child relationship, knowledge deficits in the parent or caregiver, and poor parenting skills are some reasons for inorganic failure to thrive.

Toddlers and Preschoolers

The goals of nutritional care are to foster development of good eating habits that will ensure adequate nutrient intake and minimize the risk of obesity and other health problems.

Assessment

Assessment is summarized in Table 4-1.

Nutrition for Normal Growth and Development
Developing good eating habits

Children need to consume a variety of foods from all food groups. Chronic diseases such as heart disease and type 2 diabetes may have their start in childhood, and thus it is essential that healthy eating habits be established early to provide a basis for lasting health.

Intervention and parent teaching

Parental food habits strongly influence those of children, so parents may need to make an effort to eat a balanced and varied diet and avoid voicing distaste for any foods. Both adults who smoke and their children are likely to have poorer diets than those of nonsmoking families. In families in which the parents have not been able to stop smoking, children's diets need to be carefully assessed and parents should be instructed in the principles of a healthful diet if necessary.

Young children begin to develop food likes and dislikes (Box 4-1). Parents should continue to encourage their children to eat a variety of foods, while respecting children's preferences as much as possible. Children sometimes refuse foods simply because they are unfamiliar with them, but parents should not take this refusal to be permanent. Children's opinions of particular foods improve after they are served those foods repeatedly. **Food jags,** during which children consume only one or two foods for several days, are common. Parents should avoid making an issue of food jags because this disapproval can put parents into the position of struggling with the child for control of the child's behavior. Parents should provide a variety of nutritious foods at each meal, and they should not allow the child to eat only sweets. Food jags are not usually harmful; intake over a period of several weeks balances out.

Young children want to feed themselves and need to learn the necessary skills. Although the process is messy, it should be encouraged. Overemphasis on neatness creates stress at mealtimes and could interfere with the development of good eating habits.

The American Heart Association (Steinberger and Daniels, 2003) does not recommend restricting dietary fat and cholesterol routinely before age 2. After that time, no more than 10% of the kcal should be in the form of saturated fat, cholesterol intake should not be more than 300 mg/day, and *trans*–fatty acids should be avoided as much as possible. Fried foods, peanut butter, regular luncheon meats and cheeses, and butter or margarine should be used only in moderation.

Fiber helps to reduce the risk of heart disease and improves bowel function. Children 1 to 3 years of age need 19 g of fiber daily, and those 4 to 8 years of age need 25 g daily. Whole grains, fruits, and vegetables should be an important part of the child's diet. Appendix B lists specific sources of fiber.

Box 4-1   Food Preferences of Young Children

Likes

- Crisp, raw vegetables
- Foods that can be served and eaten without help, such as finger foods (sandwiches cut into strips or shapes, raw fruit or vegetables cut into small pieces, cheese cubes) and milk and other beverages that can be poured from a child-sized pitcher
- Foods served lukewarm
- Single foods that have a characteristic color and texture; preferably, different foods should not even touch each other on the plate

Dislikes

- Strong-flavored vegetables such as cabbage and brussels sprouts; overcooked vegetables
- Highly spiced foods
- Large servings of beverages or foods
- Foods served at temperature extremes
- Combination foods (e.g., mixed vegetables) where flavors mingle and textures become similar; exceptions: pizza, spaghetti, macaroni and cheese

---

Energy intake and risk of obesity

As the growth rate slows during the toddler and preschool years, energy needs (per kg) are not as high as they were during infancy, and the appetite declines. Energy needs in early childhood are approximately 1000 kcal plus 100 kcal per year of life. That is, a 3-year-old needs about 1300 kcal/day.

Intervention and teaching

Parents may be concerned about what they perceive to be poor food intake by toddlers and preschoolers. They need to be reminded that the growth rate is slowing, and children's appetites will reflect this change. Needs for protein, vitamins, and minerals remain high; however, there is little room for "empty calories" from high-fat or high-sugar foods. Some steps that parents can take to reduce the risk of obesity are as follows:

- Avoid overwhelming the child with servings that are too large. More can be served if the child is still hungry after the initial serving.
- Keep fruits or vegetables available, include them in every meal, and offer them as snacks. Children learn to control their own energy intake when parents provide healthful foods but let the children determine the amount that they will consume. Fresh, frozen, or canned fruits and raw vegetables make better snacks than chips, cookies, or candy.
- Choose low-fat dairy and whole-grain products, as well as lean meats and poultry, because energy needs are too low to allow for consumption of many sweets or high-fat foods.
- Limit the amount of time that young children are involved in sedentary activities such as watching television and using a computer or electronic game to no more than 2 hours daily, and encourage daily activities that use large muscle groups. Excessive television watching promotes inactivity and exposes children to multiple cues to eat. Food advertisements make up more than half of all advertising during children's programming, and advertisements often promote foods with low nutrient density (those containing few nutrients in proportion to the calories provided). Parents should serve as active role models for children.
- Limit intake of fruit juice to no more than 4 to 6 fl oz (120 to 180 ml)/day for children 1 to 6 years of age (AAP, 2001). Whole fruits, a good source of fiber, should make up the remainder of the fruit servings. Water is the preferred beverage if children are thirsty. In addition to providing a significant amount of energy if consumed in excess, the fructose and sorbitol in juices (particularly juices such as pear and apple) may not be absorbed by all children. Abdominal pain, bloating, and diarrhea may result.

Mineral intake

The highest incidence of iron deficiency in the United States is found in children under age 5. Children at special risk include Mexican Americans, Native Americans, the poor, and those who consume 1 quart or more of milk per day. Milk, which is low in iron, may take the place of iron-rich foods in the diet. Iron deficiency is associated with decreased attentiveness, narrow attention span, and impaired problem-solving ability.

The recommended calcium intake for toddlers is 500 mg/day, and for preschoolers it is 800 mg/day. Development of bones and teeth depends on adequate calcium intake. Furthermore, the habit of consuming a diet rich in calcium is important for the prevention of osteoporosis in later life. Milk and cheese are the richest calcium sources in the diets of most young children. Juices, fruit drinks, and other beverages should not be allowed to replace milk in the diet.

Intervention and teaching

To ensure an adequate intake of iron, children should:

- Eat at least 2 servings of meat, poultry, fish, or legumes and 6 servings of enriched or whole-grain breads and cereals daily (Figure 4-2). Deep green, leafy vegetables can also supply some iron.
- Avoid excessive milk intake (i.e., a liter or more daily), since milk provides little or no iron and can displace iron-containing foods in the diet.
- Consume good vitamin C sources daily to improve iron absorption

To ensure adequate intake of calcium, parents should encourage children to follow these guidelines:

- Drink approximately 2 cups (240 ml) of milk daily unless the child is lactose intolerant, a condition that is less common in children than in adults. There is no significant difference in the absorption of calcium from chocolate milk and unflavored milk, so chocolate milk can be used if the child prefers it.
- Limit intake of soft drinks, which are devoid of nutrients other than energy and displace milk and other nutritious foods in the diet.
- Eat cheese often. Parents can offer cheese for snacks, use cheese in main dishes such as macaroni and cheese or Welsh rarebit, or use cheese sauce over vegetables. Low-fat or "part skim" versions of some cheeses help to reduce children's fat intake, which is often excessive.
- Eat yogurt often with meals or as a snack.

Promoting dental health

Good dental health is promoted by encouraging the child to consume a diet adequate in calcium and phosphorus. Four servings of milk daily provide the calcium and phosphorus needed. Avoid offering sticky carbohydrates such as chewy candies, cookies, and pastries, which cling to the teeth. Develop the habit of regular

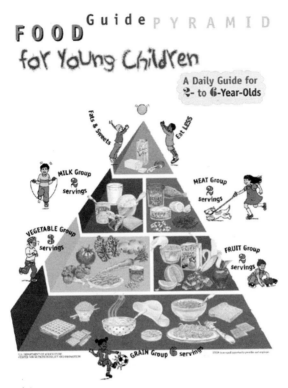

Figure 4-2
Food guide pyramid for young children.
(From USDA Center for Nutrition Policy and Promotion.)

brushing as soon as the child has teeth, and begin flossing as soon as teeth touch each other.

Fluoride makes the teeth more resistant to caries; therefore, the American Dental Association and the American Academy of Pediatrics (2003a) recommend providing some children with fluoride supplements. If the local water supply contains <0.3 ppm of fluoride, then the recommended daily supplement of fluoride is 0.25 mg before age 3, 0.5 mg between ages 3 and 6, and 1 mg from 6 to 16 years. If the water supply provides 0.3 to 0.6 ppm of fluoride, then the recommended dosage for fluoride supplementation is 0 to 3 years of age, none; 3 to 6 years, 0.25 mg; 6 to 16 years, 0.5 mg.

No supplement is routinely recommended for children of any age whose water supply provides >0.6 ppm of fluoride.

Feeding safety

All juices served to children should be pasteurized to reduce the risk of food-borne infection. Another safety concern is that most deaths resulting from asphyxiation by food occur in children under age 3. To help prevent asphyxiation, these guidelines should be followed:

- For children under age 3, avoid foods such as hot dogs, hard candy, caramels, jelly beans, gum drops, nuts or peanuts, grapes, and raw carrots, which are difficult to chew or swallow and are an appropriate size to block the airway.
- If the parent chooses to give the child foods that are likely to be aspirated, the parent should modify these foods to make them less likely to obstruct the airway. Grapes can be quartered, carrots cooked, and meat cut into very small pieces. Hot dogs can be cut lengthwise into four strips.
- Provide adult supervision for very young children while they eat.
- Insist that children sit down while they eat.
- Keep eating times as calm as possible. A child who is laughing or extremely excited could aspirate food.

School-Age Children

The goals of nutritional care are to develop sound eating habits that minimize the risk of obesity and other health problems while providing adequate amounts of all nutrients and fiber. Specifically, teaching should include choosing a balanced diet and encouraging physical activity.

Assessment

Assessment is summarized in Table 1 1.

Nutrition for Normal Growth and Development
Healthful food choices

Peers, teachers, and other significant adults begin to influence food choices during the school years, and home influences decline. As children grow older and have more money to spend, they consume more snacks and meals outside the home. Vending machines and fast-food restaurants offer foods that are likely to be high in fat, salt, and sugar and low in vitamins and minerals. Furthermore, a growing number of latchkey children may spend several hours of each day without adult supervision. Among the many issues regarding the welfare of these children is a concern about the quality of their food intake.

Intervention and teaching

Children need to consume a wide variety of fruits, vegetables, whole grains, dairy products, legumes, fish, poultry, and lean meat. Their diets should be moderate in fat, high in calcium, and adequate but not excessive in energy. The following guidelines help to achieve these goals:

- Parents can encourage children to eat a nutritious diet by involvement and example. It may take as many as ten tries to convince a child to include a new food in his/her diet, but it is worth the effort to encourage children to eat a wide variety of foods. Establish a rule that all family members eat at least one meal together daily (if at all possible). Not only does this rule encourage family interaction, but it is easier to control the amount of sodium, sugar, and fat in home-prepared foods than in items obtained outside the home.
- Involve children in obtaining or preparing food. Children can be involved in gardening if the family grows some vegetables, in choosing food at the market (with adult guidance), and in age-appropriate cooking and food preparation tasks. This involvement gives children a personal stake in the family meals and is a good way to introduce elementary nutrition.
- Make nutritious snacks available at all times to discourage the consumption of high-energy, low-nutrient foods. Good choices for snacks include fresh or dried fruits; raw vegetables; yogurt; air-popped or other low-fat popcorn; cheese, especially low-fat varieties; cottage cheese with raisins or other fruits; unsalted, dry-roasted seeds or nuts; bran or oat muffins; fruit juice frozen into pops; and peanuts or peanut butter (in moderation because of the high fat content).
- Prepare foods attractively, because meals with "eye appeal" are more likely to be enticing to youngsters. Choose appealing color combinations for foods served in a meal, and be sure that vegetables are not overcooked, to avoid causing their colors and textures to deteriorate. Bread for sandwiches can be cut with cookie cutters

into inviting shapes, and pancakes can be poured in the shape of the child's initials or other fun shapes. If vegetable intake is a problem, try incorporating vegetables into other foods (e.g., bake carrot or zucchini muffins, or add finely grated vegetables to meatballs or meatloaf).

Reducing the risk of chronic health problems

Eating habits with long-lasting effects are set during childhood. Dietary intake can influence the incidence of chronic health problems such as obesity, heart disease, cancer, and osteoporosis. A survey of U.S. children (Neumark-Sztainer et al., 2002) found that they consumed less than the recommended amounts of fruits, vegetables, and grains, and only about 30% of girls and 42% of boys consumed the recommended amount of calcium. Fat intake in the children surveyed exceeded the recommended level. Approximately 15% of children 6 to 19 years of age are overweight or obese, a substantial increase over the previous estimates (National Center for Health Statistics, 2003). This is due both to poor dietary habits and a more sedentary lifestyle that may include, for example, excessive television viewing and use of electronic games and computers. There has been an alarming increase in cases of insulin resistance and type 2 diabetes (disorders commonly associated with overweight and obesity) in children and teens. Thus, lifestyle changes to prevent overweight is one of the highest priorities in child health.

Intervention and teaching

Children need daily physical activity that involves use of large muscle groups—either team sports or individual aerobic exercises. Parent example and involvement is important. The American Heart Association recommends at least 60 minutes of moderate to vigorous physical activity every day for children and adolescents (Steinberger & Daniels, 2003). Excessive sedentary activity (more than 2 hours daily of television watching or electronic gaming) should be avoided (AAP, 2003b).

Emphasis should be placed on making healthy food choices, rather than on foods to avoid. Nutritious foods, including ample amounts of fruits, fresh vegetables, low-fat dairy products, and whole grains, should be provided for meals and snacks. The family must avoid relying regularly on fast-food meals, which tend to be high in energy, fat, and sodium and low in milk products, vegetables, and fruits. Low-fat cooking methods (grilling, baking, and stir-frying) are preferred over deep-frying.

The child's social, emotional, and family environment may contribute as much as the nutritional and physical environment to the problem of overweight. The mother who has always struggled with maintaining her weight at a stable level may put undue pressure on her child to stay slim, for example. The child's self-esteem and sense of independence can suffer as a result. Ultimately, this attitude may contribute to development of eating disorders. Parents need help from the health care team when they are too rigid in trying to control the child's behaviors or too disorganized to provide children with the structure and support they need to maintain a healthy body weight. Children benefit from counseling and modeling of behaviors that help them to improve their self-esteem and self-reliance.

Attention Deficit/Hyperactivity Disorders

Attention deficit/hyperactivity disorders (ADHDs) are characterized by focusing on irrelevant stimuli, impulsive behavior, overactivity (not in all children), inconsistency, and lack of persistence. The Feingold diet has been recommended as a treatment for ADHDs. It excludes foods containing salicylates, compounds that cross-react with salicylates, artificial flavors, colors, and preservatives. Controlled studies have not provided clear-cut evidence that this diet is effective. Positive effects from the diet may be a result of the placebo effect or of the fact that it takes pressure off the child (placing the blame for his or her behavior on the diet, rather than on the child). Unfortunately, some of the supposed salicylate-containing foods such as oranges, peaches, grapes, raisins, apples, berries, and cherries are nutritious and are commonly enjoyed by children. A modified Feingold diet, restricting only food additives, allows a more varied diet, even though it, too, increases the difficulty of food purchasing and preparation. There should be no objection if the family wants to follow such a diet, unless they substitute the diet for medication or counseling needed by the child or family or unless emphasis on the diet promotes behavioral problems by forcing the child to be "different" from his or her peers.

Sugar has also been proposed as a cause of ADHDs, but identifying the cause of ADHDs is difficult, largely because most research must depend on subjective reports by parents. Studies done so far indicate that parents expect their children to be hyperactive after consuming large amounts of sugar-containing foods, and this parental expectation may explain why children sometimes have behavioral problems after high sugar intake. Also, sugar intake tends to be high at parties and on holidays, when children are usually excited; the children's excitement over the event itself can confuse parents into thinking that sugar is causing the problem.

Adolescence

The goal of nutrition care is to help adolescents learn to make wise food choices that provide the necessary nutrients while maintaining a desirable body weight and a healthy lifestyle.

Assessment

Assessment is summarized in Table 4-1.

Nutrition for Normal Growth and Development
Healthy food and lifestyle choices

Energy needs for adolescent growth are high. Despite these needs, many adolescents do not consume an adequate diet. In a survey of U.S. children, only approximately 4% of teenage boys and 3% of teenage girls consumed the recommended number of servings from at least four of the five food groups (Muñoz et al., 1997). Fruit intake was low among both sexes, and consumption of dairy products was especially low among girls. The average fat intake among adolescents and younger children was approximately 35% of total calories, which is well above the recommended level (<30% of total calories). Snacks furnish about 40% of energy in adolescent diets. Although snacking is not bad in itself, traditional snack foods such as chips, cookies, and soft drinks are low in nutrients and high in energy. Adolescents rely heavily on fast-food restaurants, which have limited menus and serve foods that, for the most part, are high in energy (kcal), fat, and sodium.

Intervention and teaching

Fat and cholesterol. To reduce fat and cholesterol intake, these guidelines should be followed:

- Limit use of fried foods to one serving per day or less.
- Choose poultry, fish, or grain and legume main dishes often and reduce the use of red meat.

- Limit meat intake to about 5 oz/day. This is sufficient even for most athletes in training.
- Use dairy products made with skim milk whenever possible. Chapter 14 provides additional information for limiting fat and cholesterol intake.
- Fiber has a cholesterol-lowering effect. It is recommended that 9- to 13-year-old girls consume 26 g of fiber daily and boys consume 31 g. The fiber recommendation for 14- to 18-year-old girls is 36 g and for boys it is 38 g (National Academy of Sciences, 2002).

Mineral intake. Lack of calcium and iron is particularly common among teenage girls. Bone growth requires an increase in calcium intake, with a DRI of 1300 mg/day. Growth and onset of menstruation necessitate an increase in iron needs; the RDA for adolescent girls is 15 mg/day. Fast foods and traditional snack foods tend to be low in calcium and iron. Also, girls concerned about their weight often consider dairy products, which are rich sources of calcium, to be too fattening to include in their diets. To ensure adequate vitamin and mineral intake, these guidelines should be followed:

- Consume three to four servings of milk or milk products daily (especially important for adolescent girls). It is difficult to consume enough calcium in the diet without using milk products. Skim milk and yogurt, cheese, and cottage cheese made of skim milk are low in energy and may be acceptable to dieting teens. Calcium-fortified juice and cereals are reliable calcium sources, and Figure 3-1 shows other dietary calcium sources.
- Use a daily supplement if the diet is low in milk products or other good sources of calcium (see Appendix A). Calcium citrate is a well-absorbed form of calcium. Calcium carbonate, a common antacid, is 40% calcium. To improve absorption, it should be taken with foods, but preferably not with bran or whole grains.
- Eat meat; poultry; fish; legumes; enriched or whole grains; or deep green, leafy vegetables daily to receive dietary iron (see Appendix A). Even if they use a variety of these foods daily, adolescent girls may still have an inadequate or marginal iron intake. A daily supplement (15 mg) may be needed. This amount is available in many over-the-counter multivitamin-multimineral supplements. Avoid taking such supplements with milk, coffee, or tea to improve iron absorption.

Effective weight control. Approximately 15% of adolescents in the United States are overweight, and many more have the potential to become overweight as adults. To avoid excessive energy intake, these guidelines should be followed:

- Limit fat intake.
- Choose high-fiber foods (see Appendix B), because they are bulky and require more chewing than low-fiber, refined foods. The person feels full after eating less energy. Whole grains, legumes, and crisp salads without excessive additions such as dressing, eggs, meat, and bacon are nutritious, low-energy foods.
- Obtain approximately 60 minutes of moderate exercise most days of the week. Some teens wish to participate in team sports, which can be encouraged. Others need to choose individual activities that they will continue on a long-term basis. Chapter 5 shows how to calculate the target heart rate for cardiovascular fitness and includes recommendations for becoming and remaining physically fit. Excessive sedentary leisure activity (more than 2 hours daily) such as television watching, computer usage, and electronic gaming should be discouraged.
- Make sure that snacks are nutritious and low in energy, because they are such an important part of the adolescent's diet. Some examples are fresh or dried fruits; fresh vegetables with a dip made of low-fat yogurt and herbs; air-popped popcorn; bagels (plain or with low-fat cream cheese or other low-fat topping); fruit ices; and yogurt, cottage cheese, or cheese made with skim milk.
- Limit fruit juice consumption to 8 to 12 oz (240 to 360 ml) daily. It is easy to overconsume energy in this liquid form, and many juices (e.g., apple) are relatively low in nutrient density. This limit does not apply to whole fruits, which contribute a range of nutrients, as well as dietary fiber and nutraceutical components.
- Consume sugar-containing soft drinks infrequently; water is the best beverage for quenching thirst.
- Teens have such busy schedules that convenience is an overwhelming concern for them. Thus, parents need to ensure that nutritious snacks and convenience foods are readily available at home, and schools need to keep vending machines and snack bars stocked with fruits, yogurt, and other healthful items.

Inappropriate weight control practices

About three fourths of girls in high school have pursued a weight reduction diet at least once, and 40% are on diets at any one time. Fad diets are popular but are more likely to promote transient water loss than lasting changes in eating habits. Magazines aimed at adolescent girls focus on physical appearance, with thinness given extreme importance. The cultural emphasis on a slim figure contributes to the prevalence of anorexia nervosa and bulimia (see Chapter 19), eating disorders that usually develop during the teen years.

Intervention and teaching

Because teens are so interested in weight-reduction diets, they need to be taught to recognize a safe and effective eating plan. Fad diets promise and often deliver quick results, but much of the weight loss is fluid and lean body mass, rather than fat. A good plan meets the criteria outlined in Box 7-3.

Eating disorders often appear during adolescence. Magazines and television programming focused on adolescents place a priority on appearance. Adolescents who are seriously committed to certain sports or recreational activities—such as gymnastics, figure skating, wrestling, or ballet—may feel compelled to maintain unrealistically low body weights. Primary prevention of eating disorders should be the goal. Some topics to include in a primary prevention program are as follows: (1) normal physiologic, social, and psychologic changes during puberty, the normal changes in fat deposition, and the diversity that occurs among individuals; (2) general nutrition, meal skipping, and other eating habits; (3) physical activity—its importance and appropriate levels; (4) weight control—realistic and safe methods of weight control, realistic goals for weight, myths and fads about dieting, the physiologic and psychologic effects of food restriction and chronic dieting; (5) body image issues and how to determine one's appropriate body weight; (6) autonomy and self-esteem; (7) impact of nutritional habits on athletic performance; and (8) information about anorexia and bulimia. If parents observe their children to be dieting and experiencing weight loss, they need to intervene early. The prognosis is much better if intervention occurs early in the course of the illness. See Chapter 19 for a more detailed discussion.

Vegetarianism

The teen years are a time of experimentation, which may take the form of adopting vegetarianism. There are many types of vegetarians (see Chapter 1). Unless carefully planned, vegetarian diets may be nutritionally inadequate.

Plant sources of protein include legumes (soybeans; peanuts; beans such as pinto, navy, northern, or kidney; and peas such as blackeye and crowder), grains, nuts and seeds, and vegetables other than legumes. Plant sources of protein differ from animal sources such as meat, milk, and eggs in that most plant sources are not **complete proteins.** A complete protein is one that contains all of the **essential amino acids** in sufficient amounts and in proportion to one another so that it can support growth and maintenance of tissues. Essential amino acids are those that cannot be synthesized in the body in the amounts needed for the building of tissues and therefore must be provided by the diet. Most plant proteins are low in one or more essential amino acids and are therefore **incomplete proteins.** Fortunately, the amino acid patterns of the different plant protein sources vary. For example, most grains are low in the amino acid lysine but contain moderate amounts of methionine, and conversely most legumes are relatively low in methionine but contain moderate amounts of lysine. Consuming proteins from a variety of plant sources on a daily basis is the best way to ensure that the diet includes adequate amounts of all amino acids. Use of milk products also helps to ensure that the diet has high-quality protein sources, and adolescents should be encouraged to include milk, cheese, and yogurt in their diets.

Intervention and teaching

A vegetarian food guide has recently been developed for use as a teaching tool in diet planning (Messina et al., 2003). To ensure that nutritional intake is adequate, the adolescent vegetarian needs to be aware of the following:

- Consuming a wide variety of grains, legumes, nuts, and seeds allows the vegetarian to obtain adequate amounts of all amino acids. A diet including eggs and dairy products ensures that the vegetarian has complete protein in the diet, but an adequate diet without animal products is possible with careful planning.

- Whole grains; legumes; and deep green, leafy vegetables contain iron and zinc. Additional iron can be obtained from dried fruits, molasses, soy sauce, and use of iron cookware.
- Iron from plant sources is better absorbed if it is consumed with a vitamin C–containing food such as citrus fruit.
- Coffee and tea inhibit iron absorption; thus it is best not to consume these beverages with meals.
- Vegetarians who avoid dairy products often have difficulty consuming enough calcium. Furthermore, plant foods are usually lower in zinc and iron than animal products, and phytate (in whole grains) and oxalate (in chocolate, green leafy vegetables, and rhubarb) form complexes with minerals and inhibit their absorption.
- Calcium-fortified juice, cereals, tofu, and soy milk can be valuable sources of calcium for vegetarians who do not use dairy products.
- Adolescent girls, in particular, may benefit from daily use of dairy products or a calcium supplement. Dairy products are among the richest dietary sources of calcium, and lactose in dairy products stimulates calcium absorption. See Figure 3-1 or Appendix A for other good sources of calcium.
- Vitamin B_{12}–containing products must be consumed several times per week. Eggs, dairy products, and all other animal products contain vitamin B_{12}. Some soy milk and nutritional yeast is fortified with vitamin B_{12} (consult the label). If no dietary vitamin B_{12} sources are used, then the individual will need a vitamin B_{12} supplement (2 to 3 µg/day), which can be obtained as a daily multivitamin.

While the vegetarian diet can be a healthful one, as demonstrated in Table 4-4, interest in such a diet can also signal an eating disorder in an adolescent. The diets of adolescent vegetarians need to be carefully assessed to determine that they are associated with healthful eating patterns.

Nutrient supplement safety

High doses of vitamin A taken systemically, including synthetic vitamin A products used in treatment of acne (isotretinoin), can be teratogenic. Sexually active girls taking vitamin A supplements need instruction in effective methods of contraception, as do all other sexually active teens.

Table 4-4   Sample Vegetarian Diet Plan

Breakfast	
6 oz calcium-fortified orange juice	1 fruit
⅔ cup oat bran cereal	1 grain
1 sliced peach	1 fruit
1 cup fortified soy milk*	1 milk
Lunch	
2 bean burritos	1 protein + 2 grain
½ cup Spanish rice	1 grain
½ cup tomato wedges	1 vegetable
1 medium apple	1 fruit
Dinner	
1½ cups spaghetti	3 grain
1 cup sauce (tomato and textured vegetable [soy] protein)	1 protein and ½ vegetable
1 cup mixed greens	1 vegetable
½ cup broccoli florets	1 vegetable
1 cup soy milk	1 milk
Snack	
1½ cups frozen tofu dessert	1 milk
TOTAL SERVINGS	7 grain
	3½ vegetable
	3 fruit
	2 protein
	3 milk

*If at least 2 cups of vitamin B_{12}–fortified soy milk are consumed daily, no vitamin B_{12} supplement is necessary.

REFERENCES

American Academy of Pediatrics (AAP) Committee on Nutrition: Policy statement: the use and misuse of fruit juice in pediatrics, *Pediatrics* 107:1210, 2001.

American Academy of Pediatrics (AAP) Committee on Nutrition: *Pediatric nutrition handbook*, ed 5, Elk Grove Village, Ill, 2003a, American Academy of Pediatrics.

American Academy of Pediatrics (AAP) Committee on Nutrition: Prevention of pediatric overweight and obesity, *Pediatrics* 112:424, 2003b.

King CK et al: Managing acute gastroenteritis among children: oral rehydration, maintenance, and nutritional therapy, *MMWR Recomm Rep* 52(RR-16):1, 2003.

Messina V, Melina V, Mangels AR: A new food guide for North American vegetarians, *J Am Diet Assoc* 103:771, 2003.

Mofidi S: Nutritional management of pediatric food hypersensitivity, *Pediatrics* 111:1645, 2003.

Muñoz KA et al: Food intakes of US children and adolescents compared with recommendations, *Pediatrics* 100:323, 1997.

National Academy of Sciences: *Dietary reference intakes for energy, carbohydrates, fiber, fat, protein and amino acids (macronutrients),* Washington, DC, 2002, National Academy Press.

National Center for Health Statistics: Overweight children and adolescents 6-19 years of age, according to sex, age, race, and Hispanic origin: United States, selected years 1963-65 through 1999-2000. Available at http://www.cdc.gov/nchs/data/hus/tables/2002/02hus071.pdf. Accessed June 12, 2004.

Neumark-Sztainer D et al: Overweight status and eating patterns among adolescents: where do youths stand in comparison with the healthy people 2010 objectives? *Am J Public Health* 92:844, 2002.

Steinberger J, Daniels SR: Obesity, insulin resistance, diabetes, and cardiovascular risk in children: an American Heart Association scientific statement from the Atherosclerosis, Hypertension, and Obesity in the Young Committee (Council on Cardiovascular Disease in the Young) and the Diabetes Committee (Council on Nutrition, Physical Activity, and Metabolism), *Circulation* 107:1448, 2003.

Zeiger RS: Food allergen avoidance in the prevention of food allergy in infants and children, *Pediatrics* 111:1662, 2003.

SELECTED BIBLIOGRAPHY

Bachrach VR, Schwarz E, Bachrach LR: Breastfeeding and the risk of hospitalization for respiratory disease in infancy: a meta-analysis, *Arch Pediatr Adolesc Med* 157:237, 2003.

Bowman SA et al: Effects of fast-food consumption on energy intake and diet quality among children in a national household survey, *Pediatrics* 113:112, 2004.

Briefel RR et al: Feeding infants and toddlers study: improvements needed in meeting infant feeding recommendations, *J Am Dietet Assoc* 104:31, 2004.

Fluoride Recommendations Work Group: Recommendations for using fluoride to prevent and control dental caries in the United States, *MMWR Recomm Rep* 50(RR14):1, 2001.

Fulhan J, Collier S, Duggan C: Update on pediatric nutrition: breastfeeding, infant nutrition, and growth, *Curr Opin Pediatr* 15:323, 2003.

Huang JS et al: Efficacy of probiotic use in acute diarrhea in children: a meta-analysis, *Dig Dis Sci* 47:2625, 2002.

Schwartz MB, Puhl R: Childhood obesity: a societal problem to solve, *Obes Rev* 4:57, 2003.

Videon TM, Manning CK: Influences on adolescent eating patterns: the importance of family meals, *J Adolesc Health* 32:365, 2003.

Adulthood and Aging

5

A nutritious diet and regular physical activity are major factors contributing to fitness and health in the adult years. Habits that promote healthy lifestyle choices should be developed early and maintained throughout life. This chapter focuses on adulthood, but much of the content is applicable to children and adolescents as well.

Nutrition Assessment in the Adult Years

The goal of nutritional intervention in adulthood is maintenance of good health and well-being and reduction of the risk of chronic and debilitating diseases. Nutrition assessment of adults in regard to these goals is summarized in Table 5-1.

Health Promotion

Recent surveys have shown that nutrition and lifestyle practices among many adults are poor. In particular, approximately 60% are not physically active on a regular basis. Women are less active than men, and Hispanics, Native Americans, and African Americans are more sedentary than Caucasians. Sedentary habits begin to develop early in life. Activity levels decrease in adolescence, particularly among girls. At least one third of all U.S. high school students get no regular vigorous physical activity. Surveys of food intake indicate that only about 25% of adults consume the five servings of vegetables and fruits recommended in the Dietary Guidelines for Americans.

Overweight/Obesity and a Sedentary Lifestyle

Obesity and overweight are risk factors for numerous chronic illnesses including cardiovascular disease; hypertension; type 2 diabetes; and certain types of cancers, including breast (postmenopausal), colorectal, endometrial, renal cell, and gallbladder

157

Table 5-1   Assessment of the Adult

Area of Concern	Significant Findings
Overweight and Overnutrition	*History* Sedentary lifestyle; excessive energy intake *Physical examinataion* Weight >120% of desirable or BMI >25; waist circumference >102 cm (men) or >88 cm (women); TSF>95th percentile; hypertension; acanthosis nigricans* *Laboratory analysis (plasma)* ↑ Triglycerides, ↑ LDL cholesterol, ↓ HDL cholesterol, ↑ glucose
Inadequate Calcium Intake	*History* Poor intake of dairy products because of dislike of them, lactose intolerance, or belief they are fattening *Laboratory analysis* ↓ Bone mineral density
Inadequate Fiber Intake	*History* Frequent use of processed foods; low intake of fruits and vegetables, whole grains, and legumes; constipation, diverticulosis
Inadequate Antioxidant Intake	*History* Poor intake of fruits and vegetables

*Darkening of the skin, especially over the elbows, knees, and groin; associated with insulin resistance (but also linked with some gastrointestinal cancers).

cancers. Unfortunately, overweight and obesity are prevalent in the United States and Canada. The Centers for Disease Control estimate that 64% of U.S. adults are overweight or obese, if overweight is defined as a body mass index (BMI) of 25 or greater and obesity is defined as a BMI of 30 or greater. Statistics Canada reports that about half of all Canadian adults are overweight or obese. As many as 47 million individuals in the United States, and growing numbers around the world, have a disorder known as the **metabolic syndrome** (also known as the insulin resistance syndrome or syndrome X). The metabolic syndrome is characterized by obesity, hypertension, abnormal serum lipids, and **insulin resistance** (impaired responsiveness of the tissues to insulin with varying degrees of hyperglycemia). Specific criteria defining the metabolic syndrome were recently published (Table 5-2). It is clear that the metabolic syndrome is likely to be a precursor to most of the chronic illnesses mentioned earlier in this paragraph. Since overweight/obesity and a sedentary lifestyle are major contributing factors to the metabolic syndrome, these factors are key targets in efforts to prevent and correct the syndrome.

Nutrition intervention and teaching

Maintaining a healthy weight

The content in this chapter will focus primarily on prevention of overweight. Although there is some overlap with Chapter 7, that

Table 5-2   Identification of the Metabolic Syndrome[*]

Risk Factor	Defining Level
Abdominal obesity[†]	Waist circumference[‡]
Men	>102 cm (>40 in)
Women	>88 cm (>35 in)
Triglyerides	≥150 mg/dl
HDL cholesterol	
Men	<40 mg/dl
Women	<50 mg/dl
Blood pressure (systolic/diastolic)	≥130/≥85 mm Hg
Fasting glucose	≥110 mg/dl

From *Third Report of the National Cholesterol Education Program (NCEP) Expert Panel on Detection, Evaluation, and Treatment of High Blood Cholesterol in Adults (Adult Treatment Panel III),* Washington, DC, 2001, National Heart, Lung, and Blood Institute, National Institutes of Health.

[*]Any three of these findings indicates the presence of the metabolic syndrome.
[†]Overweight and obesity are associated with insulin resistance and the metabolic syndrome. However, the presence of abdominal obesity is more highly correlated with the metabolic risk factors than is an elevated body mass index (BMI). Therefore, the simple measure of waist circumference is recommended to identify the body weight component of the metabolic syndrome.
[‡]Some men exhibit the metabolic syndrome with only a borderline elevation of waist circumference (94-102 cm).

chapter deals in more detail with weight loss measures for individuals that are overweight or obese. The first step in maintaining a healthy weight is for the individual to recognize what that is. A healthy weight range for the individual is generally a weight for height that results in a BMI of 18.5 to 24.9 (see Chapter 2 or the chart inside the back cover for methods of determining the BMI). While some healthy individuals have weights that cause them to fall outside that range, health risks are statistically greater for those outside the range.

Healthy eating habits. A weight-maintaining diet includes a wide variety of foods, especially those rich in fiber and calcium and moderate in fat.

- Grains and grain products are a basis for a healthful diet. However, the focus should be on whole grains (e.g., whole-wheat, oat, and rye breads; whole-grain pasta; brown rice; oatmeal; whole-grain breakfast cereals) rather than refined products. Fiber from whole grains, along with that from fruits and vegetables, not only provides bulk that helps the individual feel full but also has beneficial effects on serum cholesterol levels and bowel function.
- Calcium intake, and particularly calcium from dairy products, has been found to have a protective effect against obesity in some studies. For every 300-mg increase in average daily calcium intake, some have estimated that body weight may be 2.5 to 3 kg (5.5 to 6.6 lb) less than in comparable individuals not consuming as much calcium (Parikh & Yanovski, 2003; Zemel, 2003). A calcium intake of at least 1000 to 1200 mg/day (equivalent to approximately three servings of dairy products plus calcium from green leafy vegetables and foods made with milk) is recommended in adulthood.
- Fat is needed in the diet to supply essential fatty acids, but more importantly for individuals trying to control their weight, it helps to promote satiety. Oils rich in monounsaturated fats (olive, canola, safflower, peanut) and polyunsaturated fats (sunflower, corn) are especially good choices due to their beneficial effects on serum cholesterol. Peanuts; tree nuts such as walnuts, pecans, pistachios, and almonds; and seeds such as sunflower, sesame, and pumpkin are good sources of monounsaturated and polyunsaturated fats and can be used in moderate amounts as cholesterol-free replacements for some of the meat servings in the diet. The risk of cancer is increased with high-fat consumption, and there-

fore limiting fat to no more than 30% of energy intake is part of a prudent diet.

- Lean meat (e.g., round or loin), fish, and poultry can be part of a healthful diet, but portion sizes are best limited to about 4 oz (120 g), about the size of a deck of cards.
- Broiling, grilling, steaming, and sautéing in small amounts of oil or with the use of nonstick cookware and vegetable cooking spray are low-fat cooking methods preferable to frying.
- Read labels carefully when shopping. "Low-fat" items (e.g., cottage cheese, milk, cold cuts, frozen meals and entrees) can be extremely helpful in controlling fat and energy intake, but "low fat" does not necessarily mean that an item provides substantially less energy than its higher-fat alternative. For example, 2 tablespoons of low-fat peanut butter provide 187 calories, while 2 tablespoons of regular peanut butter contain 191; $\frac{1}{2}$ cup light vanilla ice cream contains 111 calories, while the same amount of regular ice cream contains 133; and 2 low-fat fig cookies provide 102 calories, while 2 regular cookies provide 111.
- Keep healthful foods such as fresh fruits or vegetables (pared and cut into appropriate eating sizes if possible), low-fat dairy products, and nuts and seeds readily available as alternatives to less healthful snack choices such as chips and cookies.
- Eating out can be a special challenge to the individual trying to control body weight.
  - Avoid the temptation to "super size" items at fast-food restaurants. Choose small sandwiches and do not add cheese or bacon.
  - Select salads with low-fat dressing or grilled chicken or fish rather than burgers or fried fish.
  - Consult the nutrition information available at some fast-food restaurants and on the websites for virtually all fast-food chains to determine the wisest food choices.
  - Ask about food preparation methods before ordering at full-service restaurants if there is any question about the fat or energy content of an item, and request sauces and salad dressings to be served "on the side" so that the patron can determine how much to use.
  - Serving sizes at full-service restaurants are likely to be large. Share meals with a companion or plan to take part of the meal home for later consumption.
- Develop psychological and emotional skills for avoiding overeating.

- Eat only when hungry. Learn to recognize cues for eating that have nothing to do with hunger (e.g., situations such as watching television or movies, seeing commercials about food, emotional stresses, boredom) and avoid eating in response to those cues. Chewing sugar-free gum helps some individuals cope with the need to eat when not hungry.
- Eat slowly to allow the body to recognize satiety before overeating has already occurred.
- Avoid eating "on the run" because it is easy to overeat while focusing on matters other than eating.
- Keep a record of all food eaten to recognize the actual amounts consumed as well as times when overeating is likely. The individual may not find it necessary to do this always, but it can be helpful to do it a few days whenever weight gain occurs to identify unhealthful eating practices and provide a basis for planning changes.

Physical fitness. Regular physical activity throughout life is an extremely valuable tool for health maintenance. It not only helps to maintain muscle mass and decrease fat accumulation but also reduces the tendency to gain weight as the metabolic rate declines with age.

- *Changes in incidental activity* can improve fitness and stimulate energy expenditure. A few examples include the following: park further from the door to increase the walking needed to get into a building, take the elevator rather than the stairs whenever practical, and walk or bicycle rather than driving when running errands close to home or work.
- *Optimal exercise duration.* Moderate intensity activity for 30 minutes almost every day or a minimum of 20 minutes of vigorous intensity at least 3 days a week reduces the risk of cardiovascular disease and diabetes (National Center for Chronic Disease Prevention and Health Promotion [NCCDPHP], 2003; Knowler et al., 2002), but it is unlikely to be sufficient to prevent overweight in adults as they age. About 45 to 60 minutes of daily activity of at least moderate intensity is believed to be necessary for avoiding weight gain (Saris et al., 2003).
- *Exercise intensity.* Intensity of exercise can be judged in various ways (NCCDPHP, 2003):
  - *The talk test:* A person should be able to sing while performing light activity and carry on a conversation comfortably while

engaged in moderate activity. Exercise is vigorous if the person is too winded or breathless to talk comfortably.

- *Target heart rate:* For moderate intensity exercise, a person's heart rate should be between 50% and 70% of the maximum (HR_{max}). HR_{max} can be estimated as 220 minus the age in years. For example, for a 40-year-old, HR_{max} would be 180 bpm. To determine the target heart rate,

    $180 \times 0.5 = 90$ bpm

    $180 \times 0.7 = 126$ bpm

    Thus, the target heart rate for moderate intensity exercise at 40 years of age is 90 to 126 bpm. For vigorous intensity exercise, the target heart rate should be 70% to 85% of the HR_{max}. For the 40 year-old, the target heart rate for vigorous intensity exercise would be 126 to 153 bpm.

- *Perceived exertion (Borg scale):* The Borg scale is based on the individual's perception of how much exertion he/she is doing. The person's perception of increase in heart rate, work of breathing, sweating, and muscle fatigue may give a good indication of the actual heart rate. On this scale, a rating of 6 means no exertion at all, and a rating of 20 indicates maximal exertion. A rating of 7.5 is very light activity, 11 is light, 13 is somewhat hard, and 15 is hard. Moderate intensity exercise would be rated at approximately 12 to 14 on the scale.

- *Metabolic equivalent (MET) level:* Activities are rated according to the relative energy (oxygen) use required. One MET is the energy required while sitting quietly—for example, while reading a book. The harder the body works, the higher the MET rating for the activity (Table 5-3). The same activity may be categorized as light, moderate, or vigorous intensity, depending upon the effort put into it. In addition, at different ages, the same activity may have different intensities. A moderate activity for a woman in her 30s might be vigorous for a woman in her 60s.

- *Type of physical activity.* Almost any activity that can be performed vigorously enough to raise the heart rate to reach the target level and keep it elevated can provide aerobic benefit. Physical activity is more likely to be maintained if it is an enjoyable activity for the individual, easy to access on a daily basis, easy to fit into the daily schedule, financially reasonable, and low in negative consequences (injury, negative peer pressure, etc.).

Table 5-3   Level of Intensity of Selected Physical Activities

Light Activity* <3 METs† (<3.5 kcal/min)	Moderate Activity* 3-6 METs† (3.5-7 kcal/min)	Vigorous Activity* >6 METs† (>7 kcal/min)
Walking casually, less than 3 miles per hour (mph)	Walking at a moderate or brisk pace, 3 to 4.5 mph on a level surface	Racewalking or aerobic walking, 5 mph or faster
		Jogging or running
	Walking with crutches	Wheeling your own wheelchair
	Roller-skating or in-line skating at a leisurely pace	Backpacking
		Roller-skating or in-line skating at a brisk pace
		Mountain or rock climbing
Bicycling less than 5 mph	Bicycling 5 to 9 mph with few hills	Bicycling >10 mph or on steep uphill terrain
Stationary cycling with light effort	Stationary cycling with moderate effort	Stationary cycling with vigorous effort
Stretching exercises—slow warm-up	Yoga	Karate, judo, tae kwon do, jujitsu
	Gymnastics	Jumping rope
	Using a stair climber machine or a rowing machine at a light-to-moderate pace	Using a stair climber machine or rowing machine at a fast pace

Aerobic dancing—stretching and slow warm-up period	Aerobic dancing—high impact	Aerobic dancing—high impact
	Water aerobics	Step aerobics
Swimming—floating		Water jogging
	Swimming—recreational	Swimming—steady-paced laps
	Waterskiing	Water polo
	Snorkeling	Scuba diving
	Surfing, body or board	Downhill skiing—racing or with vigorous effort
	Downhill skiing—with light effort	Cross-country skiing
	Ice skating at a leisurely pace (9 mph or less)	Sledding
		Playing ice hockey
Gardening and yard work: pruning, weeding while sitting or kneeling, or slowly walking and seeding a lawn	Gardening and yard work: raking the lawn, bagging grass or leaves, digging, hoeing, shoveling <10 lbs/minute	Gardening and yard work: heavy or rapid shoveling (>10 lbs/minute), carrying heavy loads
		Felling trees, carrying large logs, swinging an ax, hand-splitting logs, or climbing and trimming trees

Continued

Table 5-3   Level of Intensity of Selected Physical Activities—cont'd

Light Activity* <3 METs† (<3.5 kcal/min)	Moderate Activity* 3-6 METs† (3.5-7 kcal/min)	Vigorous Activity* >6 METs† (>7 kcal/min)
Using a riding mower	Planting trees, trimming shrubs and trees, hauling branches Pushing a power lawn mower or tiller	Pushing a nonmotorized lawn mower

From U.S. Department of Health and Human Services, Public Health Service, Centers for Disease Control and Prevention, National Center for Chronic Disease Prevention and Health Promotion, Division of Nutrition and Physical Activity: *Promoting physical activity: a guide for community action*, Champaign, Ill, 1999, Human Kinetics.

*For an average person, defined as 70 kg or 154 pounds. The activity intensity levels in this chart are most applicable to men aged 30 to 50 years and women aged 20 to 40 years. Intensity is a subjective classification. For older individuals, the classification of activity intensity might be higher. For example, what is moderate intensity to a 40-year-old man might be vigorous for a man in his 70s.

†The ratio of exercise metabolic rate. One MET is defined as the energy expenditure for sitting quietly, which, for the average adult, approximates to 3.5 ml of oxygen uptake per kg body weight per minute, or approximately 1.2 kcal/min for a 70-kg individual. A 3-MET activity requires three times the metabolic energy expenditure of sitting quietly.

Walking and gardening are two of the most popular physical activities among adults, and they should be encouraged to perform them regularly and vigorously enough to obtain moderate intensity exercise.

■ *Resistance and flexibility training*. For a well-rounded exercise program, resistance and flexibility training should be performed at least 2 to 3 days per week. Resistance training consists of at least 8 to 12 repetitions (10 to 15 for elderly or very frail individuals) of 8 to 10 different exercises that condition the major muscle groups (e.g., weight training). Flexibility training stretches the major muscle groups. In the frail elderly, resistance and balance training should precede aerobic training, to ensure that aerobic exercise can be done without increased risk of injury.

Oxidative Stresses

"Free radicals" are electrically charged particles formed as the natural by-product of normal cell processes. Exposure to various environmental factors, including tobacco smoke and radiation, can lead to increases in free radical formation. In humans, the most common form of free radicals is oxygen. The oxygen radical causes damage to the DNA and other cellular molecules by binding to electrons on those molecules (thereby oxidizing the molecules). Over time, such damage may become irreversible and lead to disease, including cancer. **Carotenes** or **carotenoids** (vitamin A precursors) and vitamins E and C have antioxidant properties, meaning that they interact with free radicals to protect cell molecules. In addition, the mineral selenium is part of antioxidant enzymes. Several clinical trials have examined whether diets rich in antioxidant nutrients might decrease the risk of certain types of cancers. While some trials have shown promising results, others have not. For example, the Chinese Cancer Prevention Study, a randomized trial in people at high risk of gastric cancer, found that supplementation with beta-carotene, vitamin E, and selenium reduced the rates of gastric cancer, as well as overall cancer rates. In a study of Finnish smokers, however, beta-carotene supplementation was associated with an increase in the incidence of lung cancer.

Another disorder related to oxidative damage is age-related macular degeneration. This problem, an irreversible cause of visual loss in middle-aged and elderly individuals, appears to be less common in people with higher circulating levels of carotenoids. Two cartenoids, lutein and zeaxanthin, are found in especially high concentrations in the macula of the retina, where they protect it from damaging blue light.

Intervention and teaching

Antioxidants are abundant in fruits and vegetables, as well as in some nuts and other food sources. No study has ever found fruit and vegetable intake to be harmful, and many epidemiologic studies have shown cancer and other disease rates to be lower in individuals with the highest fruit and vegetable intakes. Therefore, there is good reason to recommend that all individuals consume more than five servings of fruits and vegetables daily. Emphasis should be on consuming a wide variety of fruits and vegetables, to increase the types of nutrients and antioxidants obtained. Specific antioxidants and good sources include the following:

- *Beta-carotene:* deep yellow vegetables and fruits such as carrots, pumpkin, and mango; deep green leafy vegetables
- *Lycopene* (a carotenoid): tomatoes, watermelon, guavas, pink grapefruit, apricots. Most of the lycopene in the American diet comes from tomatoes.
- *Lutein and zeaxanthin:* deep green leafy vegetables; corn and yellow cornmeal, broccoli, brussels sprouts, green beans, green peas, summer squash (yellow or zucchini), persimmons
- *Selenium:* grains, meats, Brazil nuts
- *Vitamin C:* many fruits and vegetables, especially citrus fruits, strawberries, melons, broccoli, cauliflower, brussels sprouts
- *Vitamin E:* oils; nuts, especially almonds; broccoli; cauliflower; spinach; mangoes
- *Anthrocyanins, polyphenols, and flavonoids (nonnutrient antioxidants, so these are **functional foods** in terms of their antioxidant role):* blueberries, blackberries, cherries, cranberries, strawberries, raspberries, red cabbage, red sweet potatoes

Bone Density

Peak bone mass is achieved by approximately age 35 in women and a few years later in men. It is especially important to have a diet rich in calcium and adequate in vitamin D to achieve the maximum possible bone density and reduce the risk of later fractures.

Intervention and teaching

A diet rich in calcium and adequate in vitamin D enhances bone mass. In addition, very thin adults usually have lower bone mass than those with greater BMI. Caucasian and Asian women are at highest risk of developing osteoporosis.

- Consume two to three servings of low-fat dairy products daily, in addition to leafy green vegetables and foods made with milk.
- Adequate amounts of vitamin K also appear to be protective against osteoporosis. Good sources of vitamin K include green tea, deep green leafy vegetables, cauliflower, broccoli, cabbage, soybeans, soybean oil, and liver.
- Participate in weight-bearing exercise daily.
- Avoid smoking and drink alcohol moderately, if at all.
- If weight loss is needed, focus on lifestyle changes such as making healthy food choices and increasing activity, rather than overly restricting intake. Develop a realistic view of body weight and strive for a healthy weight, rather than an excessively low weight.

The Aging Adult

All of the nutrition needs of younger adults, discussed earlier, also apply to the elderly. However, older adults have additional unique needs and concerns that affect nutrition status.

Assessment

The Nutrition Screening Initiative has developed a checklist that the elderly can use to screen themselves for nutritional risk (Box 5-1); friends or family members can fill out the checklist for an elderly person who is unable to complete it. Health care providers can use the information from the screening tool to target individuals who need in-depth assessment and nutrition intervention. Assessment of nutrition in the aging by the professional is summarized in Table 5-4.

The institutionalized elderly are especially vulnerable to weight loss and other nutritional problems. This is probably related to the prevalence of chronic diseases, use of multiple medications with nutritional impacts, and depression or other psychological problems. Thus, thorough assessment and appropriate nutritional

---

Box 5-1   Determine Your Nutritional Health

The warning signs of poor nutritional health are often over-
looked. Use this checklist to find out if you or someone
you know is at nutritional risk.

Read the statements below. Circle the number in the *Yes* column for those that apply to you or someone you know. For
each *yes* answer, score the number in the box. Total your
nutritional score.

	Yes
I have an illness or condition that makes me change the kind and/or amount of food I eat.	2
I eat fewer than two meals per day.	3
I eat few fruits or vegetables or milk products.	2
I have three or more drinks of beer, liquor, or wine almost every day.	2
I have tooth or mouth problems that make it hard for me to eat.	2
I don't always have enough money to buy the food I need.	4
I eat alone most of the time.	1
I take three or more different prescribed or over-the-counter drugs a day.	1
Without wanting to, I have lost or gained 10 pounds in the last 6 months.	2
I am not always physically able to shop, cook, and/or feed myself.	2
TOTAL	_____

Total your nutritional score. If it's:

0-2	Good! Recheck your nutritional score in 6 months.
3-5	You are at moderate nutritional risk. See what can be done to improve your eating habits and lifestyle. Your office on aging, senior nutrition program, senior citizens center, or health department can help. Recheck your nutritional score in 3 months.

Box 5-1   Determine Your Nutritional Health—cont'd
6 or more   You are at high nutritional risk. Bring this checklist the next time you see your doctor, dietitian, or other qualified health or social service professional. Talk with him/her about any problems you may have. Ask for help to improve your nutritional health.

Reprinted with permission by the Nutrition Screening Initiative, a project of the American Academy of Family Physicians, The American Dietetic Association, and the National Council on Aging. Inc., and funded in part by a grant from Ross Products Division, Abbott Laboratories, Inc.

intervention are especially important for elderly individuals in long-term care facilities.

Obtaining accurate values for height in the elderly can be problematic, because loss of vertebral mineralization and volume in intervertebral disks results in loss of height. Long bones, however, do not shorten with age. Knee height (length from sole of foot to anterior thigh with both ankle and knee bent at 90-degree angle) can be used to estimate height.

Women: Estimated height in cm = 84.88 + (1.83 × knee height in cm) + (−0.24 × age in yr)

Men: Estimated height in cm = 60.65 + (2.04 × knee height in cm)

Special Concerns of the Aging Adult
Physiologic and psychosocial changes

Many physiologic and psychosocial changes that affect nutritional status occur with aging. Some of these are summarized in Table 5-5.

Chronic and acute illnesses

Malnutrition is unfortunately a common finding among the elderly, and acute or chronic disease processes are often contributing factors. Disease processes may interfere with food intake or increase nutritional requirements, require modified diets that are unappealing to the individual, or require drug therapy that influences nutritional status (see Appendix H).

Table 5-4   Assessment of Nutrition in Aging

Area of Concern	Significant Findings
Underweight and Undernutrition	*History* Loss of 4.5 kg (10 lb) or more in the last 6 months; fixed income; inadequate money for food; usually eats alone; loss of spouse or friends; difficulty chewing or swallowing; pain in mouth, teeth, or gums; poor appetite; follows a modified diet; regular use of medications (particularly those that impair appetite, e.g., digoxin, especially if three or more drugs are used; has a chronic disease; avoids one or more food groups or eats inadequate servings; has more than 1 alcoholic drink per day (woman) or more than 2 drinks per day (man); difficulty getting to market or transporting purchases home; lack of food preparation skills; lack of facilities for food storage or preparation; difficulty feeding self *Physical Examination* BMI <18.5; low level of body fat, TSF <5th percentile; muscle wasting; edema; glossitis, angular stomatitis *Laboratory Analysis* ↓ Serum albumin, transferrin, prealbumin
Overweight/Obesity	*History* Gain of 4.5 kg (10 lb) or more in the last 6 months; excessive intakes, especially of fat, snack items, and sweets; increase in intake of energy dense refined foods because of difficulty chewing high-fiber foods; little physical activity

Table 5-4   Assessment of Nutrition in Aging—cont'd

Area of Concern	Significant Findings
	Physical Examination BMI >25; TSF >95th percentile
Inadequate Fluid Balance (Potential for Fluid Deficit)	*History* Altered mental status (confusion or coma) with inability to feel or express thirst; decreased thirst sensation with aging; vomiting, diarrhea, febrile illness, or extremely hot weather
	Physical Examination Poor skin turgor; dry sticky mucous membranes; rapid weight loss over 1-2 wk; oliguria; lethargy, hypotension
	Laboratory Analysis ↑ Hct, BUN, serum Na
Inadequate Calcium and Vitamin D Intake	*History* Avoids milk because of lactose intolerance, difficulty carrying milk home from the market, inadequate money, etc.; little sun exposure because of chronic illness or residing in a nursing home or other institution; vertebral or hip fractures
	Laboratory Analysis ↓ Bone density on radiographs
Impaired Vitamin B$_{12}$ Status	*History* Achlorhydria (inadequate hydrochloric acid production); meats and milk avoided because of difficulty chewing, lactose intolerance, or cost
	Physical Examination Pallor, weakness, paresthesias (abnormal sensations in feet or legs), difficulty walking

Continued

Table 5-4   Assessment of Nutrition in Aging—cont'd

Area of Concern	Significant Findings
Inadequate Zinc (Zn) Intake	*Laboratory Analysis* ↓ Hct, ↑ MCV, ↓ plasma vitamin B_{12} *History* Decrease animal protein or whole grain intake because of low income or difficulty chewing *Physical Examination* Poor sense of taste, distorted taste; dermatitis; poor wound healing; alopecia *Laboratory Analysis* ↓ Serum Zn

Coronary heart disease and type 2 (formerly referred to as non–insulin-dependent) diabetes are two nutrition-related chronic diseases that become increasingly prevalent with aging. Diet modifications used in treatment of these disorders are described in Chapters 14 and 17.

Declines in cognitive function are of great concern among seniors, and numerous investigations have been undertaken to determine whether nutritional intervention can improve cognitive ability or delay declines in functioning. Although some research indicates that antioxidant nutrients such as vitamin E may have some benefit, conclusive evidence is not available.

Intervention and Teaching
Guidelines for choosing a healthful diet

The elderly can be encouraged to choose a variety of foods from all food groups daily, including grains (especially whole grains); fruits and vegetables; lean meats, poultry, and fish or meat substitutes; and low-fat dairy products. Food is the preferred source of nutrients in the elderly, just as it is in other age groups. Unlike supplements, food provides a variety of phytochemicals and functional components that may have beneficial effects. For example, genistein, a nonnutrient component of soy, apparently reduces the risk of heart disease; soy also provides phytoestrogens (estrogenlike compounds

Table 5-5   Nutritional Implications of Changes Related to Aging

Change	Nutritional Implications
Physiologic Changes and Impairments of Physical Function	
Decreased muscle mass (sarcopenia) and increased percentage of body fat	Decline in basal metabolic rate of about 2% per decade after age 30; daily energy need declines; potential for weight gain and obesity
Decreased skin capacity for cholecalciferol (vitamin D) synthesis; decreased renal activation of cholecalciferol of the gut to stimulation of vitamin D	Impaired absorption of calcium, contribution to osteoporosis
Diminished sense of taste and smell	Disinterest in food; anorexia; some individuals salt or sugar their food heavily to compensate for loss of taste; may eat spoiled food
Poor vision, especially in dim light	Difficulty eating; food choices limited (raw or crisp fruits and vegetables and high-fiber grains often avoided; softer, low-fiber foods, which are frequently higher in energy, are substituted); can contribute to weight loss, weight gain, or constipation
Decreased secretion of hydrochloric acid (needed for absorption of vitamin B_{12}), pepsin (protein digestive enzyme), and bile (needed for fat absorption)	Potential for impaired absorption of calcium, iron, zinc, protein, fat, fat-soluble vitamins, vitamin B_{12}
Arthritis and impaired mobility	Difficulty opening food packages and preparing food

Continued

Table 5-5   Nutritional Implications of Changes Related to Aging—cont'd

Change	Nutritional Implications
Psychosocial Changes	
Fixed income	Potential for difficulty affording food or being unwilling to spend money on food, particularly foods perceived as expensive, e.g., milk, meats, fruits, vegetables, which are important sources of calcium, riboflavin, protein, iron, zinc, vitamins C and A, and fiber
Lack of socialization; loneliness	Apathy about meals; poor intake; potential for alcohol abuse
Vulnerability to advertising and food fads related to alleviation of the effects and discomforts of aging	Wasting of limited income on diet or health aids with dubious value; potential for toxic intakes of vitamins, particularly A and D
Confusion, memory loss	Potential for forgetting to eat or forgetting what has been eaten (and therefore consuming an unbalanced diet)

in plants) that are reported to reduce the risk of certain cancers and to provide some relief from menopausal symptoms.

The elderly are, like other age groups, susceptible to food fads and **nutritional quackery.** They may rely on these beliefs to treat chronic illnesses or other health problems. The elderly need instruction in ways of recognizing quackery. Some of the characteristics of quackery are heavy reliance on anecdotal and testimonial evidence, rather than clinical trials; insistence that certain foods or supplements can cure disease; and distrust of the food supply as a means of meeting nutritional needs. The National Institute on Aging (NIA) provides information on quackery and a list of reliable health information resources online at http://www.niapublications.org/engagepages/healthqy.asp. Print copies of the publication are available free from the NIA website or by mail (see Appendix I).

Most elderly individuals have no need for liquid meal replacements or other nutritional supplements, but a multivitamin-multimineral supplement may be beneficial in ensuring adequate intakes. Nutritional supplements for the elderly should not be high in iron because hemochromatosis, an iron storage disorder, is relatively common in North America, with affected people having progressive increases in their iron stores as they age, and because healthy elderly individuals do not have large losses of iron.

Achieving and maintaining desirable weight

Impaired physical function is more common among overweight and underweight elderly than among their normal-weight peers. Overweight can impair mobility and contribute to a number of chronic diseases such as heart disease and diabetes, whereas underweight is associated with debility and can predispose the individual to infectious illnesses.

Overweight

Teaching elderly patients to control their weight can include the following:

- Explain the need for controlling energy intake and/or increasing physical activity level to prevent progressive weight gain as the metabolic rate declines. Gradual weight loss or maintenance of body weight is usually possible with intakes of approximately 1200 to 1500 kcal per day for women and 1500 to 1800 calories for men.

- Assist the individual in identifying foods—such as fruits, vegetables, whole grains, and low-fat dairy products—that are relatively low in energy but that make important nutritional contributions; help the individual to create meal plans that use these foods.
- Encourage the elderly person to limit the consumption of foods of low nutrient density (sweets, snack foods) and high-fat items. Fresh, frozen, or juice-pack canned fruits can be used for desserts and snacks. Steaming, microwaving, or baking foods with little or no added fat is preferable to frying.
- Encourage the elderly person to accumulate at least 30 minutes of moderate-intensity exercise most days of the week. The elderly need to be especially careful to warm up before exercise bouts by stretching and performing light exercise and to decrease the intensity of their exercise gradually at the end of the session, allowing at least a 5- to 10-minute period to cool off. Moderate exercise can be obtained in durations as short as 10 minutes, as long as the daily total is at least 30 minutes. Walking, gardening, and water aerobics are examples of moderate-intensity physical activities that can be useful in weight control. Group activities not only motivate some individuals to maintain an exercise program but also enhance social interactions.

Underweight

Individuals with health or dentition problems or loss of the senses of smell and taste are especially likely to be underweight. If the cause of poor intake can be determined, it is possible to tailor interventions and teaching to the needs of the individual. Use the following suggestions:

- Try small, frequent feedings rather than three large meals a day if anorexia or severe weakness is present.
- Be aware of potential side effects of drugs taken regularly (see Appendix H). If medication usage appears to be decreasing the appetite, then the health care provider may be able to substitute another drug or reduce the dosage. Toxicity often develops in the older adult at lower dosages than in younger adults, and use of multiple drugs increases the risks of adverse effects.
- Assess the individual for the presence of constipation, which may cause anorexia.

- Special diets (low-cholesterol, low-sodium, etc.) may seem tasteless to the individual. Consider liberalizing diet restrictions if intake is poor because the therapeutic diet is unappealing.
- If intake is poor because of declining senses of taste and smell, experiment with low-sodium seasonings such as herbs, spices, salt-free seasoning mixes, and lemon juice to enhance the flavors of foods. Present food in an attractive manner: appealing color combinations, a variety of textures if tolerated by the individual, and not overcooked so that it loses its color or texture.
- Refer the person to social services for assistance in obtaining food stamps if financial constraints are interfering with obtaining an adequate diet, or encourage participation in the National Nutrition Program for the Elderly, which provides meals at group feeding sites.
- Encourage the individual to eat with others whenever possible. Group feeding sites (e.g., daily lunches served at senior citizen centers), church functions, or other social activities offer opportunities for socialization. Eating in a social setting can improve appetite.
- Assess the individual for dental problems and periodontal disease to determine whether this might account for poor intake, and arrange for the individual to obtain proper dental care, including well-fitted dentures, if needed.
- Involve elderly individuals in the planning of menus for extended care facilities or group feeding sites. Attempt to accommodate the culture(s) and preferences of the participants as much as possible.
- Light the dining area well so that food can be clearly seen.
- Provide assistance in eating if necessary. This may range from opening packages of condiments to feeding the person. Plates with high outer rims make it easier for the elderly with physical handicaps to scoop up food. Patience and sensitivity when feeding the individual help preserve dignity and improve intake.
- Instruct the individual in food purchasing and simple food preparation techniques, if appropriate. Elderly men who have never cooked until late in life are especially vulnerable to nutritional deficits when living alone. The county extension home economist is a good resource for food purchasing and preparation materials, and good educational materials, including simple nutritious recipes, can also be found at the following websites: http://www.agingwell.state.ny.us/eatwell/, http://www.fda.gov/opacom/lowlit/eatage, http://www.eatright.org/nfs/nfs62, and http://navigator.tufts.edu/seniors/.

- If mobility is a problem, then help the person arrange transportation to the grocery store or to feeding sites for the elderly (contact the local agency on aging or a local church or synagogue) or arrange for Meals on Wheels.

Altered gastrointestinal function

To reduce the likelihood of constipation, hemorrhoids, and diverticulosis, these guidelines should be followed:

- Encourage intake of at least 25 to 30 g of fiber daily (see Appendix B). Cooked whole grains (oatmeal, brown rice, bulgur, etc.); legumes; and cooked, canned, or very ripe raw fruits and vegetables are good choices if there is difficulty chewing. A fiber supplement (Table 5-6) can be used if dietary intake is inadequate.
- Increase physical activity as tolerated because this stimulates gastrointestinal motility.
- Encourage consumption of dried plums (prunes) and prune juice (which contain a natural laxative) regularly if they are acceptable to the individual. Avoid regular use of laxative medications, on which the individual may become dependent.

If achlorhydria is present, then the individual may need supplements of vitamin B_{12} and calcium because absorption of these nutrients is impaired by the lack of gastric acid.

Hydration

Dehydration is especially likely to occur in the ill elderly person because body water is reduced with aging (from about 55% of body weight in young adults to about 45% in people over 60). Therefore, any given volume of body fluids represents a greater percentage of body water in the elderly person than it does in the younger adult. Diarrhea, vomiting, or a febrile illness often produces dehydration in the older adult. The sensation of thirst may be diminished in old age, and immobility and confusion may hinder the elderly in getting fluids to drink, further contributing to the risk of dehydration. Some older adults have a narrow margin of safety in their state of hydration because renal or cardiac impairments make them vulnerable to fluid overload. Caregivers should adhere to the following guidelines to prevent dehydration in the elderly patient:

- Assess state of hydration regularly.
- Evaluate fluid intake of the patient receiving tube feedings or total parenteral nutrition. More fluid may be needed than is

Table 5-6 Fiber Supplements

Fiber Source	Examples of Products	Adult Recommended Daily Dose	Fiber Content Total	Fiber Content Soluble
Guar gum	Benefiber	1 tbsp (4 g) up to 5 times daily	3 g/tbsp	3 g/tbsp
Psyllium	Metamucil	2-6 capsules up to 3 times daily	0.52 g/capsule	0.34 g/capsule
		2 wafers up to 3 times daily	3.4 g/wafer	2.2 g/wafer
	Konsyl Natural Fiber	1 tbsp up to 3 times daily	3.4 g/tbsp	2.2 g/tbsp
	Rite Aid	1 tsp (6 g) up to 3 times daily	5 g/tsp	4 g/tsp
	Citrucel	1 tbsp (12 g) up to 3 times daily	3 g/tbsp	2 g/tbsp
Methylcellulose		1 tbsp (11.5 g) up to 3 times daily	2 g/tbsp	2 g/tbsp
	Fiber Choice	Up to 12 caplets daily	0.5 g/caplet	0.5 g/caplet
Fructan	FiberCon	2 caplets daily	2 g/caplet	2 g/caplet
Polycarbophil	Konsyl Bulk Forming Fiber Laxative	2 caplets daily	500 mg/caplet	*
		2 tablets up to 4 times daily	500 mg/tablet	*
	Perdiem Fiber	2 tablets up to 4 times daily	500 mg/caplet	*
	Equalactin	2 caplets up to 4 times daily	500 mg/caplet	*
Vegetable stearine	Ultra-Fiber	3 caplets up to 4 times daily	0.4 g/tablet	0.4 g/tablet

tbsp, Tablespoon (15 ml); *tsp,* teaspoon (5 ml)

Soluble fiber aids in reduction of cholesterol levels, while insoluble fiber is more important in gastrointestinal function.

*Synthetic compound that expands in water to provide bulk but is not fermented by gut bacteria as naturally occurring soluble fibers are.

included in the nutrient solutions. Extra fluid can be administered orally, as an irrigant for the feeding tube, or intravenously.

▪ Encourage intake of a minimum of 1500 ml fluid per day, unless a fluid restriction is needed. If the individual has difficulty remembering how much fluid has been consumed, it may help to fill a pitcher with the needed amount at the beginning of the day, place it in an accessible location, and instruct the person to drink it all by the end of the day.

Preserving bone density

For the person at high risk for osteoporosis (e.g., women who undergo early oophorectomy) or already showing signs of osteoporosis, certain medications reduce bone loss. Hormone replacement therapy in postmenopausal women is effective in reducing the risk of fractures from osteoporosis, but its long-term side effects include an increase in the risk of heart disease and breast and ovarian cancer. Bisphosphonates such as alendronate and risedronate reduce bone resorption without affecting the rates of heart disease or cancer. Bisphosphonates should not be taken with food or at the same time as a calcium supplement because of potential for impaired absorption. Selective estrogen receptor modulators (SERMs), such as raloxiphene and tamoxifene, appear to reduce the risk of bone loss and vertebral fractures. Calcitonin, which slows bone loss, is approved for treatment of osteoporosis in women who are at least 5 years postmenopausal, but its long-term effects on the risk of fractures is not established. Individuals taking all of these anti-osteoporosis medications should be instructed to be especially careful to consume adequate vitamin D and calcium.

▪ Encourage a calcium intake of 1200 mg/day (see Figure 3-1), especially in elderly women.
  ▪ If lactose intolerance is present, substitute cheese, acidophilus milk, yogurt, or buttermilk for milk because these products are lower in lactose than regular milk. Also, lactase enzyme–treated milk is available in some markets, or oral lactase supplements are available to take with milk.
  ▪ Use a calcium supplement (e.g., calcium citrate) if dietary calcium intake cannot be maintained at the recommended level. Box 5-2 provides guidelines for improving absorption of calcium from the diet or supplements.

Box 5-2   Improving Calcium Absorption

- Obtain adequate vitamin D. Vitamin D–fortified milk and breakfast cereals and exposure of skin to sunlight several times a week (using appropriate sunscreen) are good sources.
- Consume milk or other lactose-containing dairy products if lactose tolerance is not a problem. Lactose improves calcium absorption.
- Avoid excessive intake of phosphorus, which competes with calcium for absorption. Limit meat intake to 5 or 6 oz daily and carbonated drinks to 8 to 12 oz daily.
- Increase calcium intake if diet is high in oxalate (e.g., spinach and other deep green vegetables), phytates (e.g., bran and whole grains), or fiber, all of which inhibit calcium absorption.
- Increase calcium intake if achlorhydria is present, and consume calcium with orange juice or other acidic foods. Acid in the upper gastrointestinal tract improves absorption, and an alkaline upper gastrointestinal tract impairs absorption.
- Increase calcium intake if using corticosteroid or anticonvulsant medications, which decrease calcium absorption.

- Vitamin D is needed for the absorption of calcium. The recommended intake of vitamin D is higher for the elderly than for any other groups of individuals (10 μg/day through 70 years, and 15 μg/day after age 70). If vitamin D–fortified milk or another reliable dietary source (see Appendix A) is not consumed daily, the individual may need a supplement.
- Regular weight-bearing physical activity, at least several times weekly, helps to preserve bone.
- Consume a diet adequate in vitamins and minerals, especially vitamins K and A, to ensure that sufficient nutrients are available for bone health.

REFERENCES

Knowler WC et al: Reduction in the incidence of type 2 diabetes with lifestyle intervention or metformin, *N Engl J Med* 346:393, 2002.

National Center for Chronic Disease Prevention and Health Promotion (NCCDPHP): *Nutrition and physical activity*. Available at www.cdc.gov/nccdphp/dnpa/. Accessed November 11, 2003.

Parikh SJ, Yanovski JA: Calcium intake and adiposity, *Am J Clin Nutr* 77:281, 2003.

Saris WH et al: How much physical activity is enough to prevent unhealthy weight gain? Outcome of the IASO 1st Stock Conference and consensus statement, *Obes Rev* 4:101, 2003.

Zemel MB: Mechanisms of dairy modulation of adiposity, *J Nutr* 133:252S, 2003.

SELECTED BIBLIOGRAPHY

Denny CH et al: Surveillance for health behaviors of American Indians and Alaska Natives: findings from the Behavioral Risk Factor Surveillance System, 1997-2000, *MMWR Surveill Summ* 52(7):1, 2003.

Holmquist C et al: Multivitamin supplements are inversely associated with risk of myocardial infarction in men and women—Stockholm Heart Epidemiology Program (SHEEP), *J Nutr* 133:2650, 2003.

Lee CD et al: Physical activity and stroke risk: a meta-analysis, *Stroke* 34:2475, 2003.

Liu RH: Health benefits of fruit and vegetables are from additive and synergistic combinations of phytochemicals, *Am J Clin Nutr* 78(suppl 3):517S, 2003.

Nieves JW: Calcium, vitamin D, and nutrition in elderly adults, *Clin Geriatr Med* 19:321, 2003.

Sabate J: Nut consumption and body weight, *Am J Clin Nutr* 78(suppl 3):647S, 2003.

Short KR et al: Impact of aerobic exercise training on age-related changes in insulin sensitivity and muscle oxidative capacity, *Diabetes* 52:1888, 2003.

Zhou BF et al: Nutrient intakes of middle-aged men and women in China, Japan, United Kingdom, and United States in the late 1990s: the INTERMAP study, *J Hum Hypertens* 17:623, 2003.

Athletic Performance

6

It is clear from research done over the past two decades that nutrition has beneficial effects on athletic performance. Although most health care generalists encounter few elite athletes, many members of the general public participate in "extreme" sports and intense physical training. These individuals want and need accurate, reliable nutritional guidance to achieve their best level of performance and maintain optimal health. This chapter will summarize some of the important findings regarding nutrition for the adult athlete participating in regular, vigorous athletic training.

Assessment

Nutrition assessment is summarized in Table 6-1.

Nutrient Needs and Concerns during Training
Energy

Energy needs vary because of the intensity, duration, and frequency of exercise, as well as the effects of age, heredity, lean body mass, body size, and gender. Increased energy needs resulting from exercise can be met through a diet of regular foods. Fat is an important source of energy, and there is no evidence to recommend either an extremely low-fat or a high-fat diet for athletes. Carbohydrates maintain blood glucose concentrations during exercise and replace muscle glycogen; the amount needed depends upon factors such as the total energy needs and the type of sport performed. Males usually achieve an adequate intake of carbohydrate to maintain glycogen stores easily, but it may be more difficult for female athletes restricting their energy intakes because of concern about controlling their body fat. Excessive limitation of energy intake contributes to the immunosuppression that is prevalent among elite athletes.

Table 6-1   Assessment in Athletic Performance

Area of Concern	Significant Findings
Inadequate Energy Intake	*History* Frequent dieting to achieve and maintain low "competitive" weight; extremely strenuous exercise habits (e.g., distance running); possible eating disorder *Physical Examination* ↓ Body fat, athletic performance; TSF <5th percentile; weight for height <90% of standard or BMI <18.5 (for children or adolescents, BMI <5th percentile for age); amenorrhea; delayed growth and development (children and adolescents)
Inadequate Protein Intake	*History* Frequent dieting, energy intake so low that protein consumed is utilized for energy; physiologic state requiring ↑ protein: childhood, adolescence, pregnancy, lactation *Physical Examination* Delayed growth and development (children and adolescents); thinning of hair, changes in hair texture
Inadequate Mineral Status, Fe	*History* Frequently dieting to achieve competitive weight; vegetarian diet that may be marginal in iron provision; GI blood loss, especially in distance runners *Physical Examination* Pallor; ↓ athletic performance

Table 6-1   Assessment in Athletic Performance—cont'd

Area of Concern	Significant Findings
	Laboratory Analysis ↓ Hct, Hgb, MCV, serum Fe; ↓ serum ferritin and Fe
Volume Fluid Deficit	*History* Failure to replace fluid losses by drinking during and after athletic endeavors; fluid restriction in an attempt to achieve competitive weight; use of diuretics to achieve competitive weight or produce dilute urine in an effort to confound drug testing
	Physical Examination Dry, sticky mucous membranes; poor skin turgor; thirst; disorientation; weakness; hypotension
	Laboratory Analysis ↑ Serum sodium, Hct, BUN, serum osmolality

Teaching

Points to emphasize in teaching have recently been described in a joint report of the American College of Sports Medicine, American Dietetic Association, and Dietitians of Canada (ACSM, ADA, DC, 2000):

- Adequate energy needs to be consumed intake to prevent underweight, maximize the training effects, and maintain health. Inadequate energy intakes can reduce muscle mass, result in menstrual dysfunction, contribute to poor bone density, and increase the risk of injury. The athlete's age, sex, heredity, and sport help to determine the optimal amount of body fat, and if fat loss is necessary, it should be carried out before the competitive season.

- A moderate- to low-fat diet (20% to 25% of energy from fat) is recommended, but there is no advantage to very-low-fat diets (<15% fat) .

- Carbohydrate needs to optimize glycogen stores average about 5 to 7 g/kg body weight per day, with an increase to 7 to 10 g/kg/day for strenuously exercising endurance athletes.

■ If weight loss is needed or desirable to improve athletic performance, plan to accomplish it gradually (no more than 1 to 2 lb or 0.5 to 1 kg/week), rather than on a crash diet. Reducing intake by 10% to 20% of normal will result in a steady weight loss. Stress healthy eating choices rather than excessive restriction of intake. A registered dietitian with training in sports nutrition can provide valuable guidance.

Protein

It is commonly believed that markedly increased amounts of certain nutrients, particularly protein, are needed to build muscle mass; however, the increase in needs is actually relatively modest. The protein Dietary Reference Intake (DRI) for normal adults is 0.8 g/kg body weight/day, and the needs of most athletes are no more than 50% to 100% greater than this. Amounts close to this can be obtained in the average North American diet, which provides 80 to 110 g protein per day.

Teaching

Modest increases in protein intake over the DRI are sufficient for most athletes:

■ Endurance athletes (e.g., those involved in activities involving speed and/or distance, such as skaters, runners, and cyclists) need approximately 1.2 to 1.4 g/kg/day, a total of about 98 g for the man who weighs 75 kg (165 lb).
■ Athletes performing resistance and strength training (e.g., weight lifters and body builders) need approximately 1.6 to 1.7 g/kg/day.
■ Athletes who are vegetarians may need about 10% more protein than nonvegetarians to compensate for less complete digestion of proteins from plant sources.

Vitamins and Minerals

There is no evidence that markedly increasing vitamin and mineral intake over the Dietary Reference Intakes improves athletic performance. B-complex vitamin needs increase during vigorous activity, but they will be met by the increased energy intake needed during heavy exercise. It has been suggested that vigorous exercise increases needs for antioxidant nutrients (e.g., vitamins C and E, carotenes, and selenium), but there is no conclusive evidence for this.

Vitamin D is important for adequate calcium metabolism and thus for optimal bone mass, and vitamin D levels can be low in athletes from far southern or northern latitudes, where direct sun exposure is reduced, and those that train indoors most of the year. Inadequate intakes of calcium are common, especially among female athletes. This increases the risk of low bone mineral density and stress fractures.

Vigorous exercise increases iron needs, and iron deficiency is prevalent, especially among female athletes. Distance runners are particularly likely to have iron deficiency. Possible reasons include increased losses of iron in perspiration during prolonged physical activity, damage to red blood cells in the capillaries of the soles of the feet during running, and increased gastrointestinal blood loss, which is known to be more common in runners than in the general population. Iron deficiency impairs physical performance by interfering with oxygen delivery and allowing lactate accumulation in muscle, which makes the muscle fatigue more quickly.

Zinc nutriture may be suboptimal in the athlete. Zinc is lost in perspiration, but intakes also tend to be marginal or inadequate. The richest sources of zinc are animal products, and consumption of these is likely to be low, particularly in weight-conscious athletes or in those who have adopted a vegetarian lifestyle. Female athletes are especially prone to poor zinc intakes.

Teaching

- *Vitamin D:* If intake of fortified dairy products is low and the athlete has little regular sun exposure, a supplement providing 5 μg/day may be needed.
- *Calcium:* If consumption of dairy products is poor and the athlete is resistant to increasing consumption, a supplement providing 800 to 1200 mg daily will provide the needed calcium.
- *Iron:* Individuals participating regularly in vigorous physical exercise should be instructed in a diet that includes good sources of iron (legumes, meats, whole and enriched grains; see Appendix A), as well as vitamin C, which promotes iron absorption. Female athletes, vegetarians, and distance runners, particularly, may have difficulty maintaining adequate iron nutriture and may need a supplement. Absorption of iron from a supplement will be best if it is taken between meals or at bedtime and with fluids other than coffee, tea, or milk.
- *Zinc:* If the diet appears low in zinc, instruction in good dietary sources (see Appendix A) may be sufficient to improve intake.

A supplement providing approximately 15 mg daily can be used, but excessive intakes should be avoided because they impair copper metabolism.

Ergogenic Aids

The marketing and use of nutrition-related supplements purported to improve exercise performance is very widespread. There is little governmental control over the claims made for these supplements, and thus the athlete, coaches, and trainers must be helped to evaluate these claims. Two commonly used ergogenic aids are creatine and chromium.

Creatine phosphate is an important energy source for exercising muscle. Theoretically, increasing the muscle creatine levels should prolong the athlete's ability to perform high-intensity exercise. Some studies suggest that creatine supplements improve performance on short-term, high-intensity tasks such as sprints on stationary bicycles, squash, and elite soccer play. Creatine monophosphate, a form commonly used as a supplement, is associated with a small weight gain (approximately 1 kg in short-term studies) and fluid retention. Although there are concerns that creatine supplementation might contribute to kidney dysfunction, the risk has not yet been determined. Creatine supplementation is being explored not only in athletes but also in conjunction with exercise training in other individuals who may need to build muscle mass, such as the elderly and those with muscular dystrophy, amyotrophic lateral sclerosis, and other diseases characterized by muscle weakness.

Chromium is an essential trace mineral that is believed by many individuals to increase lean muscle mass and promote fat loss. The research done so far has not supported these beliefs. In one investigation, it appeared that chromium picolinate, a common form of chromium supplement, might actually predispose athletes to iron deficits. In animal studies, chromium picolinate causes oxidative damage and possibly mutagenesis; the implication of this for humans is not known. Other forms of chromium, such as chromium chloride, are believed to pose less risk.

Teaching

Nutritional ergogenic aids should be used with caution, and only after careful evaluation. Thorough recommendations for evaluating supplement claims have been published (ACSM, ADA, DC, 2000). In brief, consider the following points:

- *Scientific evidence:* Has the supplement undergone rigorous scientific testing? If so, were the results published in a peer-reviewed journal? Did the research use appropriate control groups, including a double-blind placebo group, if possible? Are the studies adequately described? Are the results clear, analyzed with appropriate statistics, and presented in an objective manner? Do they answer the questions of whether the supplement is effective? Do they include the incidence of adverse events among the treatment groups?

- *Claims related to the particular product:* Does the supplement make sense for the sport for which the claim is made; for example, does the advertising imply that the supplement will improve triathlon performance when the product has only shown benefit in short sprints? Is the amount of active ingredient in the supplement comparable to that used in research studies involving this particular ergogenic aid? Do the claims about the product made by the manufacturer or distributor match the scientific evidence?

- *Safety:* Is the product safe over the short and long term? Is it contraindicated for certain groups of people, such as older adults, women who may become pregnant, and those with certain health problems?

- *Legality:* Is the product banned by athletic organizations governing the sport?

The Female Athlete Triad

Physically active females, especially those in sports or dance activities where low body weight is desirable, are at risk for a syndrome known as the *female athlete triad.* The components of the triad are eating disorders, amenorrhea, and osteoporosis. Very low energy intake coupled with high energy expenditure can result in alterations of pituitary hormone secretion, with impaired secretion of luteinizing hormone and follicle-stimulating hormone. This brings about ovarian changes that result in amenorrhea and reduction in bone mass or failure to develop peak bone mass. This problem can occur in both adolescents and adult women. The minimal level of body fat for normal function is approximately 12% for females. Body building, cycling, triathlon, and running events are some of the sports in which female participants are especially likely to have low body fat.

Intervention and teaching

Coaches, trainers, and all other individuals working with female athletes need to be aware of the prevalence and signs of the female athlete triad. The triad can impair athletic performance and increase morbidity and mortality among athletes, and these facts can be used to help motivate the athlete and coaching staff to avoid unhealthy weight control practices such as excessive restriction of intake, as well as purging or use of diuretics or laxatives to maintain a low body weight. The focus should be on healthy food choices rather than body weight. Guidelines for recognizing and treating eating disorders are described in Chapter 19.

Nutrition for Athletic Events
Fluid and Electrolyte Replacement

Adequate replacement of fluid losses during exercise not only improves physical performance but also helps to maintain the health and safety of the exercising individuals. Losses from perspiration are primarily water but also include sodium (approximately 1 g/L), potassium, and other minerals. The amount of perspiration loss is affected by intensity of the exercise, temperature and humidity of the environment, and body size, but can be as great as 1.8 L/hour. It is not always possible to replace all of the fluid losses during exercise, because the maximal rate of gastric emptying is about 1 liter/hour. However, many athletes do not consume even half of the maximal possible amount. It is not necessary to include electrolytes in the fluids consumed if exercise duration is 3 to 4 hours or less. The electrolytes can be replaced in the course of normal food intake later, but including electrolytes may increase palatability of the drink and encourage adequate hydration.

Teaching

The key nutritional need during exercise is adequate fluid replacement. To maintain hydration, athletes should:

- Drink generous amounts in the 24-hour period before exercise and drink 400 to 600 ml of fluid 2 to 3 hours before exercise.
- Attempt to drink enough fluid to maintain fluid balance during exercise. If this is not possible, drink the maximum amount tolerated.
  - Make a habit of drinking 150 to 350 ml of cool fluid at 15 to 20 minute intervals throughout exercise. Gastric emptying is most rapid when there is at least 600 ml of fluid in the stomach, and regular drinking can help to keep the stomach adequately filled.

- If exercise is intense and lasts longer than 1 hour, drink beverages containing 4% to 8% carbohydrate, such as commercial sport drinks or diluted fruit juices (for most juices, dilute 1 part juice to 0.5 to 1 part water). These improve performance while maintaining efficient gastric emptying; beverages with carbohydrate contents greater than 8% can delay gastric emptying.
- Include sodium (0.5 to 0.7 g/L) in beverages if exercise lasts longer than 1 hour, both to increase fluid intake by improving palatability and to reduce the risk of hyponatremia. This level is higher than that found in most commercial sport drinks.
- Weigh before and after an exercise bout. During the first few hours after exercise, consume enough fluid to replace the weight lost. A minimum of 1 liter is needed to replace each kilogram (2.2 lb) lost, and it may be necessary to consume enough fluid to replace 150% of the weight lost (e.g., 1500 ml/kg weight loss).
- Alcohol and caffeine-containing drinks are not desirable as rehydration solutions because they promote fluid loss through diuresis.

Food Intake before and during Exercise

There is no one perfect preexercise meal, because the optimal meal varies with the event and the athlete. In general, meals before competition or strenuous endeavors should be adequate in fluid to promote hydration, low in fat and fiber to improve gastric emptying and prevent gastrointestinal discomfort, high in carbohydrate to maintain blood glucose and maximize glycogen stores, moderate in protein, and consisting of foods familiar to the athlete (to reduce the risk of intolerance of a new food).

For exercise events lasting 90 minutes or longer, there clearly is benefit to consuming carbohydrate throughout the event. For shorter periods of exercise, the effects of carbohydrate intake during the event is less clear, but there may be a benefit from carbohydrate intake during exercise, especially if glycogen stores are not high (e.g., if exercise takes place before breakfast or after only a small breakfast).

Teaching

Performance is improved if the preexercise meal supplies adequate amounts of carbohydrate. Whether carbohydrate intake during short bouts of exercise (1 hour or less) enhances performance is controversial, but it is clear that carbohydrate is beneficial when exercise lasts 90 minutes or more.

- Consume 200 to 300 g carbohydrate 3 to 4 hours before exercise to help maintain blood glucose and glycogen stores.
- For events lasting 90 min or longer, consume 0.7 g carbohydrate/kg body weight per hour (approximately 30 to 60 g/hour) starting shortly after the beginning of the event. Easy-to-digest carbohydrates that yield glucose or glucose plus fructose are more effective than those providing fructose alone. The carbohydrate can come from a sport drink, a carbohydrate gel, or a solid. Use of carbohydrate-containing beverages allows carbohydrate intake to be combined with fluid replacement. Drinking 600 to 1200 ml/hr of a solution that provides 4 to 8 g of carbohydrate/100 ml (e.g., a commercial sport drink or fruit juice diluted to half strength) will replace fluid losses and provide the needed carbohydrate.
- Following intense exercise, muscle glycogen stores need to be replaced. This process is encouraged by consumption of carbohydrate during the postexercise period. An amount often suggested is 1 to 1.5 g/kg body weight (approximately 1 cup cooked pasta and 1 cup fruit juice for an adult) every 2 hours during the waking hours, or a total of approximately 7 to 10 g/kg during the 24-hour period after exercise. Consuming protein along with the carbohydrate will provide amino acids needed for muscle synthesis and repair.

REFERENCES

American College of Sports Medicine, American Dietetic Association, Dietitians of Canada: Joint Position Statement: nutrition and athletic performance, *Med Sci Sports Exerc* 32:2130, 2000.

SELECTED BIBLIOGRAPHY

Brose A, Parise G, Tarnopolsky MA: Creatine supplementation enhances isometric strength and body composition improvements following strength exercise training in older adults, *J Gerontol A Biol Sci Med Sci* 58:11, 2003.

Burke LM: Nutritional needs for exercise in the heat, *Comp Biochem Physiol A Mol Integr Physiol* 128:735, 2001.

Burke LM et al: Guidelines for daily carbohydrate intake: do athletes achieve them? *Sports Med* 31:267, 2001.

Lawrence ME, Kirby DF: Nutrition and sports supplements: fact or fiction, *J Clin Gastroenterol* 35:299, 2002.

Lukaski HC: Magnesium, zinc, and chromium nutrition and athletic performance, *Can J Appl Physiol* 26(suppl):S13, 2001.

Maughan R: The athlete's diet: nutritional goals and dietary strategies, *Proc Nutr Soc* 61:87, 2002.

Vincent JB: The potential value and toxicity of chromium picolinate as a nutritional supplement, weight loss agent and muscle development agent, *Sports Med* 33:213, 2003.

Obesity and
Weight Control

7

Approximately 60% of adults in the United States and nearly half of the adults in Canada are now overweight or obese (Mokdad et al., 2003; Statistics Canada, 2003). In addition, overweight and obesity affects one third or more of children between 5 and 14 years of age. Because of the prevalence of obesity and the health risks associated with it, it is probably the most serious nutritional problem among developed countries.

Pathophysiology
Diagnosis of Obesity and Overweight

In the clinical setting, several practical methods are used to determine whether obesity is present:

1. *Calculation of the body mass index (BMI).* This is one of the simplest methods, and the BMI correlates well with health risks from obesity. A chart for determining BMI can be found inside the back cover of this book, or BMI can be calculated as shown in Box 2-1.

2. *Comparison of weight with tables of ideal body weight (IBW) or desirable weight for height* (see Appendix C).

   % of IBW = (Actual body weight ÷ ideal body weight) × 100

   Overweight is considered to be 110% to 120% of the desirable or ideal body weight (IBW). With this method, obesity can be divided into three degrees: (1) mild, 120% to 140% of IBW; (2) moderate, 141% to 200% of IBW; and (3) severe or morbid, more than 200% of IBW.

3. *Measurement of abdominal girth.* Visceral, or abdominal, fat (the so-called "apple" shape, or android fat pattern) is a predictor of cardiovascular disease risk. Fat in the hips and thighs ("pear" shape, or gynecoid fat pattern), on the other hand, is much less

likely to be associated with health risk. The National Institutes of Health (2000) have suggested that the waist circumference be used as an indicator of abdominal fat in individuals with BMI less than 35. Men are considered at high risk if the waist circumference is >102 cm (40 in), and women are at high risk if the waist circumference is >99 cm (35 in). When BMI is greater than 35, abdominal measurement is no longer necessary because health risks are high enough that abdominal obesity is no longer an independent predictor of cardiovascular risk. Abdominal circumference is measured at the top of the iliac crest, at the end of an exhalation.

4. *Measurement of subcutaneous fat.* It is estimated that as much as 50% of the fat can be found in the subcutaneous area. Therefore, skinfold (fatfold) measurements can be an indicator of the amount of body fat. Much variability can occur between skinfold measurements performed by two different examiners. To reduce error, only well-trained individuals should measure skinfolds.

5. *Measurement of body composition.* The most accurate way in which to diagnose overweight and obesity is to use a reliable method for measuring body composition. Underwater weighing is generally considered to be among the most accurate methods, but it is not practical for the majority of individuals. Computerized tomography (CT) and magnetic resonance imaging are very informative, but their cost, the fact that young children usually have to be sedated for the scans, and the radiation exposure from CT limits their usefulness. Bioelectrical impedance is gaining wide acceptance as a reasonably priced method that is practical for use in the clinical area. The reliability of bioelectric impedance is impaired by altered tissue fluid, such as edema and ascites.

Etiology

Most cases of obesity are multifactorial in etiology. Some of the factors are described in the following sections.

Environment

The widespread availability of appealing food and a lifestyle with little need for physical activity are conducive to overweight. Familial influences (e.g., using food as a reward, withholding dessert until the plate is clean) help develop eating habits that contribute to overweight. Portion sizes in fast food and full service restaurants, as well as individual packaging (e.g., soft drinks, chips, and other snack foods), have increased in recent years, contributing to excessive intake.

Energy expenditure

Energy expenditure can be divided into three parts: **resting energy expenditure (REE), thermic effect of food (TEF),** and the energy expended in physical activity (see Chapter 2). REE, the energy required for vital body processes such as operation of the heart and lungs, accounts for 60% or more of energy expenditure for most individuals. REE appears to be normal in the obese. TEF, the energy required for digestion, absorption, and disposition of the nutrients in food, is normally about 10% of the total energy expenditure. The obese have been reported to have low TEF, but this abnormality probably is insufficient to be the cause of most cases of obesity. Physical activity, the most variable component of energy expenditure, accounts for about 20% to 30% of the daily energy expenditure for most individuals. The obese tend to be more sedentary than normal-weight people, but this is partially balanced by the fact that the obese require more energy to perform the same tasks as normal-weight individuals. Overall, both adults and children in the United States and Canada obtain less physical activity than is optimal.

Genetics

Children of obese parents are three to eight times as likely to be obese as children of normal-weight parents, even if they are not reared by their natural parents. Some individuals may have an inherited metabolic makeup that allows them to store fat more efficiently than other individuals do. **Leptin** is released by adipose tissue, and it appears to provide a mechanism for the adipose tissue to communicate with the central nervous system and contribute to the control of food intake and energy metabolism (Figure 7-1). In some animal models of obesity, leptin formation or the receptor for leptin is defective. Leptin levels are high in most obese individuals, so obese people apparently have no defect in leptin formation. It may be that some obese individuals are resistant to the effects of leptin. At this point, however, no abnormalities in leptin or its metabolism have been found that could explain most cases of human obesity. Other hormones released by the fat cells, including

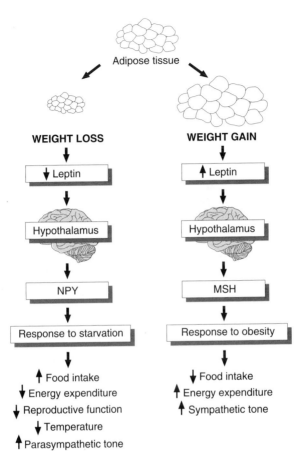

Figure 7-1

Leptin provides a mechanism so that the body can maintain stable fat stores. The adipose, or fat, tissue releases leptin. A loss of body fat (weight loss or starvation) reduces leptin release, and an increase in body fat enhances leptin production. It is believed that the binding of leptin to receptors in the hypothalamus, a brain region known to be involved in regulation of body weight, causes the release of neurotransmitters that act to keep the fat stores relatively stable. Neuropeptide Y (NPY) is released in response to decreased levels of leptin, and melanocyte-stimulating hormone (MSH) is released in response to increased leptin.

(Modified from Friedman JM: *Leptin, leptin receptors, and the control of body weight,* Nutr Rev 56(2):S40, 1998. ©1998 International Life Sciences Institute, Washington, DC) adiponectin and resistin, have a role in regulation of body weight. Ghrelin, a hormone released by the stomach, is also involved in appetite control.

Neuroendocrine

Hypothyroidism, Cushing's syndrome, and polycystic ovary syndrome are some of the neuroendocrine disorders that can lead to overweight and obesity. Prader-Willi syndrome, associated with excessive appetite, inappropriate food-seeking behaviors, and mental retardation, can lead to massive obesity, but it is quite rare. Overall, neuroendocrine disorders are responsible for less than 1% of all cases of obesity.

Psychology

Overeating may occur as a response to loneliness, grief, or depression. Overeating may also result from a learned response to external cues such as food advertising or the fact that it is mealtime, rather than the internal cue of hunger.

Physiology

Energy expenditure declines with aging, and thus body weight often increases during middle age. Women are especially vulnerable to excess weight gain during pregnancy and the perimenopausal years.

Health Risks Associated with Obesity

Obesity is associated with numerous health risks, which are summarized in Table 7-1. Health risks increase progressively with the severity of obesity. In the past, moderate weight gain with aging was believed to be associated with little health risk, but recent data indicate that deaths from heart disease and cancer are increased in women who gain 10 kg (22 lb) or more after the age of 18. Among women, the lowest risk was reported in nonsmokers who were at least 15% below average weight (those who had a BMI <19).

Weight cycling, or "yo-yo" dieting, occurs when individuals repeatedly lose and regain weight. There is some concern that this process may accelerate arteriosclerosis or aggravate other health problems, but conclusive data are lacking. The health risks of obesity are so great that the obese should not avoid trying to lose weight because of fears of weight cycling.

Table 7-1   Health Problems Caused or Worsened by Obesity

Type of Problem	Disease, Symptom, or Difficulty
Cardiovascular or respiratory	Hypertension, coronary heart disease, varicose veins, sleep apnea
Endocrine or reproductive	Type 2 diabetes mellitus, insulin resistance, amenorrhea, infertility, preeclampsia
Gastrointestinal	Gallstones, fatty liver
Musculoskeletal and skin	Osteoarthritis, skin irritation and infections, especially in fat folds, striae
Malignancies	Cancer of the colon, rectum, prostate, gallbladder, breast, uterus, and ovaries
Psychosocial	Social discrimination, poor self-image

Treatment and Nutritional Care

Figure 7-2 provides a treatment algorithm for weight loss. All individuals with a BMI greater than 30 are advised to implement a weight loss strategy. For individuals with a BMI between 25 and 29.9, weight loss is indicated for women with a waist circumference greater than 88 cm (>35 inches) and men with a waist circumference greater than 102 cm (>40 inches) if they have two or more risk factors (summarized in Box 7-1) for subsequent mortality. Adults with a BMI 25 to 29.9 without concomitant risk factors should also be encouraged to lose weight if they desire to do so.

When overweight and obesity are identified, and the patient and clinician determine that weight loss is needed, the goals of intervention are as follows: (1) decrease body fat, (2) develop more healthy eating and physical activity habits, (3) prevent loss of lean body mass (LBM) during weight reduction, and (4) maintain weight loss.

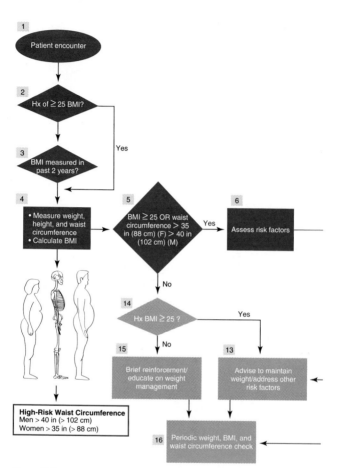

Figure 7-2

Treatment algorithm for overweight and obesity. BMI, waist circumference, presence of health risk factors and comorbidities, and patient willingness to lose weight guide decision making.

(From National Institutes of Health, National Heart, Lung, and Blood Institute, and the North American Association for the Study of Obesity: *The practical guide: identification, evaluation, and treatment of overweight and obesity in adults,* Washington, DC, 2000, NIH.)

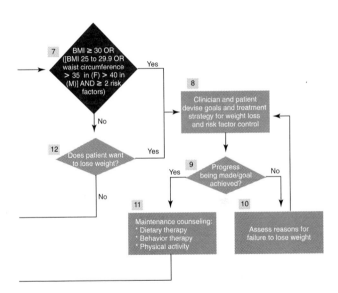

7 BMI ≥ 30 OR ([BMI 25 to 29.9 OR waist circumference > 35 in (F) > 40 in (M)] AND ≥ 2 risk factors)

Yes

8 Clinician and patient devise goals and treatment strategy for weight loss and risk factor control

No

12 Does patient want to lose weight?

Yes

9 Progress being made/goal achieved?

Yes

No

11 Maintenance counseling:
* Dietary therapy
* Behavior therapy
* Physical activity

10 Assess reasons for failure to lose weight

No

Examination

Treatment

This algorithm applies only to the assessment for overweight and obesity and subsequent decisions based on that assessment. It does not reflect any initial overall assessment for other cardiovascular risk factors that are indicated.

Box 7-1   Assessment in Obesity and Weight Control

Anthropometric and Body Composition Data
- Body mass index (BMI)
- Waist circumference
- Body fat (bioelectric impedance, dual x-ray electron absorptiometry, air displacement plethysmography) (optional)[*]

Health History

Risk factors or comorbidities associated with obesity
- Very high risk: established coronary heart disease (CHD), including a history of myocardial infarction, angina pectoris, and coronary artery surgery or other procedures; other atherosclerotic diseases, including peripheral arterial disease, abdominal aneurysm, or symptomatic carotid artery disease; type 2 diabetes; and sleep apnea.
- High risk for cardiovascular disease: cigarette smoking; hypertension (systolic blood pressure 140 mm Hg or greater or diastolic blood pressure 90 mm Hg or greater) or current use of antihypertensive medications; serum low-density lipoprotein (LDL) cholesterol concentration of 160 mg/dl or greater or a borderline LDL concentration (130 to 159 mg/dl) plus two or more other risk factors; serum high-density lipoprotein (HDL) cholesterol less than 35 mg/dl; impaired fasting glucose (fasting plasma glucose between 110 and 125 mg/dl); family history of premature CHD (myocardial infarction or sudden death experienced by the father or other first-degree male relative at or before 55 years of age or experienced by the mother or other first-degree female relative at or before 65 years of age); or age 45 years or older for men or 55 years or older for women (or postmenopausal).
- Other risk factors: physical inactivity, elevated serum triglycerides (a marker of cardiovascular risk in obese individuals).

Readiness to Lose Weight
- Reasons and motivation for weight loss
- Previous attempts at weight loss

Box 7-1   Assessment in Obesity and Weight Control—cont'd

- Support expected from family and friends
- Understanding of risks and benefits
- Attitudes toward physical activity
- Time availability
- Potential barriers, including financial limitations, to adoption of change

Diet History

- Usual food intake: meal and snack patterns, portion sizes, food preparation methods
- Activity patterns: type, amount, intensity

---

*In clinical management of adult patients, body composition measurements add little information that cannot be obtained from the BMI.

From National Institutes of Health, National Heart, Lung, and Blood Institute, and the North American Association for the Study of Obesity: *The practical guide: identification, evaluation, and treatment of overweight and obesity in adults*, Washington, DC, 2000, NIH.

Assessment

Assessment is summarized in Box 7-1.

Intervention and Teaching

Weight reduction is achieved by consuming less energy than required to meet energy needs. Methods for achieving weight reduction include diet, behavior modification, and increased physical activity, as well as medications and surgery. All of these methods are discussed in this chapter.

Preventing development of overweight and obesity

It is easier to prevent weight gain than to reduce excess weight. The following points are useful in helping adults avoid weight gain:

- Health risks are increased even at moderate degrees of overweight.
- Anticipate the likelihood of weight gain with aging and make lifestyle changes (increase activity level and evaluate and improve eating habits) as needed.
- Be alert to times when weight gain is likely (when quitting smoking, undergoing unusual stress, or in the perimenopausal period,

for example), and plan strategies in advance to prevent weight gain.

Establishing a weight goal

A weight that is no more than 20% greater than desirable (see Appendices C and D), or a BMI between 18.5 and 25 for adults, is associated with the least health risks. Especially in the severely obese individual, however, achieving a weight within the desirable range for height may seem overwhelming. Moreover, even a modest weight loss can have health benefits (Box 7-2). Therefore, setting a goal of a 5% to 10% weight loss over 6 months may achieve better results than setting a goal of achieving an ideal body weight. Once the 5% to 10% weight loss has been achieved, and the individual is successful in maintaining the weight loss, it may be possible to set another weight loss goal. If the obese individual participates in setting personal weight goals, he or she is more likely to be successful in losing weight.

Low-energy weight reduction diets

A weight loss of 0.5 to 1 kg (1 to 2 lb) a week is achievable and safe for most adults. To determine energy needs for weight reduction, subtract 500 to 1000 kcal/day from the estimated energy needs for maintenance of current body weight. This results in loss of approximately 0.5 to 1 kg per week because 0.5 kg of body fat is equivalent to approximately 3500 kcal.

To calculate daily maintenance energy needs, follow these steps:

- Determine ideal body weight (IBW) in kilograms; if IBW is in pounds, divide by 2.2.
- Estimate daily energy needs for weight maintenance: multiply IBW in kilograms by 20 to 25 kcal to estimate basal energy needs, then add sufficient energy to allow for activity. For sedentary individuals, add 30% to basal energy needs; for moderately active individuals, add 50%; for very active individuals, add 100%.
  Example: A moderately active woman who is 5'5" has an IBW of 100 lb + (5 × 5 lb) = 125 lb (from the rules of thumb on p. 53, or see Appendix C).
- IBW in kg = 125 lb ÷ 2.2 = 57 kg
- Basal needs = 57 kg × 20 kcal/kg/day = 1140 kcal/day
- Needs for weight maintenance (basal plus activity needs) = 1140 kcal/day × 150% = 1710 kcal/day

Box 7-2   Potential Health Benefits of a 10 kg (22 lb) Weight Loss by an Obese Individual

Mortality

20% to 25% decrease in total mortality
30% to 40% decrease in mortality from diabetes
40% to 50% fall in obesity-related cancer deaths

Blood Pressure

10 mm Hg decrease in systolic pressure
20 mm Hg decrease in diastolic pressure

Angina

Symptoms reduced by 91%
33% increase in exercise tolerance

Serum Lipids

10% decrease in total cholesterol
15% decrease in low-density lipoprotein (LDL) cholesterol
30% decrease in triglyceride levels
8% increase in high-density lipoprotein (HDL)[*] cholesterol

Diabetes

>50% reduction in the risk of developing diabetes
30% to 50% decrease in fasting blood glucose
15% decrease in hemoglobin A1c[†]

From Jung RT: Obesity as a disease, *Br Med Bull* 53:307, 1997. Used with permission.

[*]Increases in HDL are inversely related to risk of heart disease.
[†]Elevated levels are evidence of elevated blood glucose over an extended period of time.

- Needs for loss of approximately 0.5 kg or 1 lb/week = 1710 kcal/day – 500 kcal/day = 1210 kcal/day

Caution: If the calculation yields a value less than 1000 to 1200 kcal/day, it is better to maintain an intake of at least 1000 to 1200 kcal/day and increase the activity level to encourage weight loss. It is difficult to maintain an adequate nutritional intake with lower energy intakes. For most adult women, an energy intake of 1000 to 1200 kcal/day should be selected, and for men 1200 to 1600 kcal/day should be chosen. Very active women and those who weigh more than 75 kg (165 lb) may need 1200 to 1600 kcal/day, also (National Institutes of Health, 2000).

The optimal balance of carbohydrate, fat, and protein in a weight reduction diet is a subject of great debate. There is some evidence that low-carbohydrate diets result in slightly greater weight loss than low-fat diets (Bravata et al., 2003; Foster et al., 2003; Samaha et al., 2003). However, an equally important question is which type of diet is more effective in helping the dieter to maintain weight loss, and thus far there is no evidence that either type of diet is superior in this regard. Obese individuals are often found to have poor diets, frequently skipping breakfast and consuming foods of low nutrient density. The eating habits established during weight loss and maintenance efforts should change the quality of the diet in a positive way. There are a variety of ways to plan a healthful low-energy diet based on common foods. Most adults or adolescents can learn to use the *Exchange Lists for Meal Planning* available from the American Diabetes Association and the American Dietetic Association, which allow flexibility and are easier than calorie counting. The DASH diet (Chapter 1), with an emphasis on making healthful, low-energy choices (e.g., dairy products made with skim milk, whole grains and other good sources of fiber, and ample servings of fruits and vegetables, lean meats, fish, or poultry), can also be used as a tool for wise food selection. Individuals may want to use other diet plans that are found in magazines or books or supported by various commercial or community organizations. Box 7-3 provides guidelines for evaluating weight loss programs.

Practical suggestions for weight loss

Some practical suggestions for the person attempting to make diet changes include the following:

- Weigh or measure foods initially in order to learn to recognize portion sizes.
- Consume foods rich in fiber. High-fiber foods take longer to consume than low-fiber ones, and satiety (fullness or satisfaction) may be achieved with a reduced energy intake when consuming high-fiber foods.
- Broil, bake, or steam rather than frying foods. Use herbs, spices, lemon juice, or other low-energy seasonings rather than butter, margarine, olive oil, or salt pork. Choose skim milk and dairy

Box 7-3   Characteristics of a Safe and Effective Weight Control Program

1. The diet plan includes more than 800 kcal/day.
2. The diet plan includes foods from all food groups. A plan that relies on regular foods, rather than special proprietary products, is likely to be more effective in retraining eating habits. Very few servings from the fats, oils, and sweets group should be included.
3. No magical "fat-burning" or appetite-reducing products are recommended.
4. Claims for weight loss are no more than an average of 1 kg (~2 lb) per week.
5. Exercise is encouraged.
6. Behavior changes are incorporated.
7. The plan can be adapted to the lifestyle of the individual.
8. The cost of the plan is reasonable.

products made with skim milk. Limit foods with "hidden" fat, such as doughnuts, pie crust, croissants, muffins, and other quick breads. If desserts are desired, choose fruit ices, fresh fruit, or low-fat cookies (gingersnaps, newtons) rather than ice cream, cake, pie, or higher-fat cookies.

■ Do not expect rapid, easy weight loss. Weight gain is usually a gradual process, and so is weight reduction. When lapses occur, do not become depressed; simply resume proper eating habits and physical activity patterns.

■ Include occasional high-energy treats in the eating plan. This approach helps to prevent feelings of deprivation that may lead to binge eating and reduces guilt over indulging in a favorite high-calorie food. It may be necessary to eat high-energy favorite foods under the supervision of a counselor, health care provider, or trusted family member or friend initially, to avoid losing control.

Overweight in childhood

In dealing with obese children, frequently the goal is to achieve weight maintenance; as the child grows in stature, weight for height then becomes more appropriate. One teaching technique for preschool and young school-age children is the "traffic light" plan. Foods less than 20 kcal/serving are green, or GO, foods and can be used freely. Green foods include seasonings and a few vegetables, such as asparagus and lettuce. Yellow foods are the primary foods in the diet; they can be eaten with CAUTION. Examples are corn, oranges, grilled chicken, skim milk, and English muffins. Red, or STOP, foods are high in energy. No more than four servings of red foods are to be eaten per week. Some examples of red foods are scalloped potatoes, fruit in heavy syrup, fried chicken, whole milk, and doughnuts. A modification of the traffic light plan categorizes foods based on their fat content, since the foods highest in fat tend to be the ones highest in total energy. Foods with 0 to 3 g fat/serving are considered green foods, those with 4 to 5 g fat/serving are yellow, and those with >5 g fat/serving are red foods according to this categorization. Parents need to be made aware how important it is for them to make available nutritious food choices and model healthy eating and activity habits. Schools are another important influence on children's eating and exercise, and cafeteria meals and vending machines should provide nutritious, low-energy food choices. The increasing use of fast food (300% increase in children's consumption during the last two decades) and sweetened soft drinks are a special concern. Children who consume soft drinks regularly receive 188 kcal/day more than those who do not (St-Onge et al., 2003), and the American Academy of Pediatrics (2004) has recommended that the sale of these drinks be restricted in schools.

Very-low-calorie diets

Very-low-calorie diets (VLCDs) are those providing 400 to 800 kcal/day; they should be used only as medically directed. Special diet formulas (usually flavored drinks) are available, with the energy being mostly in the form of high-quality protein. This diet is sometimes called a *protein-sparing modified fast*. The usual regimen is to follow the VLCD for 12 to 16 weeks, followed by a gradual reinstitution of regular foods over a period of 3 weeks or longer. Losses of 1.5 to 2.3 kg (3.3 to 5.1 lb) per week occur during the VLCD, with the higher losses occurring in men.

These diets are usually reserved for individuals who are morbidly obese. They are designed to preserve LBM, but some LBM is lost during the dieting period. The severely obese not only contain more body fat but also have a greater LBM and thus tolerate severe energy restriction better than less obese individuals. However, even among the morbidly obese, these diets pose a risk for excess loss of critical tissues (e.g., myocardium), with serious morbidity and even death.

A VLCD should be begun only after a thorough medical examination, and dieters should have regular measurement of serum electrolytes and examinations by a physician. Intake of noncaloric fluids should be at least 2 L/day to prevent dehydration. Unsupervised dieting can lead to dehydration, electrolyte imbalance, elevation of uric acid, fatigue, dizziness, and headache; over the long term, there is a potential for ventricular dysrhythmias as well as binge eating after the severely restricted diet is ended. Rates of gallbladder disease are also reported to be higher among individuals consuming VLCD than the general population.

Counseling and behavior modification is essential because one half to two thirds of the weight loss is rapidly regained without it; lifestyle modification can reduce the amount of weight regained to about one third of that lost.

Fad diets

Diets that promise quick weight loss are popular. Unfortunately, these diets tend to be undesirable for one or more of the following reasons: (1) they are nutritionally inadequate; (2) they require expensive foods or time-consuming food preparation; (3) they are medically unsafe; (4) they do not help the individual change poor eating habits, and thus the weight lost is usually regained; and (5) much of the weight lost is fluid or lean body mass, rather than fat. All weight reduction diets should be evaluated with the criteria in Box 7-3 before beginning the program. In particular, the prospective dieter should remember that weight loss can be achieved without the purchase of expensive diet aids, very rapid weight loss can pose health risks, diet plans that focus heavily on one or a few foods can be nutritionally inadequate, and retraining of eating habits (i.e., recognition of appropriate serving sizes and focusing on healthful food choices) is a key component of a successful weight reduction regimen.

Behavior modification

Behavior modification, in conjunction with a balanced weight reduction diet, helps promote lasting weight loss. It should be a part of all weight loss programs. The following techniques are the primary features of behavior modification programs:

- *Self-monitoring:* recording exercise, food intake, and emotional and environmental circumstances at the time of food consumption to provide a basis for planning changes and for continued monitoring of adherence to lifestyle changes.
- *Stimulus control and environmental management:* acquiring techniques to help break learned associations between environmental cues and food intake.
- *Positive reinforcement:* a reward system to encourage changes in behavior.
- *Contracts:* signed contracts between the therapist and the individual seeking to modify behavior, outlining the consequences if various changes are made or are not made.

Box 7-4 provides suggestions for behavioral modification strategies designed to promote weight loss and maintenance. The individuals who are most successful in losing weight and maintaining weight loss tend to be those who develop personalized methods of controlling food intake and increasing energy expenditure. As an example, overly rapid food consumption is one cause of overeating. The feeling of satiety takes 20 minutes or more to develop in a hungry person, and the person who eats a meal in less time may overeat simply because he or she does not yet feel full. To slow the eating rate, the individual can eat with friends or family and talk with them during meals, lay utensils down after each bite, chew each bite thoroughly, and eat many leafy salads and other bulky foods.

Physical activity

Activities involving gross movements of large muscles promote fat loss while conserving LBM. Aerobic exercise is especially effective in reducing visceral fat. Many individuals on weight reduction diets find that, after an initial period of weight loss, their weight plateaus. The primary reason is that energy expenditure decreases as weight decreases. An increase in physical activity can prevent this plateau from occurring. Moderate physical activity for 30 minutes most days of the week is sufficient to achieve cardiovascular benefits, but more exercise is required to promote weight loss. For best results, the dieter must exercise most days of the week, expending a total of at least 1500 to 2000 kcal a week (Saris et al., 2003). Table 5-3 provides a guide to energy expenditure during exercise.

Although a regular exercise regimen is invaluable, increasing energy expenditure in the activities of daily living can also facilitate

---

Box 7-4   Modifying Behavior to Promote Weight Loss or Maintenance

1. Chew food slowly, and put utensils down between bites.
2. Never shop for food on an empty stomach.
3. Make out a grocery shopping list before starting, and do not add to it as you shop.
4. Leave a small amount of food on your plate after each meal.
5. Fill your plate in the kitchen at the start of the meal; do not put open bowls of food on the table.
6. Eat in only one or two places (e.g., the kitchen and dinning room table).
7. Never eat while involved in any other activity, such as watching television.
8. Do not eat while standing.
9. Keep a diary of when and where you eat and under what circumstances (e.g., boredom, frustration, anxiety). Be aware of problem circumstances, and substitute another activity for eating.
10. Keep low-calorie snacks available at all times.
11. Reward yourself for weight loss (e.g., buy new clothes, treat yourself to concert tickets or a trip). Establish a stepwise set of goals with a reward for achieving each goal.
12. If you violate your diet on one occasion, do not use that as an excuse to go off the diet altogether. Acknowledge that setbacks happen, and return to your weight control program.
13. When confronted with an appealing food, remember that this will not be your last chance to have the food. Content yourself with a small portion.

---

weight loss and maintenance. For example, park farther from the door, use stairs rather than the elevator, and bicycle or walk rather than driving on errands when possible.

Medications

Most medications used for weight loss suppress the appetite through effects on the central nervous system. Drugs fall into two general categories, those with anorexic properties, generally stimulators of the sympathetic nervous system, and those that reduce nutrient absorption. The prescription drug sibutramine (Meridia) suppresses appetite and also increases energy expenditure, as does phenylpropanolamine (in over-the-counter products such as Acutrim and Dexatrim). Orlistat (Xenical) acts by inhibiting the release of gastric and pancreatic lipases and thereby blocking the digestion and absorption of approximately one third of the fat consumed. Only sibutramine and orlistat are approved in the United States for use for more than a short time (a few weeks).

Weight loss medications are usually used in conjunction with other methods (low-energy diets, exercise programs, behavior modification) to stimulate weight loss. Medications increase the likelihood that the obese will lose at least 10% of their initial body weight, and therefore they reinforce the effects of lifestyle changes designed to promote weight loss; however, the total amount of weight loss caused by medications by themselves is only moderate—2 to 10 kg (4 to 22 lb) in most reports—and the weight plateaus after about 6 months. Weight regain is common after medications are stopped. Because obesity is a long-term problem, there is little benefit from short-term use of medications. Long-term use of medications is currently recommended only for carefully selected patients, particularly those who have obesity-related health problems, and not in the general obese population.

Orlistat can reduce absorption of fat-soluble vitamins (A, D, E, and K) and carotenoids. People using this medication should take a multivitamin containing the fat-soluble vitamins daily, and they should take it at least 2 hours before or after taking orlistat. Other side effects of orlistat include oily spotting, increased flatus, oily or fatty stools, fecal urgency, increased number of bowel movements, and fecal incontinence. These are usually temporary, but they may be worsened by a high-fat diet (greater than 30% of energy intake) or a very-high-fat intake at a single meal or snack.

Bariatric surgery

An individual with a BMI >40, or a BMI >35 and a serious obesity-related complication, who has failed to lose weight via more conventional methods may be considered for obesity surgery. Two strategies are used: restrictive procedures, which limit the capacity of the stomach to store food and cause the individual to feel full quickly, and malabsorptive procedures that bypass a portion of the intestine. In the increasingly popular gastric banding procedure, an inflatable band is placed around the stomach to create a 15 to 30 ml pouch; the size of the pouch outlet can be adjusted by altering the amount of fluid in a reservoir attached to the band (Figure 7-3, *A*). In gastroplasty (or gastric stapling; Figure 7-3, *B*), the stomach is partitioned to create a small pouch (30 to 60 ml). The use of a vertical band around the pouch outlet (vertical banded gastroplasty) reinforces it and reduces the risk of stretching the outlet. Gastric bypass (Figure 7-3, *C*) combines the restrictive approach with some degree of malabsorption. A gastric pouch is created and connected to the jejunum, bypassing the distal stomach and the duodenum. The biliopancreatic diversion technique (Figure 7-3, *D*) uses a larger gastric pouch (200 to 250 ml), with bypass of much of the small bowel, maintaining a food channel of 50 to100 cm of ileum. The standard biliopancreatic diversion creates an anastomosis of the ileum to the stomach, while the biliopancreatic diversion with duodenal switch creates an anastomosis of the ileum to the duodenum.

Overall, bariatric surgeries are successful in reducing excess weight by approximately 30% to 60%, sufficient to reduce the symptoms of diabetes, cardiovascular disease, hypercholesterolemia, obstructive sleep apnea, and hypertension, as well as many other complications of obesity, in most individuals (Fisher & Schauer, 2002; Kim et al., 2003). Gastric bypass and biliopancreatic diversion procedures produce the greatest weight loss. Weight loss usually ceases within 12 to 24 months after surgery, but it may continue for longer if patients participate in a follow-up program that emphasizes lifestyle practices for weight control. Losses of 50% or more of the excess weight may be maintained for as long as 10 to 15 years, especially by individuals who have a malabsorptive procedure.

Diet and behavior modification promote weight loss following obesity surgery. The surgical procedures in themselves can produce disappointing results unless combined with lifestyle changes to promote weight loss. Especially with the restrictive procedures, it is possible to gain weight by continually sipping high-energy liquids. Three small solid meals daily appear to yield the best results.

Complications after bariatric surgery

The malabsorptive procedures are especially likely to be associated with nutritional problems. Some of the most common concerns are as follows:

Text continued on p. 218

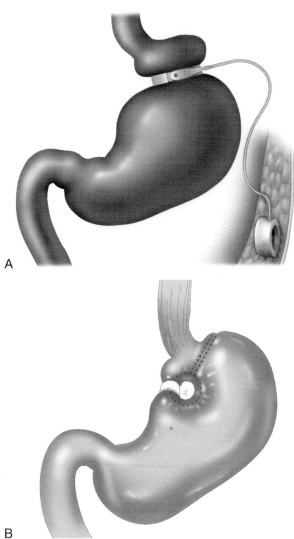

A

B

Figure 7-3
Surgical approaches to weight control. **A,** Gastric banding.
B, Vertical banded gastroplasty.

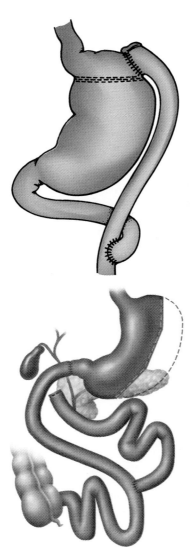

C

D

Figure 7-3, cont'd

C, Roux-en-Y gastric bypass. The stomach is stapled completely horizontally; the jejunum is resected from the duodenum and connected to the upper gastric pouch; the distal duodenal stump is connected to the jejunum to permit drainage of intestinal secretions. **D,** Biliopancreatic diversion.

- *Dumping syndrome.* Consumption of simple carbohydrates is likely to cause dumping syndrome after gastric bypass or biliopancreatic diversion, because of the rapid movement of osmotically active particles into the small bowel. The symptoms of dumping syndrome include dizziness, sweating, nausea, abdominal cramping, weakness, tachycardia, and diarrhea. Limiting intake of simple sugars, such as candy and sugar-sweetened beverages, reduces the likelihood of dumping syndrome.

- *Iron.* Gastric acid promotes iron absorption, and the small gastric pouch produces less acid; in addition, iron is normally absorbed in the duodenum and upper jejunum, which are partially or totally bypassed. Patients need a supplement (iron sulfate 325 mg/day) to avoid iron deficiency.

- *Calcium.* Calcium malabsorption is especially likely with the biliopancreatic diversion because it is associated with steatorrhea. A supplement providing the DRI for calcium will help to avert deficiency and osteoporosis.

- *Vitamin B_{12}.* Vitamin B_{12} deficiency may occur because the stomach produces less acid and intrinsic factor—both of which are required for vitamin B_{12} absorption—than normal. Oral supplements of pharmacologic amounts of vitamin B_{12} may be absorbed well enough to prevent deficiency.

- *Protein-energy malnutrition.* This is particularly likely following the biliopancreatic diversion, with steatorrhea (3 to 5 loose stools daily) being a common finding.

A variety of problems not related to nutrition are encountered with these surgeries. Wound infections, wound dehiscence, and venous and pulmonary thrombosis are relatively common in the early postoperative period. With gastric banding, gastric prolapse is possible but infrequent. With the other surgeries, leaks along the staple lines or at the sites of anastomosis can occur. Hernia and ulcers are two of the most common complications with the biliopancreatic diversion. Patients need to be followed for the rest of their lives to detect complications and monitor weight control.

Weight maintenance

After weight is lost, by whatever means, the goal becomes maintenance of the loss. Instead of thinking of weight control in terms of dieting, which is a temporary practice, the individual must think of it as a permanent lifestyle change. He or she can never return to old eating habits, or the weight will be regained. A study of individuals successful in maintaining a loss of at least 13.6 kg (30 lb) revealed that successful maintainers had certain common characteristics: frequent self-monitoring of their weight and dietary intake (i.e., keeping food records), adherence to a low-fat diet, participation in regular physical activity, and consumption of breakfast (Wing and Hill, 2001). Weight maintenance does become easier over the long term; 3 to 5 years after weight loss, fewer weight control strategies were required than during or immediately after weight loss.

REFERENCES

American Academy of Pediatrics Committee on School Health: Soft drinks in schools, *Pediatrics* 113:152, 2004.

Bravata DM et al: Efficacy and safety of low-carbohydrate diets: a systematic review, *JAMA* 289:1837, 2003.

Fisher BL, Schauer P: Medical and surgical options in the treatment of severe obesity, *Am J Surg* 184:9S, 2002.

Foster GD et al: A randomized trial of a low-carbohydrate diet for obesity, *N Engl J Med* 348:2082, 2003.

Kim JJ, Tarnoff ME, Shikora SA: Surgical treatment for extreme obesity: evolution of a rapidly growing field, *Nutr Clin Prac* 18:109, 2003.

Mokdad AH et al: Prevalence of obesity, diabetes, and obesity-related health risk factors, 2001, *JAMA* 289:76, 2003.

National Institutes of Health, National Heart, Lung, and Blood Institute, and the North American Association for the Study of Obesity: *The practical guide: identification, evaluation, and treatment of overweight and obesity in adults*, Washington, DC, 2000, NIH.

Samaha FF et al: A low-carbohydrate as compared with a low-fat diet in severe obesity, *N Engl J Med* 348:2074, 2003.

Saris WH et al: How much physical activity is enough to prevent unhealthy weight gain? Outcome of the IASO 1st Stock Conference and consensus statement, *Obes Rev* 4:101, 2003.

St-Onge MP, Keller KL, Heymsfield SB: Changes in childhood food consumption patterns: a cause for concern in light of increasing body weights, *Am J Clin Nutr* 78:1068, 2003.

Statistics Canada: *Overweight and obesity in Canada*. Available at http://www.hc-sc.gc.ca. Accessed December 30, 2003.

Wing RR, Hill JO: Successful weight loss maintenance, *Annu Rev Nutr* 21:323, 2001.

SELECTED BIBLIOGRAPHY

Krebs NF, Jacobson MS, American Academy of Pediatrics Committee on Nutrition: Prevention of pediatric overweight and obesity, *Pediatrics* 112:424, 2003.

Pi-Sunyer FX: The obesity epidemic: pathophysiology and consequences of obesity, *Obes Res* 10(suppl 2):97S, 2002.

Proctor MH et al: Television viewing and change in body fat from preschool to early adolescence: The Framingham Children's Study, *Int J Obes Relat Metab Disord* 27:827, 2003.

Riebe D et al: Evaluation of a healthy-lifestyle approach to weight management, *Prev Med* 36:45, 2003.

Yackel EE: An activity calendar program for children who are overweight, *Pediatr Nurs* 29:17, 2003.

Yanovski SZ, Yanovski JA: Obesity, *N Engl J Med* 346:591, 2002.

NUTRITION SUPPORT

II

Nutrition support is the use of oral, enteral, or parenteral feedings as a part of the therapeutic regimen. **Enteral feedings** are those given into the gastrointestinal tract, either by mouth or by tube. **Parenteral,** or intravenous, **feedings** may be given via a central venous catheter or peripheral vein. Enteral feedings are preferred over parenteral feedings if they are at all feasible. It is commonly said, "If the gut works, use it." Enteral feedings are generally less expensive and, in selected groups of patients, may pose less risk for development of sepsis than parenteral feedings. Enteral feedings in experimental animals help to prevent atrophy of the intestinal mucosa and "translocation" of microorganisms from the intestinal lumen across the intestinal wall. Studies in humans have not yet clearly demonstrated that enteral feedings maintain intestinal structure or prevent bacterial translocation better than parenteral feeding. Nevertheless, enteral feedings have some theoretical physiologic advantages. Enteral feeding stimulates the release of gastrointestinal hormones involved in nutrient metabolism and allows the liver "first-pass" extraction of nutrients, before they are presented to other tissues. The liver plays an important role in metabolism of many nutrients, control of blood glucose, storage of carbohydrates as glycogen, and protein synthesis. Patients who require parenteral feedings also are often given enteral feedings, even if only small amounts of enteral feedings are tolerated, in order to receive the benefits of both types of feedings. The choice of route and type of nutrition support are based on the individual patient's needs. Figure II-1 shows an example of a decision tree that might be used for determining the appropriate form of nutrition support.

Nutrition support is a specialized treatment modality, and multidisciplinary groups of health care professionals have been developed to deliver this treatment in the safest, most efficacious,

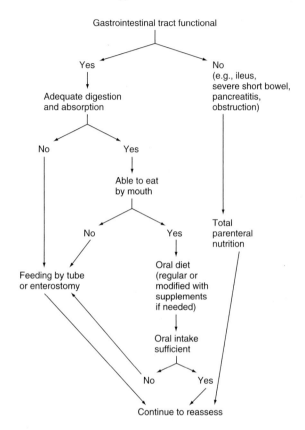

Figure II-1
Determining the optimal form of nutrition support. Caregivers continually reassess the individual and change the type of nutrition support as needed.

and most cost-effective manner possible. These groups are called *nutrition support services* or *teams.* They often include one or more physicians, nurses, dietitians, and pharmacists (and sometimes other professionals such as physical therapists and social workers) with advanced skills in nutrition assessment and delivery of nutrition support.

Enteral Nutrition

8

Enteral feedings can be delivered in three ways: (1) diets of regular or modified foods delivered orally, (2) nutritional supplements given by mouth, and (3) tube feedings.

Modified Diets

Modified diets are used by individuals with specific difficulties in consuming, digesting, absorbing, or metabolizing foods usually included in regular, unmodified diets. Some typical modified diets are summarized in Appendix J. Additional information is given in the chapters in Section III.

Oral Supplements

Oral supplements are useful for individuals who can digest and absorb nutrients. They are most effective for people who are consuming some foods but cannot take in enough because of anorexia or increased metabolic demands resulting from trauma, burns, infection, or other causes.

Types of Supplements

Some individuals prefer home-prepared foods such as shakes and eggnogs. Commercial formulas, or medical nutrition products, that contain protein, carbohydrates, fat, vitamins, and minerals may also be used and may be more appropriate for individuals requiring dietary modification (Table 8-1). Some medical nutrition products are available in the form of fortified bars, soups, coffee, frozen desserts, cookies, cereals, or puddings.

Modular products (Table 8-2) providing specific nutrients (usually carbohydrates, lipids, or protein) can be added to such foods as cooked or dry cereals, mashed potatoes, applesauce, juices, tea,

Text continued on p. 233

Table 8-1   Enteral Feeding Formulas

Product* and Manufacturer	kcal/ml	Osmolality (mOsm/kg H₂O)	Nonprotein kcal: N Ratio	Pro/CHO/ Fat (g/L)	Water Content (ml/L)	Fiber (g/L)	Approximate ml Needed to Meet Vitamin/ Mineral DV†
Polymeric Formulas							
Oral Supplements for Clear Liquid Diets							
Boost High Protein Drink[3]	1.01	540–605	80:1	61/139/23	833	—	946
Enlive!6	1.25	840	163:1	42/271/0	776	—	‡
Forta Drink6	0.52	410–502	71:1	33/87/<6	NA	—	1500
NuBasics Juice Drink4	1.0	990	132:1	40/209/0.6	820	—	‡
Resource Fruit Beverage5	1.06	750	152:1	9/54/0	817	—	‡
Oral Supplements, Lactose-Free Unless Stated That They Contain Milk							
Boost Drink3	1.01	610–670	125:1	43/173/18	833	—	1180
Boost High Protein Powder3 (in skim milk)	1.09	950	63:1	79/180/3	833	—	1060
Boost High Protein Powder3 (in water)	0.75	640	77:1	47/135/1	900	—	1060
Boost Plus3	1.52	720	139:1	59/200/58	780	<4	946
Carnation Instant Breakfast4 (in 2% milk)	0.93	661–747	105:1	45/147/19	804	—	1065

Enfamil Kindercal[3] (children)	1.06	440-520	200:1	30/135/44§	850	—	946
Great Shake[2]	1.7	NA	183:1	50/233/67	708	6.7	800
NuBasics Drink[4]	1.0	480-490	154:1	35/132/37	840	—	1000
NuBasics Plus[4]	1.5	620	154:1	52/176/65	764	—	650
Resource[5]	1.06	600	149:1	38/170/25	830	—	1180
Resource Benecalorie[5]	7.0	NA	255:1	155/0/733	880	—	‡
Resource Plus[5]	1.5	870	148:1	55/220/46	754	—	946
Resource Shake Plus[5]	2.0	1430	175:1	62/288/67		—	686
Scandishake[1] (in soy milk)	1.65	1094	163:1	13/68/30	711	—	‡
VHC 2.25[4]	2.25	950	131:1	90/197/122	672	—	‡
Oral or Tube Feeding, Lactose-Free							
Deliver 2.0[3]	2.0	640	144:1	75/200/101	700	—	1000
Ensure[6]	1.06	590	153:1	35/167/25	800	—	960
Novasource 2.0[5]	2.0	790	116:1	90/220/88§	692	—	948
Nutren Junior[4] (children)	1.0	350	183:1	30/128/42§	850	—	1000
Nutren Junior with Fiber[4] (children)	1.0	350	183:1	30/128/42§	844	6	1000
Pediasure Enteral[6] (children)	1.0	335	185:1	30/110/50§	844	—	1000-1300
Pediasure Enteral with Fiber[6] (children)	1.0	345	185:1	30/114/50§	844	5	1000-1300

Continued

Table 8-1   Enteral Feeding Formulas—cont'd

Product* and Manufacturer	kcal/ml	Osmolality (mOsm/ kg H₂O)	Nonprotein kcal: N Ratio	Pro/CHO/ Fat (g/L)	Water Content (ml/L)	Fiber (g/L)	Approximate ml Needed to Meet Vitamin/ Mineral DV†
Promote[6]	1.0	340	75:1	62/130/26§	837	—	1000
Resource Just for Kids[5]	1.0	390	185:1	30/110/50§	853	—	1000
Resource Just for Kids with fiber[5]	1.0	390	185:1	30/110/50§	853	6	1000
TwoCal HN[6]	2.0	730	125:1	84/219/92§	692	—	947
Tube Feeding, Lactose-Free							
Compleat[5]	1.07	300	114:1	43/140/37	781	6	1500
Compleat Pediatric[5]	1.0	380	142:1	38/130/39§	844	4.4	900
Comply[3]	1.5	460	134:1	60/180/61§	830	—	830
Enfamil Kindercal TF[3] (children)	1.06	345	200:1	30/135/44§	850	—	946
Enfamil Kindercal TF with fiber[3] (children)	1.06	345	200:1	30/135/44§	850	6.3	946
Fibersource HN[5]	1.2	490	115:1	53/160/39§	814	10	1165
Isocal[3]	1.06	270	168:1	34/135/44§	840	—	1890

Isocal HN[3]	1.06	270	125:1	44/124/45§	850	—	1180
Jevity 1.5 Cal[6]	1.5	525	122:1	64/50/216§	766	22	1500
Nutren 2.0[4]	2.0	745	131:1	80/196/106§	690	—	750
Osmolite[6]	1.0	300	153:1	37/151/35§	841	—	1887
Ultracal[3]	1.06	300	124:1	45/142/39§	830	14.4	1120
Elemental Formulas							
Criticare HN[3]	1.06	650	149:1	38/220/5	850	—	1890
f.a.a.[4]	1.0	700	100:1	50/176/112§	824	—	1000
Glutasorb[2]	1.0	575	96:1	52/186/7	732	—	1800
L-Emental[2]	1.0	630	137:1	38/206/3	NA	—	NA
Pediatric Peptinex DT[5]	1.0	290	189:1	30/138/39§	852	—	1000
Pediatric Peptinex DT with Fiber[5]	1.0	290	189:1	30/138/39§	852	—	1000
Peptamen 1.5[4]	1.5	550	131:1	68/188/56§	771	—	1000
Peptamen Junior[4] (children)	1.0	260–360	183:1	30/138/38§	850	—	1000
Peptamen PreBio[4] (with FOS and inulin)	1.5	290	131:1	40/127/39§	844	4	1500
Peptamen VHP[4]	1.5	300–430	75:1	62/104/39§	844	—	1500
Peptinex DT[5]	1.0	460	115:1	50/164/17§	830	—	1500
PRO-Peptide[2]	1.0	270	131:1	40/127/39§	NA	—	1500
PRO-Peptide for Kids[2]	1.0	350	187:1	32/132/41§	NA	—	2000

Continued

Table 8-1   Enteral Feeding Formulas—cont'd

Product* and Manufacturer	kcal/ml	Osmolality (mOsm/kg H₂O)	Nonprotein kcal:N Ratio	Pro/CHO/Fat (g/L)	Water Content (ml/L)	Fiber (g/L)	Approximate ml Needed to Meet Vitamin/Mineral DV†
Reabilan HN[4]	1.33	490	117:1	58/158/54§	800	—	1500
Vital HN[6]	1.0	500	125:1	42/185/11§	867	—	1500
Vivonex Pediatric[5]	0.8	360	200:1	24/130/24§	893	—	1000-1170
Vivonex T.E.N.[5]	1.0	630	149:1	38/210/3	853	—	2000
Disease-Specific Formulas							
Gastrointestinal Disease/Fat Malabsorption							
Advera[6]	1.28	680	108:1	60/216/23§	802	8.9	1184
(AIDS/HIV infection)							
Lipisorb Liquid[3]	1.35	630	125:1	57/161/57§	800	—	1180
Modulen IBD[4]	1.0	370	149:1	36/108/46§	800	—	2000
Portagen[3] (children <2 y)	0.676	230	157:1	23/76/32§	880	—	—
Subdue[3]	1.0	330-525	100:1	50/130/34§	840	—	1180
Hepatic Failure							
HepaticAid II[2]	1.2	560	142:1	44/168/36	750	—	‡
NutriHep[4]	1.5	790	209:1	40/290/21§	760	—	1000

Hyperglycemia or Diabetes							
Choice DM Beverage[3]	0.93	400	129:1	39/101/43	850	11	1310
Choice DM Tube-Feeding[3]	1.06	300	125:1	45/119/51	850	14.4	1120
Diabetisource AC[5]	1.2	350	95:1	60/100/59§	818	10	1250
Glucerna[6]	1.0	355	125:1	42/96/54	853	14.1	1420
Glytrol[4]	1.4	380	114:1	45/100/48§	847	15	1400
Resource Diabetic[5]	1.06	300	79:1	60/100/47	847	12.8	1180
Resource Diabetishield[5] (clear liquid)	0.63	380	76:1	30/126/0	921	—	‡
Pulmonary Disease or Ventilator Dependence							
Novasource Pulmonary[5]	1.5	650	116:1	75/150/68§	764	8	933
Nutrivent[4]	1.5	330–450	116:1	68/100/94§	781	—	1000
Oxepa[6]	1.5	493	125:1	62/106/94§	785	—	960
Pulmocare[6]	1.5	475	125:1	63/106/93§	785	—	946
Respalor[3]	1.5	400	102:1	75/146/68§	780	—	1000
Renal Failure							
Magnacal Renal[3] (dialysis)	2.0	570	144:1	75/27/101§	710	—	1000
Nepro[6] (dialysis)	2.0	665	154:1	70/223/96	699	—	960
Novasource Renal[5] (dialysis)	2.0	700	140:1	74/200/100§	709	—	1000
NutriRenal[4] (dialysis)	2.0	650	154:1	70/205/104§	704	—	750

Continued

Table 8-1   Enteral Feeding Formulas—cont'd

Product* and Manufacturer	kcal/ml	Osmolality (mOsm/ kg H$_2$O)	Nonprotein kcal: N Ratio	Pro/CHO/ Fat (g/L)	Water Content (ml/L)	Fiber (g/L)	Approximate ml Needed to Meet Vitamin/ Mineral DV†
Renalcal[4] (undialyzed)	2.0	600	339:1	34/290/82§	704	—	1000
Re/Neph[6] (dialysis; snack beverage)	2.1	NA	170:1	32/258/44	583	—	‡
Suplena[6] (undialyzed)	2.0	600	393:1	30/255/96	713	—	960
Trauma/Wound Healing/Burns/Critical Illness							
AlitraQ[6]	1.0	575	94:1	52/165/16§	846	—	1500
Crucial[6]	1.5	490	67:1	94/135/8§	771	—	1000
Impact with Fiber[5]	1.0	375	71:1	56/140/28§	868	10	1500
Impact Recover[5]	1.0	830	49:1	72/110/28§	775	3	1185
Intensical[3]	1.3	550	75:1	81/150/42§	800	—	1000
Optimental[6]	1.0	540	97:1	51/138/28	835	—	1422
Nutrifocus[6] (oral supplement for prevention/treatment of decubitus ulcer)	1.5	NA	125:1	62/21/49	754	2.5	‡
NutriHeal[4]	1.0	480	75:1	62/112/33	883	—	1000
Perative[6]	1.3	385	97:1	67/177/37	789	—	1155

Protain XL[3]	1.0	340	86:1	57/145/30§	830	9.1	1250
Replete[4]	1.0	300-350	75:1	62/113/34§	845	—	1000
Replete with Fiber[4]	1.0	310-390	75:1	62/113/34§	835	14	1000
TraumaCal[3]	1.5	560	91:1	82/142/68§	780	—	2000

*This is only a representative sample of the available products and is not meant to imply endorsement of these products.

†DV are for adults, unless product is designed for children. Children's formulas are for ages 1 to 10 years.

‡Not intended to provide complete nutrition.

§Contains MCT (medium-chain triglyceride).

Immune-enhancing; contains fish oil (omega-3 fatty acids) and increased amounts of antioxidant nutrients, may have increased arginine and glutamine, may contain nucleotides.

NA, Not available; *CHO*, carbohydrate; *FOS*, fructooligosaccharides (fermentable fiber conducive to growth of beneficial gut flora).

Manufacturers: [1] Axcan Scandipharm, Birmingham, Alabama; [2] Hormel HealthLabs, Plymouth, Minnesota; [3] Mead Johnson & Co, Evansville, Indiana; [4] Nestle Clinical Nutrition, Glendale, California; [5] Novartis, Minneapolis, Minnesota; [6] Ross Products, Columbus, Ohio.

Table 8-2   Modular Components for Enteral Feeding

Product and Manufacturer	Nutrient Content
Protein Modules	**Protein Content per gram Powder**
Casec[3]	0.9 g
ProMod[6]	0.76 g
ProPass[2]	0.75 g
ProRight[7]	0.7 g
Resource Beneprotein[5]	0.86 g
Carbohydrate Modules	**kcal Content per gram Powder**
Moducal[3]	3.8
Polycose[6]	4 (2 kcal/ml liquid)
Fat Modules	**kcal/ml**
MCT Oil[3]	7.7 (8.3 kcal/g)
Microlipid[3]	4.5
Protein and Carbohydrate Modules	**Protein/Carbohydrate/kcal Content per gram Powder**
Hi ProCal[2]	0.37 g/0.56 g/3.7 kcal
Multimix Protein Supplement[2]	0.38 g/0.44 g/3.3 kcal
Protein and Energy Modules	**Protein/Carbohydrate/ Fat/kcal Content per gram Powder**
Additions[4]	0.32 g/0.47 g/0.26 g/5.3 kcal
Fiber Modules	**Fiber/kcal Content per gram Powder**
Fiberbasics Instant Soluble Fiber[1]	0.38 g/3.8 kcal
Resource Benefiber[5]	0.75 g/4 kcal
UniFiber[8]	0.43 g/2 kcal

kcal, Kilocalorie.

Manufacturers: [1]Axcan Scandipharm, Birmingham, Alambama; [2]Hormel HealthLabs, Plymouth, Minnesota; [3]Mead Johnson & Co., Evansville, Indiana; [4]Nestle Clinical Nutrition, Glendale, California; [5]Novartis, Minneapolis, Minnesota; [6]Ross Products, Columbus, Ohio; [7]Leahy IFP, Northbrook, Illinois; [8]Niche Pharmaceuticals, Roanoke, Texas.

coffee, shakes, soups, salad dressings, and sandwich fillings. Modular carbohydrates are especially versatile because they can be added to most soft foods or liquids without altering their flavor or texture. Modular products are especially useful for enhancing the protein or energy provided by infant formulas.

Delivery of Oral Supplements

Liquid supplements are best tolerated if consumed slowly, taking 180 to 360 ml over 15 to 45 minutes. Liquid supplements contain readily digested carbohydrate. As a result, they can cause **dumping syndrome,** with abdominal cramping, weakness, tachycardia, and diarrhea, if they are consumed rapidly. Most liquid supplements taste best if they are chilled or served over ice. Fat is an important energy source; supplements containing at least a moderate amount of fat (~30% of energy) are desirable unless contraindicated or poorly tolerated, as with acute pancreatitis or massive small bowel resection.

Enteral Tube Feedings

Enteral tube feedings may be needed for the following reasons:

- Inability to consume adequate food because of mechanical problems with eating, psychologic disorders, or unconsciousness. Tube feedings may be used to supplement or replace oral feedings; examples include head and neck tumors, esophageal stricture or obstruction, coma, anorexia of chronic illness, anorexia nervosa, hyperemesis gravidarum, and neurologic disorders interfering with swallowing.
- Increased nutritional requirements that may not be met by oral feedings alone; examples include severe trauma, burns, congenital heart disease.
- Maldigestion or malabsorption requiring unpalatable modified formulas or making continuous feedings necessary to maintain adequate nutritional status; examples include pancreatic or biliary insufficiency, short bowel syndrome, inflammatory bowel disease, and protracted diarrhea with malnutrition.

Types of Tube Feeding Formulas
Polymeric or intact protein formulas

When the gastrointestinal (GI) tract is functional, nutritionally complete **polymeric formulas** can be used. These contain proteins such as casein or lactalbumin; carbohydrates in the form of sugars, hydrolyzed starches, or dextrins; and varying amounts of fat. Most commercially prepared formulas are lactose-free because lactose intolerance is common among adults, especially individuals of African or Asian descent, as well as individuals with malabsorption. The optimal ratio of nonprotein kcal to nitrogen in healthy adults is approximately 150 kcal to 1 g of nitrogen. In critically ill and metabolically stressed individuals, nitrogen needs are increased, and the ratio is reduced. In children, the ratio is higher than in adults, to provide the energy needed for growth. Adults with renal and hepatic failure may also need a higher ratio to ensure that adequate fat and carbohydrate are available to meet energy needs, so that the nitrogen in the feeding is available for tissue synthesis.

Fiber is included in some polymeric formulas as an aid to the control of bowel function. Insoluble forms of fiber such as wheat bran and psyllium increase the fecal mass and thus reduce the likelihood of constipation. Soluble forms of fiber such as modified guar gum decrease serum cholesterol and postprandial blood glucose concentrations. In addition, some of the soluble fiber is fermented to short-chain fatty acids by colonic bacteria. The short-chain fatty acids are absorbed along with sodium and water in the colon, and evidence suggests that this action reduces the likelihood of diarrhea. An increase in soluble fiber is not recommended in patients with diarrhea until infectious causes (e.g., pseudomembranous colitis) are ruled out.

The fat in polymeric formulas is usually in the form of vegetable oils or a combination of vegetable oils and **medium-chain triglycerides (MCTs).** MCTs contain fatty acids 8 to 12 carbons in length. They are used as a calorie source because they are easily digested and absorbed, compared with the long-chain triglycerides (LCTs) found in vegetable oils. MCTs do not provide the essential fatty acids, and thus it is necessary that formulas provide at least a small amount of fat (approximately 3% of total energy intake) in the form of long-chain essential fatty acids.

Fat digestion and absorption

Fat is a key nutrient to consider when planning enteral feedings for the patient with impaired digestion or absorption. LCTs in particular require adequate lipase enzyme to remove fatty acids from the glycerol backbone of the triglyceride, bile salts, and absorptive area in the small intestine (see Figure 1-4). The following ingredients are necessary for absorption of fat:

- *Lipase:* LCTs are too large and too insoluble in the watery intestinal secretions to be absorbed intact. Usually the two outer fatty acids are removed, leaving the inner fatty acid attached to glycerol and creating a monoglyceride (one fatty acid attached to glycerol). Lipases released in the mouth and the stomach may be important in infancy. Most fat digestion in adults and older children is performed by lipase released by the pancreas, however. Release of pancreatic lipase is likely to be low in individuals with diseases of the pancreas such as cystic fibrosis and pancreatitis. Because MCTs are smaller and more water-miscible than LCTs, lipase activity is less important with MCTs.

- *Bile salts:* Bile salts (produced in the liver and stored in the gallbladder) combine with fatty acids and monoglycerides to form **micelles**, forming an emulsion of the fats with the digestive secretions in the bowel. Bile salts can cause micelle formation because they have both water-soluble and fat-soluble components. The fatty acids and the fat-soluble part of the bile salt are in the center of the micelle, and the water-soluble portion of the bile salt and the glycerol portion of the monoglycerides are on the outer part of the micelle. Long-chain fatty acids are relatively insoluble in water, but by forming an emulsion with the bile salts, their solubility is improved enough to allow them to pass through the unstirred water layer that lies just over the intestinal mucosal cells. Because medium-chain fatty acids are smaller and more soluble in water than long-chain fats, they do not require thorough micelle formation to pass through the unstirred water layer.

- *Bowel surface area for absorption:* The jejunum is responsible for much of the fat absorption, and the ileum is needed for bile salt reabsorption. Reabsorbed bile salts are returned to the liver for reuse. Conditions such as surgical removal of the jejunum, inflammatory bowel disease, or radiation damage to the bowel can interfere with fat absorption. Ileal resection or damage impairs bile salt reabsorption and can deplete the body's pool of bile salts. Because absorption of MCTs is less dependent on bile salts than absorption of LCTs, MCTs can be useful in treating fat malabsorption that occurs when bowel surface area is diminished.

The absorption of MCTs is more similar to the absorption of protein and carbohydrate than it is to the absorption of LCTs (see Figure 1-4). Not only is micelle formation less important for MCTs than for LCTs, but also MCTs do not have to be packaged with proteins and phospholipids as chylomicrons in order to be soluble enough to enter the circulation. The majority of fatty acids from MCTs are released directly from the intestinal cells into the portal vein blood, just as the amino acids and monosaccharides are, instead of entering the lymph system with the LCTs.

Elemental (predigested) formulas

Many individuals with maldigestion and malabsorption tolerate polymeric formulas, particularly those containing MCTs; however, **elemental** or **predigested formulas** are also available. The nitrogen source in elemental formulas is in the form of protein hydrolysates, peptides, and/or free (crystalline) amino acids (see Table 8-1). Free amino acids and small peptides are absorbed via different mechanisms, and thus total nitrogen absorption may be greater if the formula contains both forms of nitrogen. Elemental formulas are either very low in fat or provide much of their fat in the form of MCTs to reduce fat malabsorption. These formulas are more expensive than the polymeric ones. They are appropriate for selected patients with short bowel syndrome or other malabsorptive disorders, such as severe enteropathy associated with acquired immune deficiency (AIDS), pancreatitis, and inflammatory bowel disease.

Disease- or condition-specific formulas

Specialized formulas have been developed for many different disease or metabolic conditions, including acquired immune deficiency syndrome (AIDS), glucose intolerance or diabetes, hepatic encephalopathy, pulmonary disease, renal failure, trauma and critical illness, and wound healing (see Table 8-1). It is important to evaluate patients carefully to determine whether there is a real need for a specialized product. These condition-specific products can be characterized in the following manner:

- *AIDS and severe malabsorption:* concentrated in energy, low in fat (e.g., Advera) or very high in MCT (e.g., Lipisorb) to reduce fat malabsorption. These formulas are typically taken by mouth and thus are flavored.
- *Glucose intolerance:* fiber-containing (10 to 15 g/L) to help reduce the blood glucose response to feeding; high in monounsaturated fatty acids and low in saturated fat to reduce serum triglycerides and the risk of heart disease. These formulas are high in fat

(40% to 49% of total energy) and moderate to low in carbohydrate (30% to 45% of energy) to try to reduce hyperglycemia. In comparison, the American Diabetes Association (ADA, 2004) recommends that most diabetic individuals consume a diet supplying less than 30% fat, with 55% to 60% of energy as carbohydrate. However, these recommendations are primarily intended for individuals eating a diet of regular foods, where high-fat diets are likely to be associated with excessive energy, cholesterol, and saturated fat intake. In the formulas for glucose intolerance, monounsaturated fat and carbohydrate together provide approximately 60% to 70% of total energy, and protein provides 15% to 20%, consistent with the ADA (2004) recommendations for diabetic individuals without renal failure. Individualized assessment is required to determine whether these formulas meet the needs of a patient with renal impairment. High-fat diets may exacerbate the delay in gastric emptying in individuals with diabetic gastroparesis, and it may be necessary to choose a formula with a lower fat content in this circumstance.

- *Hepatic encephalopathy:* concentrated in energy to allow fluid restriction, low protein (11% to 15% of total energy), high in branched-chain amino acids (approximately 50% of the protein equivalent vs. the 20% in standard formulas) and low in aromatic amino acids and methionine, low in sodium, low to moderate in fat (13% to 27%) to compensate for impaired fat absorption; not indicated for patients without encephalopathy.

- *Pulmonary disease:* concentrated in energy to allow fluid restriction; moderate to low in carbohydrate to reduce carbon dioxide production; contain MCT to enhance fat absorption; fortified with antioxidants (vitamins A, C, beta-carotene, and possibly selenium) to reduce oxidative damage during oxygen therapy. Although carbohydrate does result in greater carbon dioxide production than fat, these formulas have not been demonstrated to improve outcome in patients with pulmonary disease. Excessive energy intake is a greater risk for carbon dioxide production than a high-carbohydrate diet in these patients. Oxepa, a specialized product for patients with acute respiratory distress syndrome (ARDS), contains increased levels of omega-3 fatty acids and antioxidants. In clinical trials, ARDS patients receiving this formula spent significantly less time on a ventilator and less time in the intensive care unit, with a decreased incidence of new organ failure (Gadek et al., 1999), as well as improved oxygenation and reduction in inflammatory cytokine concentrations in the bron-choalveolar fluid (Pacht et al., 2003).

- *Renal disease:* concentrated in energy to allow fluid restriction; predialysis products are low in protein (6% to 7% of total energy) with emphasis on essential amino acids, dialysis products are moderate in protein (approximately 15% of total energy); moderate to low in vitamins A and D and high in folic acid and vitamin B_6; restricted in sodium, potassium, phosphorus, and magnesium; contain carnitine to improve fat metabolism. Protein status of patients should be carefully evaluated. The renal formulas may be inadequate in protein for some dialysis patients.

- *Surgery, trauma, stress, and critical illness:* high protein (>20% of total energy intake), low nonprotein kilocalorie–to–nitrogen ratio. These formulas are generally enriched in antioxidants and nutrients especially important in healing (including some or all of the following: vitamins A, C, and E; beta-carotene; selenium; and zinc) and may contain increased levels of branched-chain amino acids, glutamine, and omega-3 fatty acids, as well as nucleotides. Immune-enhancing formulas are enriched in arginine, as well as constituents previously listed. They contain only low levels of omega-6 fatty acids, which have proinflammatory properties. Although immune-enhancing formulas reduced the length of hospital stay and the length of stay in the intensive care unit in trauma patients in a number of studies, there was no significant reduction in infectious complications or mortality. For critically ill patients in general, the formulas did not reduce mortality, and indeed there was a possible increase in mortality among septic patients (reviewed in A.S.P.E.N., 2002; Heyland et al., 2003). Since most of these formulas contain several factors that might foster the immune response, it is impossible to determine what impact each individual factor might have in the critically ill. Thus far no benefits of vitamin and mineral supplementation have been identified in individuals without deficiencies of these nutrients.

Other formula characteristics

Energy density and fluid content

Many formulas provide 1 kcal/ml because adults need approximately 1 ml of water per kilocalorie consumed, or approximately 30 ml/kg/day. However, energy-dense formulas containing 1.5 to 2 kcal/ml are available for individuals needing fluid restrictions. The hydration status of patients receiving these concentrated formulas must be closely monitored, with more free water given as required.

Table 8-3 provides a guideline for calculating fluid requirements for maintenance needs; these must be adjusted based on estimated losses from wounds, ostomies, vomiting, diarrhea, gastrointestinal drainage, and so forth. Careful intake and output records are essential in estimation of these losses. Intermittent fever does not alter fluid requirements very much, but prolonged fever increases fluid needs about 12% for every degree above 37° C (or 7% for every degree above 98.6° F). If a deficit in fluid intake occurs in adults and adolescents, the volume of replacement fluid needed (in addition to that needed to maintenance) can be calculated from the ratio of the normal serum sodium concentration (approximately 140 mEq/L [140 mmol/L]) to the patient's actual serum sodium, as follows:

Fluid deficit in liters = 0.6 × Body weight (kg) − [(Normal serum sodium/Patient sodium) × 0.6 × Body weight (kg)]

In infants and young children, the most accurate method of estimating fluid deficit is by weight loss:

Fluid deficit in liters = Usual weight (kg) − Present weight (kg)

Where the usual weight is unavailable or unclear, clinical signs (see Table 2-7) can be used for estimation of the amount of fluid deficit.

Table 8-3   Maintenance Fluid and Electrolyte Requirements*

Infants, Children, and Adults	Water (ml)	Na+ (mEq/kg)[†]	K+ (mEq/kg)[†]
Infants/ Children		2-4	1-3
≤10 kg	100/kg		
11-20 kg	1000 + 50/kg over 10 kg		
>20 kg	1500 + 20/kg over 20 kg		
Adults	1500 + 20/kg over 20 kg	2-3	2-3

*Must be increased when losses are greater than normal.
[†]1 mEq Na+ (sodium) = 23 mg; 1 mEq K+ (potassium) + 39 mg.

Osmolality

Osmolality refers to the number of osmotically active particles per kilogram of water in a solution. A formula is considered to be isotonic or isosmolar if its osmolality is similar to that of plasma (approximately 300 mOsm/kg). It is hypertonic or hyperosmolar if its osmolality is greater than that of plasma. It was once thought that hyperosmolar solutions were a common cause of diarrhea. For this reason, formulas were diluted to quarter- or half-strength when tube feedings were initiated, and the strength was gradually increased. Evidence now indicates that hyperosmolality by itself is unlikely to cause diarrhea and that use of diluted formula only delays the delivery of adequate nutrients to the patient. In some patients with other causes for diarrhea, use of a hyperosmolar formula might worsen diarrhea, however.

Feeding Tubes

Routes for tube feedings

Tube feedings may be given into the esophagus, stomach, or small intestine. Figure 8-1 illustrates the gastric and intestinal locations. Nasogastric (NG) and nasoduodenal (ND)/nasojejunal (NJ) tubes are often used for short-term feedings, and esophagostomy, gastrostomy, and jejunostomy are frequently chosen for long-term feedings. Percutaneous endoscopic gastrostomies (PEGs) are especially popular because they can be performed without general anesthesia.

Nasogastric (NG) tubes (or orogastric in infants)

Advantages: Tube easily inserted; allows use of almost all of the GI tract; suited to intermittent feedings.

Disadvantages: Tube easily dislodged, especially with altered sensorium; potential for pulmonary aspiration and for development of sinusitis and otitis media.

Nasoduodenal (ND) or nasojejunal (NJ) tubes

Advantages: Theoretically decreases the likelihood of pulmonary aspiration, although clinical investigations to date have not found a significant difference in rates of aspiration between gastric and small bowel feedings; useful in individuals with delayed gastric emptying; allows for simultaneous gastric decompression and small bowel feeding.

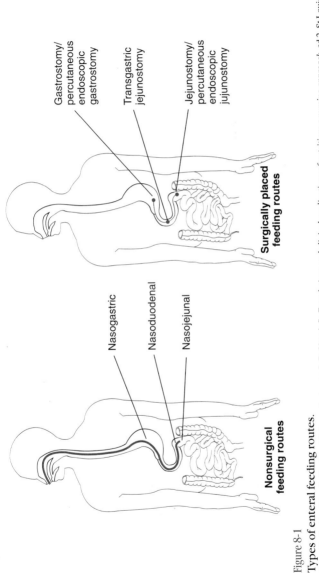

Figure 8-1

Types of enteral feeding routes.
(From Rolin Graphics. In Grodner M, Long-Anderson S, DeYough S: *Foundations and clinical applications of nutrition: a nursing approach,* ed 2, St Louis, 2000, Mosby.)

Disadvantages: More difficult to insert tube than NG; bypasses the stomach, a barrier to infection; usually necessitates continuous feedings given with a pump; can cause dumping syndrome; tube easily dislodged; potential for development of sinusitis and otitis media.

Gastrostomy

Advantages: More difficult to dislodge tube than NG; usually has a larger diameter than NG, allowing use of more viscous formulas (e.g., home blended); easily hidden by clothing (and gastric button device fits flush against the skin, with no tube protruding except during feedings); conventional surgical gastrostomies can bypass esophageal obstruction, but placement of PEG tubes requires a patent esophagus; a jejunostomy tube can be inserted via a gastrostomy.

Disadvantages: Potential for irritation of skin around insertion site caused by leakage of gastric secretions; bleeding and infection of the insertion site (usually in the immediate postinsertion period).

Jejunostomy

Advantages: Same as for ND/NJ; can bypass upper GI obstruction; more difficult to dislodge tube than with ND/NJ.

Disadvantages: Requires surgical insertion; potential for erosion of skin around insertion site from leakage of intestinal contents (containing digestive enzymes); bypasses the stomach, a barrier to infection; usually requires continuous feedings given via pump; feedings can cause dumping syndrome; bleeding and infection of the insertion site (usually in the immediate postinsertion period).

Selection of feeding tubes

Nonreactive tubes are soft, nonirritating tubes made of polyurethane, silicone rubber, or similar materials. Tubes for NG and ND/NJ feedings range in size from 5 to 12 french (F) (1 F ≈ 0.34 mm). Insertion of these pliable tubes is sometimes difficult, but stylets are available to facilitate insertion. Nonreactive tubes can be left in place for several weeks without stiffening. Some tubes have weighted tips designed to facilitate ND/NJ intubation and to help to maintain the tube's position in the intestine; however, studies suggest that unweighted tubes actually pass through the pyloric sphincter more readily than weighted ones and that tube position is better maintained with unweighted tubes.

Insertion of NG and ND/NJ tubes (Figure 8-2)

1. Select an appropriately sized tube. Generally, 8 F tubes, often called "small-bore" or "fine-bore," are suitable for adults and children. If thick fluids are to be used, then a 10 to 12 F tube may be needed. Most infants can use 6 or 8 F tubes, but premature infants may need 5 F tubes.

2. Explain the procedure to the individual. Patients may be reassured by the information that tube insertion is not painful, although it may cause gagging. Have the person sit up, if possible, and lean the head forward.

3. Determine the length of tube to be inserted (Beckstrand et al., 1990; Hanson, 1979). For adults, use the following equation:

Length for NG insertion = ([Nose to ear to xiphoid process
measurement (cm) − 50 cm] ÷ 2) + 50 cm

For children, one suggested method is as follows:

Length for NG insertion = 6.7 + 0.226 (Height in cm) + 3 cm +
Distance from distal tip to feeding pores on tube (cm)

4. Lubricate the tip of the tube with water-soluble lubricant. Gently advance the tube through the nostril parallel to the roof of the mouth and then down the esophagus. Inhalable nasal decongestants used before tube insertion can make the process more comfortable. The patient can help by sipping fluids, unless they are contraindicated, or swallowing while the tube is being advanced.

5. If the individual begins to cough or choke during the insertion, the tube may be in the trachea. Remove it and try again.

6. When the proper length of tube has been inserted, secure the tube to the nose with tape.

7. If ND/NJ placement is desired, insert a sufficient length of tubing (85 cm appears adequate for most adults). Prokinetic agents such as metoclopramide or erythromycin administered *before* beginning the insertion of the tube increase the likelihood that the tube will pass spontaneously through the pylorus. A variety of techniques have also been recommended by experienced practitioners, including rotating the tube slightly while advancing it gradually through the stomach, placing the individual in the right lateral decubitus position, insufflation of air into the

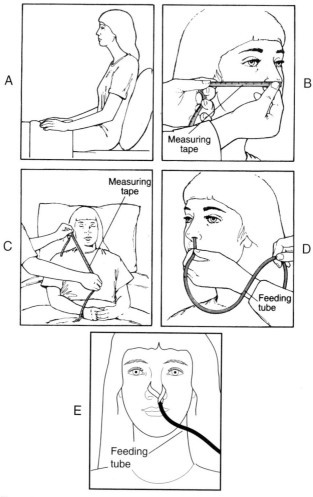

Figure 8-2

Insertion of a feeding tube. **A,** Place the patient in Fowler's position before tube insertion, if possible, so that gravity can facilitate passage of the tube. **B** and **C,** Measure the distance nose to ear and then to xiphoid process and calculate length of tube needed. **D,** Encourage patient to sip fluids or chew ice chips while the tube is gently advanced. **E,** Tape tube securely in place.

(**A-D,** From Beare PG, Myers JL, editors: *Principles and practice of adult health nursing*, St Louis, 1990, Mosby. **E,** Redrawn from Beare PG, Myers JL, editors: *Principles and practice of adult health nursing*, St Louis, 1990, Mosby.)

stomach while advancing the tube, and use of an external magnet in conjunction with a metal-tipped tube. For a discussion of this topic, see Cresci and Martindale (2003). Fluoroscopic or endoscopic techniques may be used to place the tube if the aforementioned techniques are unsuccessful.

8. Confirm tube placement before administering feedings.

Methods of confirming tube placement

- *Abdominal radiograph:* This method is recommended because it is the most accurate. Disadvantages include the cost and exposure of the patient to radiation.
- *pH and bilirubin of fluid obtained from the tube:* The combination of the two measurements is a sensitive indicator of tube placement (Metheny, Smith, and Stewart, 2000). If pH is >5 and bilirubin is <5 mg/dl, this indicates probable respiratory tract placement. A pH <5 and bilirubin <5 mg/dl indicate that the tube tip is in the stomach. A pH >5 and bilirubin >5 mg/dl indicate intestinal placement of the tube tip.
- *Other methods:* Auscultation over the left upper quadrant of the abdomen while insufflating air through a nasogastric tube is sometimes used, but this method cannot be recommended because of the potential for hearing air when the tube tip is positioned in the respiratory system.

Delivery of tube feedings

Continuous feedings

Continuous feedings, feedings delivered over the entire day or some portion of the day (usually 10 to 12 hours), are used in certain circumstances:

- Duodenal or jejunal feedings because continuous feedings reduce the risk of dumping syndrome.
- Decreased absorptive area (chronic diarrhea, short bowel syndrome, acute radiation enteritis, and severe malnutrition with atrophy of the villi) because continuous feedings may increase the total amount tolerated.
- Some cases of severe stress with normal GI function. (Burn patients, for instance, have been found to have less diarrhea and more adequate intake if given continuous, rather than intermittent, feedings.)

Although continuous NG or gastrostomy feedings may be beneficial in certain situations, they keep the gastric pH continuously high and have been associated with increased risk of pneumonia in very ill patients. It is suggested that the less acid gastric pH allows increased growth of bacteria and yeast in the stomach and that these organisms can colonize the trachea and cause pneumonia. In addition, aspiration pneumonia related to reflux of feedings or gastric fluid is relatively common in seriously ill and elderly patients. While transpyloric feedings (delivered into the small bowel) have a theoretical advantage over intragastric feedings in reducing the risk of aspiration, there is little evidence that this is the case in practice (A.S.P.E.N., 2002). To reduce the risk of pneumonia during tube feedings, use aseptic or scrupulously clean technique in administering tube feedings and administer feedings in closed feeding sets. Keep the patient in a semirecumbent position (head elevated 30 to 45 degrees) as much as possible. Patients who must remain flat in bed such as those with head or neck injuries are at risk of aspiration, as are those with neurologic deficits. During mechanical ventilation, the mouth and upper airway can become colonized with pathogenic organisms. Scrupulous mouth cleansing, as well as frequent suctioning of subglottic secretions, has been suggested to reduce the risk of pneumonia.

It has long been thought that gastric residuals should be aspirated from the feeding tube and measured on a regular schedule; however, the nonreactive tubes tend to collapse when suction is applied to them and often do not yield accurate residuals. Moreover, regular aspiration of residuals increases the likelihood of clogging the tube because gastric acid can coagulate the protein in the formula. Therefore, measuring gastric residuals is currently undergoing critical examination by many clinicians. If residual volumes are measured, the tube should be thoroughly flushed with water afterward. The practice of stopping feedings for large residuals (defined in different ways in different institutions and by individual practitioners) interferes with adequate nutrient delivery. Occasional large residuals are common even among patients who tolerate feedings well, although a trend toward consistently large residuals may indicate delayed gastric emptying due to sepsis, poorly controlled hyperglycemia, or other clinical problems. Once the correctable causes of delayed gastric emptying have been addressed, use of prokinetic medications such as metoclopramide can be effective in improving feeding tolerance in patients who still exhibit problems. Erythromycin has prokinetic effects, but concerns about antibiotic resistance limit its routine use for this purpose. Monitoring the patient frequently for gastric distension, bloating, and increase in abdominal girth is an important part of care.

Intermittent feedings

Feedings given every 2 to 4 hours are preferred for certain patients:

- Confused individuals who, if left unattended, are in danger of dislodging the tube.
- Stable long-term patients, especially home patients, in whom continuous feedings interfere with normalization of lifestyle.

Intermittent feedings are usually better tolerated if given by slow drip rather than by rapid bolus infusion. Usually 300 to 400 ml can be tolerated several times daily if each feeding is infused over at least 20 to 30 minutes. Abdominal discomfort, diarrhea, tachycardia, and nausea during or shortly after feedings signal that the flow is too rapid or the volume too large.

Promoting comfort

The most common complaints of tube-fed individuals are thirst, being deprived of tasting food, sore nose or throat, and dry mouth. Comfort can be increased by the following methods:

- Encourage intake of food and fluids if not contraindicated. (Many people are initially afraid that they cannot eat while the tube is in place.)
- Provide adequate fluid. Most formulas for adults provide 1 kcal/ml. This ratio may not provide adequate fluid for some patients. If the individual cannot drink fluid and is not fluid restricted, then provide extra water by tube. For example, irrigate the tube after each feeding or every 4 to 6 hours with 30 to 60 ml or more of water.
- Provide regular mouth care and stimulation of saliva flow. Important comfort measures include rinsing the mouth with water or mouthwash; brushing the teeth; sucking hard candy or chewing gum in moderation, if not contraindicated; and gargling with warm saltwater to relieve sore throat.
- Use nonreactive tubes, and use the tube with the smallest possible diameter.

■ Tape the tube in place securely so that it does not move back and forth.

Assessing Response to Nutrition Support

Anthropometric measurements, physical assessment, and hematologic and biochemical measurements are used in assessing response to nutrition support (Table 8-4).

Preventing and Correcting Complications of Enteral Nutrition

Enteral nutrition support is sometimes perceived as less risky than total parenteral nutrition, but tube feedings are associated with several serious and challenging complications. Measures for the prevention or correction of tube feeding complications are described in Table 8-5.

Malnourished individuals receiving either enteral or parenteral feedings are at risk of developing the **refeeding syndrome.** One major contributor to the refeeding syndrome is hypophosphatemia. As muscle and fat are lost in starvation, fluid and minerals, including phosphorus, are also lost. During refeeding, especially with high-carbohydrate feedings, insulin levels rise and cellular uptake of glucose, water, phosphorus, potassium, and other nutrients is stimulated. Serum levels of phosphorus subsequently fall, which can lead to cardiac dysrhythmias; congestive heart failure; hemolysis; muscular weakness; seizures; acute respiratory failure; and a variety of other complications, including sudden death. Hypokalemia, hypomagnesemia, and vitamin (thiamin) deficiency may occur for similar reasons. Glucose intolerance and fluid overload often accompany the refeeding syndrome. Caregivers should be aware of patients who are at risk for refeeding syndrome, especially those with kwashiorkor or marasmus (see Chapter 2), anorexia nervosa, morbid obesity with recent massive weight loss, and prolonged fasting. In these individuals, it is especially important to monitor blood levels of electrolytes, phosphorus, glucose, and magnesium carefully, particularly during the first week of refeeding; keep careful records of fluid intake and output; record weight daily; and monitor heart rate frequently. Severely malnourished patients are often bradycardic. With overfeeding and an increase in the intravascular volume, heart rate increases; a rate of

Text continued on p. 256

Table 8-4 Assessing Response to Nutrition Support

Parameter	Frequency of Measurement*	Purpose/Comments
Anthropometric Measurements		
Weight	Daily	Indicator of efficacy; patients should have steady gain or weight maintenance, as appropriate; use usual or IBW for guide to desirable weight; a gain of >0.1-0.2 kg (0.25-0.5 lb) a day usually indicates fluid retention
Length or height (pediatrics only)	Monthly	Indicator of efficacy; see growth charts (see Appendix D) for expected growth pattern
Physical Assessment		
State of hydration, intake and output	Daily	Overhydration: check for edema of dependent body parts, shortness of breath, rales in lungs, fluid intake consistently >output; dehydration: look for poor skin turgor, dry mucous membranes, complaints of thirst, output >intake (measure stool volumes if liquid), >10% difference between blood pressure when lying and standing

Continued

Table 8-4   Assessing Response to Nutrition Support—cont'd

Parameter	Frequency of Measurement*	Purpose/Comments
Gastrointestinal motility (tube-fed individuals) (i.e., presence of bowel sounds, signs of abdominal distension, passage of flatus or stool, nausea or vomiting)	Every 2-4 hr during initiation of feedings; every 8 hr when stable	Indicators of GI motility and feeding tolerance
Hematologic and Biochemical Measurements		
Serum glucose	3 times daily until stable, then 2-3/wk	Assess glucose tolerance; determine need to adjust infusion rate of enteral or parenteral feeding or administer insulin
Serum electrolytes	Daily until stable, then 2-3/wk	Indicates need for modification of fluid/electrolyte intake
BUN	1-2/wk	Increased: inadequate fluid intake, renal impairment, or excessive protein intake; decreased: inadequate protein intake is possible
Serum Ca, P, Mg	1-2/wk	Ensure stability; avoid refeeding syndrome

Complete blood count	1/wk	Indicator of adequacy of Fe, protein, folate, and vitamin B_{12}; see Chapter 2 for more information
Serum triglycerides (during TPN)	After each ↑ in lipid dosage; 2-3/wk when stable	Elevated levels indicate inadequate lipid clearance and possibly a need for reduction in lipid dosage
Serum transferrin or prealbumin[†]	1/wk	Indicator of efficacy in maintaining or improving protein nutriture

IBW, Ideal body weight; *BUN*, blood urea nitrogen; *Ca*, calcium; *P*, phosphorus; *Mg*, magnesium; *Fe*, iron.

*These are suggested frequencies only. Individual patients may need more or less frequent assessment. Stable home patients need laboratory analyses on a much less frequent schedule.

[†]Altered by the acute-phase reaction, overhydration or underhydration, renal or liver disease. Therefore they have limited value in critically ill patients or those with organ failure. However, they can be useful markers during nutritional rehabilitation.

Table 8-5 Management of Tube Feeding Complications

Complication	Possible Cause	Suggested Intervention
Pulmonary aspiration*	Feeding tube in esophagus or respiratory tract	Confirm proper placement of tube before administering any feeding; check placement at least every 4-8 hr during continuous feedings.
	Regurgitation of formula	Consider giving feeding into small bowel rather than stomach; keep head elevated 30-45 degrees during feedings; stop feedings temporarily during treatments such as chest physiotherapy.
Diarrhea	Antibiotic therapy	Antidiarrheal medications may be ordered if the possibility of infection with *Clostridium difficile* has been ruled out; *Lactobacillus* or *Saccharomyces boulardii* are sometimes given enterally in an effort to establish benign gut flora.
	Hypertonic medications (e.g., KCl or medications containing sorbitol)	Dilute enteral medications well; evaluate sorbitol content of medications.
	Malnutrition/hypoalbuminemia	Use continuous rather than bolus feedings; consider a formula with MCT and/or soluble fiber.

	Bacterial contamination	Use scrupulously clean formula preparation and administration techniques; refrigerate home-prepared, reconstituted, or opened cans of formula until ready to use, and use all such products within 24 hr.
	Predisposing illness (e.g., short bowel syndrome, inflammatory bowel disease, AIDS)	Use continuous feedings; consider a formula with MCT and/or soluble fiber.
	Lactose intolerance	Use a lactose-free formula.
	Fecal impaction	Perform digital examination to rule out fecal impaction with seepage of liquid stool around the obstruction.
	Intestinal mucosal atrophy	Consider use of formula containing soluble fiber and MCT.
Constipation	Lack of fiber	Consider fiber-containing formula; ensure that fluid intake is adequate; stool softeners may be ordered.
Tube occlusion	Administration of medications via tube	Avoid crushing tablets and administer medications in elixir or suspension form whenever possible; irrigate feeding tube with water before and after giving medications; never mix medication with enteral formulas because this may cause clumping of formula.

Continued

Table 8-5   Management of Tube Feeding Complications—cont'd

Complications	Possible Cause	Suggested Intervention
	Sedimentation of formula	Irrigate tube with water† every 4-8 hr during continuous feedings and after every intermittent feeding; irrigate tubes well if gastric residuals are easured, since gastric juices left in the tube may cause precipitation of formula in the tube; instilling pancreatic enzyme into the tube may clear some occlusions.
Delayed gastric emptying	Serious illness, diabetic gastroparesis, prematurity, surgery, high-fat content of formula, hyperglycemia	Consult with physician regarding whether feedings can be administered into the small bowel, a lower-fat formula can be used, or metoclopramide can be administered to stimulate gastric emptying; improve glycemic control if hyperglycemia exists.

| Hyperglycemia | Excessive glucose in feedings/fluids, glucose intolerance due to stress/sepsis, concomitant disease (e.g., diabetes), drug therapy (e.g., corticosteroids) | Monitor serum glucose several times daily until stable and regularly thereafter, correct underlying illness if possible, reduce enteral or parenteral feedings if excessive, consider use of insulin, consider higher fat/lower carbohydrate formula. |

MCT, Medium-chain triglycerides.

*Signs and symptoms of pulmonary aspiration include tachypnea, shortness of breath, hypoxia, and infiltrate on chest radiographs.

†Fluids such as cranberry juice or Coca-Cola are sometimes used as irrigants, in the belief that they are better than water at preventing tube occlusion. However, research has shown cranberry juice to be inferior to and Coca-Cola no better than water.

A variety of metabolic complications (hypernatremia and hyponatremia, hyperkalemia and hypokalemia, hypercalcemia and hypocalcemia, hyperphosphatemia and hypophosphatemia, etc.), as well as deficiencies of vitamins and minerals, occur in patients receiving enteral and parenteral nutrition. For this reason, adequacy of electrolytes, calcium, phosphate, magnesium, zinc, and other nutrients must be assessed regularly (frequently during the early stages, less frequently in stable long-term patients) for the duration of nutrition support.

80 to 100 beats/minute in a previously bradycardic patient may be a sign of significant cardiac stress.

Home Care

A discharge planner or social worker should be involved in preparation for home care, assisting in arranging for supply sources and third-party coverage of costs. Teaching of the individual and family who are going to deliver tube feedings at home includes the following:

- Clean technique
- Caring for the access device (if applicable: insertion of feeding tube and care of the tube, care of the feeding stoma site; irrigation of tube after feeding)
- Preparation of the enteral formula, if necessary
- Safe administration of the formula, including operation of the enteral feeding pump if one is used
- Appropriate feeding schedule and volume
- Obtaining the necessary formula and supplies
- Signs and symptoms of complications; measures to take if these occur
- Self-monitoring; including measuring weight regularly and evaluating state of hydration

REFERENCES

American Diabetes Association: Evidence-based nutrition principles and recommendations for the treatment and prevention of diabetes and related complications, *Diabetes Care* 27(suppl 1):S36, 2004.

A.S.P.E.N. Board of Directors and Clinical Guidelines Task Force: Guidelines for the use of parenteral and enteral nutrition in adult and pediatric patients, *J Parent Ent Nutr* 26(suppl):90SA, 2002.

Beckstrand J et al: The distance to the stomach for feeding tube placement in children predicted from regression on height, *Res Nurs Health* 13:411, 1990.

Cresci G, Martindale R: Bedside placement of small bowel feeding tubes in hospitalized patients: a new role for the dietitian, *Nutrition* 19:843, 2003.

Gadek JE et al: Effect of enteral feeding with eicosapentaenoic acid, gamma-linolenic acid, and antioxidants in patients with acute respiratory distress syndrome, *Crit Care Med* 27:1409, 1999.

Hanson R: Predictive criteria for length of nasogastric tube insertion for tube feeding, *J Parent Enter Nutr* 3:160, 1979.

Heyland DK et al: Canadian clinical practice guidelines for nutrition support in mechanically ventilated, critically ill adult patients, *J Parent Enter Nutr* 27:355, 2003.

Metheny NA, Smith L, Stewart BJ: Development of a reliable and valid bedside test for bilirubin and its utility for improving prediction of feeding tube location, *Nurs Res* 49:302, 2000.

Pacht ER et al: Enteral nutrition with eicosapentaenoic acid, γ-linolenic acid, and antioxidants in patients with acute respiratory distress syndrome, *Crit Care Med* 31:491, 2003.

SELECTED BIBLIOGRAPHY

Alpers DH: Enteral feeding and gut atrophy, *Curr Opin Clin Nutr Metab Care* 5:679, 2002.

Bourgault AM et al: Prophylactic pancreatic enzymes to reduce feeding tube occlusions, *Nutr Clin Prac* 18:398, 2003.

Crook MA, Hally V, Panteli JV: The importance of the refeeding syndrome, *Nutrition* 17:632, 2001.

Jeejeebhoy KN: Enteral feeding, *Curr Opin Gastroenterol* 18:209, 2002.

Marik PE, Zaloga GP: Gastric versus post-pyloric feeding: a systematic review, *Crit Care* 7:R46, 2003.

McCowen KC, Bistrian BR: Immunonutrition: problematic or problem solving? *Am J Clin Nutr* 77:764, 2003.

Metheny NA: Risk factors for aspiration, *J Parent Enter Nutr* 26:S26, 2002.

Metheny NA, Stewart BJ: Testing feeding tube placement during continuous tube feedings. *Appl Nurs Res* 15:254, 2002.

Vanek VW: Ins and outs of enteral access: Part 2: long-term access— esophagostomy and gastrostomy, *Nutr Clin Prac* 18:50, 2003.

Vanek VW: Ins and outs of enteral access: Part 3: long-term access— jejunostomy, *Nutr Clin Prac* 18:201, 2003.

Parenteral Nutrition

9

The term *parenteral nutrition* describes a continuum of intravenous (IV) nutrient delivery. At its simplest, parenteral feeding may involve only IV provision of fluid and electrolytes. At the other end of the continuum lies total parenteral nutrition (TPN), or delivery of all nutrients by IV infusion.

Intravenous Fluid and Electrolytes

Water makes up approximately 60% of body weight in healthy adults. The intracellular compartment contains about two thirds of body water, and the extracellular compartment contains the remaining one third. Interstitial fluid and lymph make up the majority of extracellular fluid, with the blood, or intravascular space, accounting for approximately one third. Other extracellular body fluids such as peritoneal, synovial, cerebrospinal, and pleural fluids, as well as gastrointestinal secretions, total only about 1 liter of fluid at any one time. However, the daily flux (secretion and reabsorption) of gastric secretions amounts to 6 to 8 liters or more. Elderly adults and obese people contain less water per kg body weight than younger, nonobese individuals and therefore can become dehydrated more quickly. Infants contain a greater proportion of water than adults (70% to 80% of body weight).

The body fluids contain solutes, which can be divided into electrolytes (ions that will conduct an electric current) and nonelectrolytes such as glucose and urea. The predominant extracellular electrolytes are sodium and chloride, and these are contained in many IV solutions. The predominant intracellular electrolytes are potassium and phosphate. Other important electrolytes include calcium, magnesium, and bicarbonate (or total CO_2). Deficits or excesses of electrolytes can result from inadequate or excessive levels in IV and TPN solutions, as well as clinical disorders (Box 9-1).

Caretakers should be alert to signs of these disorders in patients receiving IV therapy.

There are two primary types of IV solutions: colloids and crystalloids. The colloids contain cells, proteins, or synthetic macromolecules that do not cross the capillary membrane readily, and therefore they primarily expand the intravascular volume. Blood products are the most commonly used colloids. The crystalloids contain dextrose (glucose) and/or electrolytes (Table 9-1); these can cross the capillary membrane and therefore can increase the volume of other fluid compartments, in addition to the blood volume. Isotonic electrolyte solutions (e.g., normal saline) can enter all of the extracellular fluid. Patients receiving colloids and isotonic electrolyte solutions should be monitored for fluid overload. In addition to expanding the extracellular fluid, hypotonic saline solutions (0.45% saline) and solutions of dextrose in water contribute fluid to the intracellular space. This is known as providing "free water," and fluids that have this ability can replace deficits of total body water. Hypotonic fluids should not be administered in the presence of increased intracranial pressure or third-space fluid shift (loss of fluid into a body compartment where it is unavailable to either the intracellular or extracellular fluid, e.g., ascites, abnormal sequestration of fluid in the interstitial space in burns or trauma, trapping of fluid due to lymphatic or venous obstruction).

Fluids and electrolytes are needed for maintenance (to replace ongoing excretion in urine, normal feces, and sweat, as well as insensible losses through skin and lungs) and to replace any abnormal losses. Maintenance losses are normally replaced with crystalloid solutions such as 0.45% saline, even though this solution does not contain electrolytes other than sodium and chloride. Thus other electrolytes must be monitored and replaced as needed. In normal adults, daily urine output is approximately 1.5 liters and skin (sweat and insensible), gastrointestinal, and lung losses total approximately 1.2 liters. Maintenance needs (per unit of body weight) are higher in infants and small children than in adults (see Table 8-3). In particular, caring for low-birth-weight infants under radiant warmers can greatly increase insensible losses; insensible losses are essentially electrolyte free, requiring hypotonic replacement fluids (see Table 9-1). Where there are abnormal fluid losses (polyuric renal failure, osmotic diuresis with diabetic ketoacidosis, burns, severe diarrhea, fistula drainage, etc.), the composition of the fluid lost determines the appropriate composition of replace-

---

Box 9-1   Summary of Electrolyte Disorders

Hyponatremia

- Possible causes: increased renal sodium excretion (diuretic use, chronic renal failure, adrenal insufficiency); syndrome of inappropriate antidiuretic hormone secretion (SIADH), excess free water intake
- Signs/symptoms: weakness, fatigue, muscle cramps, confusion, anorexia, nausea, vomiting, headaches, seizure, coma

Hypernatremia

- Possible causes: gastrointestinal fluid losses (copious diarrhea, vomiting, nasogastric suction), fluid loss in excess of sodium loss (osmotic diuresis, e.g., in hyperglycemia; diuretics; excessive sweating), hyperaldosteronism, Cushing's syndrome
- Signs/symptoms: thirst, agitation, lethargy, tachycardia, decreased blood pressure, fever, oliguria, dry sticky mucous membranes, flushed skin

Hypokalemia

- Possible causes: intracellular shift (acute alkalosis, administration of glucose and insulin, anabolism), increased losses (vomiting, diarrhea, small bowel or biliary fistula), excessive renal excretion (diuretic or glucocorticoid treatment, hyperaldosteronism, magnesium deficiency)
- Signs/symptoms: weakness, paralytic ileus, cardiac conduction defects (flattened T wave, depressed ST segment, prominent U wave)

Hyperkalemia

- Possible causes: tissue destruction (hemolysis, massive tissue injury, tumor lysis, catabolism), acidosis, renal failure, adrenal insufficiency, heparin therapy (especially combined with potassium-sparing diuretics, angiotensin-converting enzyme inhibitors, or nonsteroidal antiinflammatory drugs)
- Signs/symptoms: weakness, cardiac toxicity (peaked T waves, prolonged PR interval and widened QRS, loss of P wave, progressing to ventricular fibrillation)

Box 9-1   Summary of Electrolyte Disorders—cont'd

Hypocalcemia

- Possible causes: thyroidectomy or parathyroidectomy, acute pancreatitis, hyperphosphatemia, magnesium depletion, chronic renal failure, chronic vitamin D deficiency; transient hypocalcemia can occur in sepsis, burns, acute renal failure, massive transfusions
- Signs/symptoms: muscle spasms, carpopedal spasm, facial grimacing, laryngeal spasm, convulsions, prolonged QT interval, dysrhythmias, poor responsiveness to digitalis

Hypercalcemia

- Possible causes: malignancy, hyperparathyroidism, excess of vitamins A or D
- Signs/symptoms: bone pain, weakness, lethargy, confusion, paresthesias, renal stones, cardiovascular alterations (QT interval shortened in moderate hypercalcemia; QT lengthened in severe hypercalcemia)

Hypophosphatemia

- Possible causes: intracellular anabolic shifts (recovery from malnutrition and burns), diabetic ketoacidosis (during treatment), alcoholism, renal loss (hypomagnesemia, hypokalemia, recovery from acute renal failure), prolonged vomiting, diarrhea, vitamin D deficiency, respiratory alkalosis
- Signs/symptoms: acute muscular weakness, occasionally with respiratory muscle paralysis; ataxia; confusion; seizures; coma; hemolysis; platelet dysfunction with bruising

Hyperphosphatemia

- Possible causes: renal failure, hyperthyroidism, intracellular to extracellular shifts (rhabdomyolysis, sepsis, malignant hyperthermia, chemotherapy)
- Signs/symptoms: soft tissue calcifications, e.g., in kidney

Continued

Box 9-1   Summary of Electrolyte Disorders—cont'd

Hypomagnesemia

■ Possible causes: gastrointestinal losses (malabsorption from pancreatic insufficiency, short bowel syndrome, inflammatory bowel disease, etc.; prolonged nasogastric suction or vomiting; fistulas), poor intake (alcoholism, protein-energy malnutrition), increased urinary losses (diabetic ketoacidosis or poorly controlled hyperglycemia, drugs that increase urinary excretion such as loop diuretics, cisplatin, amphotericin, aminoglycosides, cyclosporine)
■ Signs/symptoms: muscle spasms, tetany, weakness, hypocalcemia, hypokalemia resistant to correction, tachycardia, atrial fibrillation

Hypermagnesemia

■ Possible causes: renal failure, adrenocortical insufficiency (Addison's disease), hypothermia, excessive intake of magnesium-containing antacids, enemas, and laxatives or magnesium sulfate
• Signs/symptoms: nausea, vomiting, flushing, diaphoresis, muscular weakness or paralysis, hypotension, soft tissue calcification, loss of patellar reflex

---

ment fluids. The composition of some common body fluids is given in Table 9-2.

IV glucose and electrolyte solutions are nutritionally inadequate. If an adult's oral nutrient intake is inadequate or is expected to be inadequate for more than 5 to 7 days, enteral or parenteral feedings providing nitrogen as protein or amino acids, vitamins, minerals, and adequate amounts of energy and electrolytes are needed.

Total Parenteral Nutrition

TPN is usually recommended when oral or tube feedings are expected to be contraindicated or inadequate for more than 5 to 7 days in adults and children. A neonate with an illness that delays oral or enteral feedings should receive parenteral nutrition as soon after birth as possible (A.S.P.E.N., 2002). TPN is most commonly used for one of two reasons:

Text continued on p. 268

Table 9-1   Common Crystalloid Solutions

Solution	Glucose (g/l)	kcal/L	Electrolyte Composition (mEq/L)		Osmolality (mOsm/kg)*	Provides Free Water	Uses/ Comments
			Na⁺	Cl⁻			
Dextrose in water							Used to replace total body water losses (ECF and ICF) and treat hypernatremia, does not provide any electrolytes; $D_{10}W$ is hypertonic when infused, but the glucose is rapidly metabolized, and the solution is then hypotonic to cells
5% (D_5W)	50	170	—	—	278	Yes	
10% ($D_{10}W$)	100	340	—	—	556	Yes	
Saline 0.45%	—	—	77	77	154	Yes	Used to replace hypotonic fluid losses, e.g., increased sweating or insensible losses,

Continued

Table 9-1 Common Crystalloid Solutions—cont'd

Solution	Glucose (g/l)	kcal/L	Electrolyte Composition (mEq/L) Na+	Electrolyte Composition (mEq/L) Cl−	Osmolality (mOsm/kg)*	Provides Free Water	Uses/ Comments
0.9% (normal saline)	—	—	154	154	308	No	osmotic diuresis in diabetic ketoacidosis (used after initial restoration of ECF volume in ketoacidosis); used as a maintenance solution although it does not replace all electrolytes Used to expand intravascular volume and replace ECF losses, e.g., initial correction of hypovolemia in diabetic ketoacidosis; contains Na+ and Cl− in excess of

Dextrose in saline						
5% in 0.2% (D_5 ¼ NS)	50	170	38.5	8.5	355	Yes	plasma concentrations; the only IV fluid that can be infused with blood products
5% in 0.45% (D_5 ½NS)	50	170	77	77	432	Yes	Similar in usage to the saline-only products
5% in 0.9% (D_5 NS)	50	170	154	154	586	No	
Multiple electrolyte solutions							
Ringer's	—	—	147	156	309	No	Similar in electrolyte composition to normal plasma except they contain no magnesium Contains (in mEq/l): 4 K^+ and 5 Ca^{++}; contains more Cl^- than plasma; used to expand intravascular volume and replace ECF losses

Continued

Table 9-1   Common Crystalloid Solutions—cont'd

Solution	Glucose (g/l)	kcal/L	Electrolyte Composition (mEq/L)			Osmolality (mOsm/kg)*	Provides Free Water	Uses/Comments
			Na+	Cl-				
Lactated Ringer's	—	—	130	109		274	No	Closely resembles electrolyte composition of plasma; contains (in mEq/l): 4 K+, 3 Ca++, 28 bicarbonate (as lactate); used to treat losses from burns and lower gastrointestinal tract; should not be used in lactic acidosis

Na+, Sodium; *Cl-*, chloride; *K+*, potassium; *Ca++*, calcium; *mOsm/kg*, milliosmoles per kg water; *ECF*, extracellular fluid; *ICF*, intracellular fluid.

Normal plasma concentrations are: sodium, 135-145 mEq/l; chloride, 95-105 mEq/l; 1 mEq = 1 mmol for sodium and chloride.

*Solutions with osmolality between 240 and 340 mOsm/kg are considered isotonic; those with osmolality less than 240 are hypotonic, and those with osmolality greater than 340 are hypertonic.

Table 9-2   Electrolyte Composition of Various Body Fluids (mEq/L or mmol/L)

Fluid	Sodium	Potassium	Chloride	Bicarbonate
Gastric	65 (20-80)	10 (5-20)	100 (90-150)	0
Bile	150 (120-160)	4 (3-8)	100 (80-120)	35 (30-40)
Pancreatic	140 (120-150)	7 (5-15)	80 (75-120)	75 (60-110)
Small bowel				
Mid bowel	140 (80-150)	6 (5-15)	100 (90-130)	30 (20-40)
Terminal ileum	140 (80-150)	8 (5-30)	60 (20-115)	70
Diarrhea	50 (10-90)	35 (10-80)	40 (10-110)	50 (30-55)
Sweat	45	5	580	

Data from Feldman M, Friedman LS, Sleisenger MH: *Sleisenger and Fordtran's gastrointestinal and liver disease*, ed 7, Philadelphia, 2002, Saunders; Behrman RE, Kliegman RM, Arvin AM: *Nelson textbook of pediatrics*, ed 16, Philadelphia, 2000, Saunders; Way LW, Doherty GM, editors: *Current surgical diagnosis and treatment*, ed 11, New York, 2003, McGraw-Hill.

Values are mean, with approximate range, where available, in parentheses.

1. The gastrointestinal (GI) tract is unable to digest or absorb adequate nutrients. Examples include intractable vomiting, severe diarrhea, prematurity, some cases of abdominal trauma, prolonged ileus, and massive small bowel resection.
2. There is a need for bowel rest. Examples include enteral fistulae and acute inflammatory bowel disease that does not respond to other therapies.

In most instances, initiation of TPN is contraindicated when the gastrointestinal tract is functional, enteral feedings are expected to be adequate within 5 days, or death from the underlying disease is imminent.

Routes and Devices for Delivery of Parenteral Nutrition

Parenteral nutrition may be delivered via peripheral or central veins. Use of peripheral parenteral nutrition (PPN) depends on the adequacy of peripheral venous access. Blood flow through the peripheral veins is not as great as that through the large central veins, and thus PPN is not as rapidly diluted into the blood stream as centrally delivered TPN is. This limits the concentrations of the glucose and amino acid solutions used in PPN. TPN delivered into the central veins can contain higher concentrations of glucose and amino acids, but it requires the placement of an indwelling central venous catheter, which is associated with more serious infectious and mechanical complications than peripheral venous vascular access devices.

Peripheral venous catheters

These catheters are usually inserted in the upper extremities, although lower extremity veins are used frequently in infants. Hypertonic (hyperosmolar) fluids are irritating when delivered via small peripheral veins (discussed in the following text). A rough estimate of the osmotic concentration (in mOsm/kg) of a parenteral nutrition solution can be obtained from the following formula (Davis, 1997):

$$(100 \times \text{Amino acid percentage}) + (50 \times \text{Carbohydrate percentage}) + (2 \times \text{Total electrolyte additives in mEq})$$

Short catheters (7.6 cm [3 in] or less)

Advantages: Few mechanical or infectious complications, other than the risk of superficial phlebitis; inexpensive and easy to place at the bedside.

Disadvantages: Requires good peripheral venous access; not useful for prolonged therapy; may be difficult to deliver adequate energy to stressed individuals or those with high energy needs because peripheral veins do not tolerate solution concentrations >900 mOsm/kg (although with simultaneous infusion of lipid emulsions as much as 1000 to 1200 mOsm/kg may be tolerated), which limits dextrose concentrations to about 10% and amino acid concentrations to 5%; not suitable for TPN in patients needing fluid restriction; in adult patients, the catheters should be removed and replaced routinely (no more frequently than every 72 to 96 hours) to reduce the risk of infection and phlebitis, but no recommendation is made for routine replacement in children (Centers for Disease Control and Prevention [CDC], 2002).

Midline catheters (7.6 to 20.3 cm [3 to 8 in])

These catheters are inserted in the antecubital fossa into the basilic or cephalic veins; they do not enter a central vein and thus are peripheral catheters.

Advantages: Similar to short cannulas and less likely to cause phlebitis; longer life than the short catheters (no recommendation is made for routine replacement of midline catheters, and they have lasted as long as 2 to 4 weeks); preferred over short catheters when IV therapy will likely last 6 days or longer (CDC, 2002).

Disadvantages: Fluid, dextrose, amino acid, and osmolality limitations are similar to those of short catheters; site infections and phlebitis possible; some anaphylactoid reactions have occurred with catheters made of elastomeric hydrogel.

Central venous catheters

Central venous catheters (CVCs) are usually inserted into the superior or inferior vena cava via the subclavian, internal or external jugular, or femoral veins. They may be 20 cm (8 in) or longer, depending on patient size. These catheters provide a reliable intravenous route for long-term access (weeks to years), and they allow use of extremely hypertonic solutions (≥1800 mOsm/kg) with high dextrose and amino acid concentrations. Most of the catheters are made of Teflon, silicone rubber, or polyurethane. A variety of types are available.

Nontunneled CVCs

These catheters are primarily for temporary use (up to a few weeks). They are available in either single- or multi-lumen styles. Most catheter-related blood stream infections occur with these catheters, but it must be noted that they are used frequently in critically ill patients with a variety of risk factors for infection.

Advantages: Can be inserted at the bedside; easily removed. Multi-lumen catheters reduce the risk of drug incompatibilities when more than one medication must be given at once and allow for blood sampling via the CVC. Multi-lumen catheters are best suited to adults and older children because they are generally too large in diameter for infants and small children.

Disadvantages: Complications include pneumothorax, air embolism, central vein thrombosis, superior vena cava syndrome, catheter-related sepsis, and catheter embolization (rare); not as appropriate as other CVCs for home patients.

Peripherally inserted central catheters

Peripherally inserted central catheters (PICCs) are long (51 cm [20 in] or longer in many adults) catheters threaded through peripheral veins, usually the basilic, cephalic, or brachial, into the superior vena cava.

Advantages: Can be inserted at the bedside or in the clinic; allow delivery of very hypertonic solutions without the risk of pneumothorax; less costly than central venous catheter placement; can be used for long-term patients and at home; less risk of infection than the nontunneled CVCs.

Disadvantages: Complications include phlebitis and potential central vein thrombosis, catheter-related sepsis, and catheter fracture (with potential for embolization).

Tunneled CVCs

These catheters are inserted into the subclavian, internal jugular, or femoral veins, and the proximal end is tunneled under the skin away from the insertion site (Figure 9-1). A cuff on the catheter encourages the subcutaneous tissues to adhere to the catheter.

Advantages: Infection rate is lower than with nontunneled CVCs; not easily dislodged after the subcutaneous tissues have had

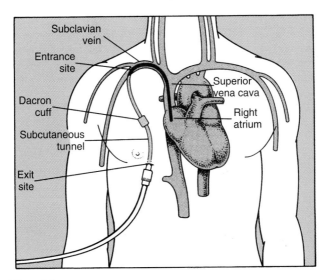

Figure 9-1
Hickman central venous catheter. The proximal end is tunneled under the subcutaneous tissue to increase stability. A Dacron cuff on the catheter provides a roughened surface, which encourages subcutaneous tissue to adhere to the catheter and further secure it.
(From Beare PG, Myers JL, editors: *Principles and practice of adult health nursing,* St Louis, 1990, Mosby.)

time to adhere to the cuff; easier for the patient to care for than nontunneled CVCs and well suited to home use; may not require a dressing once the insertion site has healed.

Disadvantages: Complications are the same as for nontunneled CVCs, except for the lower risk of infection. More difficult to remove than nontunneled CVCs.

Totally implantable catheter

The totally implantable catheter is a tunneled catheter with a subcutaneous infusion port attached. Before each infusion, a noncoring needle is inserted through the skin and into the septum on the port.

Advantages: Useful for intermittent therapy (e.g., chemotherapy, selected patients needing intermittent fluid therapy or TPN);

require flushing only every 28 days if not in use; no routine site care and no dressing is needed; lower infection rates than non-tunneled catheters; more cosmetically appealing than other CVCs; long lasting (predicted life span of the port is approximately 2000 punctures); well suited to home patients.

Disadvantages: All of the disadvantages of CVC, except need for site care; requires a needle to access the port, thus some pain is associated with access; risk of extravasation of infusate if the needle slips out of the port; a tunneled CVC or PICC line is preferable when therapy is continuous rather than intermittent; requires a surgical procedure for removal of the catheter.

Umbilical catheters

These catheters, used in newborns, are inserted into either an umbilical artery or an umbilical vein.

Advantages: Access easy to establish. Use of an arterial catheter allows access for monitoring blood gases as well as parenteral feeding/fluid administration.

Disadvantages: Risk of infection/sepsis, bleeding, obstruction of circulation to the lower extremities (removal of the catheter is recommended with any sign of vascular insufficiency). The recommended life span of these catheters is short, with arterial catheters being removed in 5 days or less and venous catheters in 14 days or less (CDC, 2002).

Catheter Care

Insertion

Insertion of peripheral catheters can be done with clean technique (i.e., clean but not sterile gloves) and no mask. Central catheters, including PICC lines, require sterile technique with full barrier precautions (gown, mask, gloves, and drapes).

The skin should be thoroughly disinfected prior to catheter insertion. Chlorhexidine 2% is preferred for adults and older children, but povidone iodine, tincture of iodine, or 70% alcohol can also be used. The patient should be questioned about allergies before using these preparations, particularly iodine-containing solutions. The safety of chlorhexidine in infants less than 2 months of age is not established, and other disinfectants should be used in this age group at this time (CDC, 2002).

Catheter dressings

Peripheral and central catheters can be covered by a gauze and tape or transparent semipermeable polyurethane dressing. Either type of dressing should be replaced if it becomes damp, soiled, or loosened. There is no apparent advantage of one dressing over the other in terms of infection control, but gauze and tape dressings require more frequent routine changes (every 2 days versus weekly for semipermeable) and thus more time for care. The transparent dressings have the additional advantage of allowing visual inspection of the insertion site. However, because of their absorbent nature, gauze and tape dressings may be preferable for patients with diaphoresis or oozing of blood at the insertion site. The catheter should not be submerged in water, but showering can be permitted if the catheter is protected with a waterproof covering. Dressings on tunneled and totally implanted catheters should be changed weekly until the insertion site heals, after which no dressing may be needed.

Good hand cleansing prior to any contact with the dressing or infusion sets is essential. Clean gloves can be worn during changes of peripheral catheter dressings, while sterile gloves are needed for central catheter (including PICC) dressing changes. During dressing changes, the skin should be cleaned with a disinfectant, as for catheter insertion. No topical antibiotic ointment or cream should be used at the catheter insertion site, because this raises the risk for growth of fungi and antibiotic-resistant bacteria.

Monitoring and maintaining the catheter

Consistent, well-trained nursing staff reduces the risk of infection. The catheter site should be monitored routinely through the dressing, with the frequency depending on the patient's status (e.g., critical care versus stable home patient). Pain on palpation, purulent drainage, and fever of unexplained origin in a patient with a CVC suggest catheter-related infection and deserve further evaluation. Peripheral catheters should be removed at any sign of phlebitis (erythema, warmth, tenderness, or palpable hardness of the vein) or infection at the site.

CVCs are normally flushed with a heparin-containing solution when not in use. Routine flushing of the catheter while in use may reduce the risk of thrombosis (CDC, 2002). CVC catheters with a heparin-bonded coating are also available. Some CVC catheters are permeated with antimicrobial or antiseptic substances (e.g., chlorhexidine/silver sulfadiazine, silver/platinum, minocycline/ rifampin). Chlorhexidine catheters are not approved for infants weighing 3 kg or less because of uncertainty about safety in that population. While the antibiotic-containing catheters raise concerns about antibiotic-resistant microorganisms, they do appear to reduce the risk of catheter-related blood stream infections in critical care patients (Alonso-Echanove J et al., 2003).

Parenteral Nutrition Solutions

The estimated nutrient needs of stable patients needing TPN are shown in Table 9-3. Crystalline amino acids provide the nitrogen (protein) needed. Specialized amino acid solutions are available for use in renal and hepatic failure and for infants. Renal solutions contain the essential amino acids only. Patients with renal failure need both essential and nonessential amino acids, and therefore use of these special formulations should be limited to short periods. Amino acid formulations for hepatic failure are low in aromatic amino acids and methionine and higher in branched-chain amino acids than the standard formulations. They should be used only for patients with hepatic encephalopathy. Standard adult amino acid solutions are not ideal for infants. In particular, they contain too little tyrosine, glutamine, and cysteine for optimal growth. The amino acid solutions for infants are designed to resemble the amino acid composition of human milk. The proper age to switch from an infant to an adult amino acid solution is not established, but most institutions use the infant formulation until the child is at least 1 year of age.

Glucose (dextrose) is an important energy source, but adults cannot oxidize glucose more rapidly than approximately 5 mg/ kg/minute. If glucose is infused at a faster rate, then the excess may be used to form lipids. Thus, a 70-kg adult should receive no more than about 500 g of glucose daily. Lipid is given as a source of essential fatty acids and energy, as well as to provide balance to the nutritional intake. PPN solutions are similar to those delivered centrally in their electrolyte, mineral, and vitamin composition but, as described earlier, are restricted in the amount of glucose and amino acids they may contain.

Lipid emulsions, containing triglycerides (fat), phospholipids, and glycerol, are available as 10%, 20%, and 30% preparations. These contain 10, 20, or 30 g fat/100 ml and provide 1.1, 2, or

Table 9-3 Estimated Daily Nutrient Needs of TPN Patients[a]

Component	Adults (per kg per Day)	Term Infants (per kg per Day)	Children over 1 yr (per kg per Day)
Amino acids (g)	0.8-1 (maintenance) 1.2-2 (catabolic)	2-2.5	1.5-2 (children) 0.8-2 (adolescents)
Energy (kcal)[b]	25-30[c]	90-120 (<6 mo) 80-100 (6-12 mo)	75-90 (1-7 yr) 60-75 (7-12 yr) 30-60 (>12-18 yr)
Fluid (ml)	25-40	100	See note on p. 277
	(total)	(per kg per day)	(per kg per day)
Electrolytes and Minerals			
Na (mEq)	≥60	2-3	3-4
K (mEq)	≥60	1-2	2-4
Mg (mEq)	8-20	0.3-0.7	0.2-0.3
Ca (mg)	200-300	60-70[d]	20-60
Phosphate (mg)	600-1200	50-55[d]	40-45
Zinc (mg)	2.5-5[e]	0.25 <3 mo 0.10 >3 mo	0.05 (max 5/day)
Copper (mg)	0.3-0.5	0.02	0.02 (max 0.3/day)
Chromium (µg)[f]	10-15	0.2	0.2 (max 5/day)

Continued

Table 9-3   Estimated Daily Nutrient Needs of TPN Patients[a]—cont'd

Component	Adults (total)	Term Infants (per kg per Day)	Children over 1 yr (per kg per Day)
Manganese (μg)[g]	60-100	1	1 (max 50/day)
Selenium (μg)	40-80	2	2 (max 30/day)
Molybdenum (μg)	—	0.25	0.25 (max 5/day)
Vitamins (per Day)[h]	(total)	(total)	(total)
A (retinol) (mg)[i]	1	0.7	0.7
D (ergocalciferol or cholecalciferol) (μg)	5	10	10
E (alpha-tocopherol) (mg)	10	7	7
K (phylloquinone) (μg)	150	200	200
C (ascorbic acid) (mg)	100	80	80
Folic acid (μg)	600	140	140
Niacin (mg)	40	17	17
Thiamin (B$_1$) (mg)	6	1.2	1.2
Riboflavin (B$_2$) (mg)	3.6	1.4	1.4
Pyridoxine (B$_6$) (mg)	6	1	1

Cyanocobalamin (B$_{12}$) (µg)	5	1	1
Pantothenic acid (mg)	15	5	5
Biotin (µg)	60	20	20

From *Federal Register* 65(no. 77):21200, 2000; National Advisory Group on Standards and Practice Guidelines for Parenteral Nutrition: Safe practices for parenteral nutrition formulation, *J Parent Ent Nutr* 22:49, 1998; Shils ME et al: *Modern nutrition in health and disease*, ed 9, Philadelphia, 1999, Lippincott Williams & Wilkins.

[a]Amounts of constituents must be individualized; the levels listed are "usual" ranges.

[b]Glucose monohydrate, used in IV solutions, contains 3.4 kcal/g.

[c]Estimated range only. See Box 2-5 for the Harris-Benedict equations for calculation of energy needs. Indirect calorimetry provides the most accurate estimate.

[d]Calcium and phsophate not to exceed 500 to 600 mg/L and 400 to 450 mg/L, respectively, to prevent precipitation.

[e]For maintenance needs; add 2 mg daily during acute periods of hypermetabolism; add 12 mg for each liter of small bowel losses and 17 mg/kg of stool or ileostomy losses.

[f]Decrease or omit with increasing severity of renal dysfunction.

[g]Excreted in bile; omit in patients with obstructive jaundice and cholestasis.

[h]Adult vitamin dosages are for individuals 11 years of age and older.

[i]1 mg of vitamin A = 3300 USP units; 0.7 mg = 2300 USP units.

Note: Children's approximate fluid needs are based on body weight as follows: ≤10 kg, 100 ml/kg/day; 11-20 kg, 1000 ml + 50 ml/kg over 10 kg; >20 kg, 1500 ml + 20 ml/kg over 20 kg.

3 kcal/ml, respectively. It is recommended that intravenous lipid be limited to 2.5 g/kg/day for adults and no more than 4 g/kg/day for children. Lipid emulsions may be administered separate from or mixed with the glucose–amino acid solutions. The latter is known as a total nutrient admixture or *3-in-1 solution*. Lipid emulsions support the growth of *Candida* species and many bacteria better than glucose–amino acid solutions do and thus should be administered with scrupulous aseptic technique. The 20% lipid emulsion is preferred over 10% for neonates because the 10% solution has a higher phospholipids-to-triglyceride ratio than the 20% emulsion, which is of concern in the neonate.

TPN solutions also include multivitamin mixtures, minerals, and trace elements. Iron is not typically included. Most patients receive TPN for 3 months or less, and deficiency is unlikely if iron stores were adequate before beginning TPN. Long-term TPN patients and those with poor stores who cannot absorb oral iron must receive parenteral iron. Three forms are available: iron dextran, sodium ferric gluconate, and iron sucrose. The latter two are approved by the U.S. Food and Drug Administration only for hemodialysis patients receiving erythropoietin therapy. All three preparations can be delivered intravenously, and iron dextran can also be administered via deep (Z-track) intramuscular injection. Iron dextran requires a test dose before administering a full dose because of the risk of anaphylactoid reaction. It is the only preparation that has been added to TPN solutions. Iron should not be added to lipid-containing solutions because it can destabilize the lipid preparation, causing the small particles to coalesce into large droplets and creating a risk of fat embolus. When iron dextran is added to glucose–amino acid mixtures, there is a risk of precipitate formation. If it is included in a TPN solution, iron should be added immediately before the solution is administered, the solution should be visually inspected for precipitate before administration and periodically during infusion, and a 0.2 or 1.2 μm filter should be used. Molybdenum is not usually administered to adults receiving TPN, and other elements believed to have a role in human nutrition (boron, tin, etc.) are also omitted, largely because of lack of knowledge of absolute requirements and concern for possible toxicity. Careful ongoing monitoring of physical signs and symptoms is essential in identifying micronutrient deficiencies that may occur, particularly in long-term TPN patients and those who receive or absorb little or no oral intake. Electrolytes are included in TPN and may be modified as needed to replace losses or compensate for electrolyte retention.

Carnitine, a derivative of the amino acid lysine, stimulates passage of long-chain fatty acids into the mitochondria so that they can be oxidized as an energy source. Carnitine is found in foods of animal origin and is synthesized by healthy adults and children, but TPN solutions do not contain carnitine unless supplemented with it. Infants, especially preterm infants, and older children and adults who receive long-term TPN may not synthesize adequate amounts of carnitine. Signs of deficiency include cardiomyopathy, muscle weakness, lethargy, hypoglycemia, encephalopathy, delayed growth, and seizures. Carnitine supplements are available to be given orally or added to TPN solutions when deficiency is suspected or anticipated.

TPN solutions may include numerous nonnutritive additives, particularly drugs used to prevent or control the potential complications of TPN. Common additives are insulin, heparin (used both to reduce the likelihood of thrombosis and to stimulate lipoprotein lipase [the enzyme responsible for removing fatty acids from triglycerides, allowing them to be utilized by cells, and thus improving utilization of lipid emulsions]) and histamine-H_2 blockers (used because gastric acid secretion is frequently increased in TPN patients, especially those with short bowel syndrome).

Administration of TPN

TPN may be infused continuously or cyclically. Continuous infusions are used for the critically ill and most other hospitalized patients. Cyclic TPN is usually infused for several hours, then discontinued until the next day (e.g., 12 hours on TPN, then 12 hours off). Cyclic TPN allows the long-term patient more flexibility and freedom and may improve liver function; it is especially well suited to home patients. In administering either continuous or cyclic TPN, follow these guidelines:

- Examine TPN solutions and lipid emulsions for precipitation, separation, or signs of contamination (e.g., fungal growth) before hanging them.
- Handle TPN solutions, administration sets, and the peripheral or central catheter with aseptic technique.
- A filter with 0.22 μm pores can be used for amino acid–glucose mixtures, and a filter with 1.2 to 5 μm pores can be used for

lipid-containing solutions. Filters have not been proven to be necessary for infection control, because solutions can be filtered to remove contaminants and particulates in the pharmacy in a more cost-efficient manner (CDC, 2002). However, an air-eliminating filter may reduce the risk of air embolus.

- Administer TPN within 10% of the ordered rate. A constant infusion rate minimizes rapid changes in blood glucose and insulin levels. A flow rate too low can result in hypoglycemia and inadequate nutrient delivery. A flow rate too high can cause hyperglycemia and excessive delivery of energy, protein, fluid, and other nutrients.
- Some clinicians recommend that the rate be tapered before TPN is discontinued. For instance, the rate may be reduced 50% for 1 to 2 hours before stopping the infusion. The glucose content of the solution causes increased insulin secretion, and tapering the TPN infusion rate helps to prevent hypoglycemia from occurring by allowing insulin levels to begin to decline before the infusion is stopped altogether.

Assessing Response to TPN

Anthropometric measurements, physical assessment, and hematologic and biochemical measurements are used in assessing response to nutrition support (see Table 8-4). Hyperglycemia, imbalances of electrolytes, and acid-base disturbances are common complications of TPN delivery. Fluid and electrolyte status must be carefully monitored. In the long-term patient, adequacy of vitamin and trace mineral status must be assessed regularly by thorough physical examination as well as use of appropriate biochemical testing (see Table 2-2). A positive nitrogen balance occurs when there is nitrogen retention within the body, presumably for protein synthesis, and is an indicator of adequate protein delivery. Nitrogen balance determination requires a 24-hour record of protein intake (the amino acids delivered in TPN plus the protein consumed in enteral and/or oral feedings), in addition to 24-hour collection of urine and feces. If fecal losses are low, skin and fecal losses together are often estimated as 4 g/day. Nitrogen losses from unusual sources (e.g., large exudative skin lesions, ungrafted burns, fistula drainage) must be measured or estimated.

$$\text{Nitrogen balance} = [\text{24-Hour protein intake (g)} \times 0.16] - [\text{24-Hour urine urea nitrogen (g)} + \text{Fecal nitrogen (g)}]$$

Preventing and Correcting Complications of Parenteral Nutrition

Table 9-4 summarizes complications of parenteral nutrition and lists measures for their prevention or correction. In addition to the complications listed, excess or deficits of electrolytes (see Box 9-1) and acid-base disorders are relatively common and require close monitoring. The refeeding syndrome, which can occur in malnourished patients given either enteral or parenteral nutrition, is described in Chapter 8.

Long-term TPN patients are susceptible to the development of a number of serious complications, including biliary dysfunction (acalculous cholecystitis, bile sludging, and cholelithiasis), hepatic steatosis, and metabolic bone disease. Cholecystitis may occur because of inadequate stimulation of gallbladder contraction in individuals with little or no food intake. The most important measure to prevent the problem is to encourage oral intake if indicated. Stimulation of the gallbladder with cholecystikinin injections is also effective (Koretz et al., 2001). Steatosis, or fatty liver, may occur because of overfeeding but also appears to be associated with elevation of the inflammatory cytokines. Avoiding overfeeding; providing an appropriate balance of protein, carbohydrate, and fat; and correcting underlying inflammatory processes, if possible, are proposed remedies. Oral or enteral intake, if tolerated, is beneficial in preventing steatosis; cycling of TPN (e.g., 12 hours on and 12 hours off) has also been used in an effort to decrease the risk of steatosis. Metabolic bone disease, including osteomalacia and osteopenia, occurs primarily in long-term TPN patients. The etiology is not definitely known, but possible contributors include vitamin D toxicity, inadequate provision of calcium in TPN because of the difficulty in including enough of both calcium and phosphorus without causing precipitation of calcium phosphate, chronic metabolic acidosis, aluminum contamination of parenteral nutrition components, and the patient's underlying disease or treatment (e.g., corticosteroids). Correction of metabolic acidosis if present and use of acidic amino acid mixtures (which increase the solubility of calcium and phosphorus in the TPN solution) reduces the risk of bone disease. The U.S. Food and Drug Administration has placed limits on the amount of aluminum that can be contained in products for use in TPN.

Table 9-4   TPN Complications

Complication	Signs/Symptoms	Prevention/Intervention
Catheter site infection	Erythema, warmth, inflammation, and pus at the catheter insertion site	Insert catheter with maximal barrier precautions (gown, mask, gloves, drapes) and strict aseptic technique; use aseptic technique in maintaining the insertion site; monitor insertion site regularly; culture site and administer antibiotics as appropriate if infection is apparent
Catheter-related sepsis	Fever, chills, glucose intolerance, positive blood culture; bacterial colony counts in blood from the catheter 5-10 times higher than in blood obtained from a peripheral site	Insert catheter with maximal barrier precautions (gown, mask, gloves, drapes) and strict aseptic technique; maintain an intact dressing; change if contaminated by vomitus, sputum, etc.; use aseptic technique whenever handling catheter, IV tubing, and TPN solutions; hang a single bottle of TPN no longer than 4 hr and lipid emulsion no longer than 12 hr; a 0.22-μm filter with solutions that contain lipids; avoid using single-lumen nontunneled catheter for blood sampling and infusion of non-TPN solutions if possible
Air embolism	Dyspnea, cyanosis, tachycardia hypotension, possibly death	Use Luer lock system or secure all connections well; Groshong catheter, which has valve at tip, may reduce risk of air embolism; use an inline 0.22-μm air-

		eliminating filter if solutions do not contain lipids or 1.2 μm or larger if solutions contain lipids; have patient perform Valsalva's maneuver during tubing changes; if air embolism is suggested, place patient in left lateral decubitus position and administer oxygen; immediately notify physician, who may attempt to aspirate air from the heart
Central venous thrombosis	Unilateral edema of neck, shoulder, and arm; development of collateral circulation on chest; pain in insertion site	Follow measures to prevent sepsis; repeated or traumatic catheterizations are most likely to result in thrombosis; treatment usually includes anticoagulation; if symptoms are not too severe, thrombolytic therapy may be attempted, but catheter removal is usually necessary
Catheter occlusion or semiocclusion	No flow or sluggish flow through the catheter; or infusion through the catheter possible, but blood cannot be aspirated from the catheter	Flush catheter with heparinized saline if infusion is stopped temporarily; if catheter appears to be occluded, attempt to aspirate the clot; thrombolytic agent may restore patency if clotted or occluded by fibrin sheath; hydrochloric acid, 0.1 N, has been used to clear drug precipitates and 70% ethanol to clear lipid precipitates

Continued

Table 9-4 TPN Complications—cont'd

Complication	Signs/Symptoms	Prevention/Intervention
Hypoglycemia	Diaphoresis, shakiness, confusion, loss of consciousness	Do not discontinue TPN abruptly, taper rate over several hours; use pump to regulate infusion so that it remains ±10% of ordered rate; if hypoglycemia is suggested, then administer oral carbohydrate; if oral intake is contraindicated or patient is unconscious, a bolus of IV dextrose may be used
Hyperglycemia	Thirst, headache, lethargy, increased urination	Monitor blood glucose frequently until stable; TPN is usually initiated at a slow rate or with a low dextrose concentration and increased over 2-3 days to avoid hyperglycemia; the patient may require insulin added to the TPN if the problem is severe
Hypertriglyceridemia	Serum triglyceride concentrations elevated (especially serious if >400 mg/dl); serum may appear turbid	Monitor serum triglycerides after each increase in rate and at least 3 times weekly until stable in patients receiving lipid emulsions; reduce lipid infusion rate or administer low-dose heparin with lipid emulsions if elevated levels are observed

Preparing the Patient and Family for Home Parenteral Nutrition

Preparation for home TPN is a multidisciplinary process, usually involving the physician, nurse, dietitian, pharmacist, and social worker. Topics that must be covered in patient teaching include the following:

- Aseptic technique
- Caring for the access device, including irrigation and heparinization of the catheter, site care, and dressing changes, if applicable
- Making additions to the TPN solution (if necessary)
- Initiating, administering, and discontinuing the TPN infusion, including operation of the infusion pump
- Signs and symptoms of complications and management of those complications; self-monitoring (e.g., monitoring of blood glucose, regular weighing, checking body temperature as needed, evaluating state of hydration, etc.)
- Financial, third-party payer, and supply issues related to delivery of home TPN

References

Alonso-Echanove J et al: Effect of nurse staffing and antimicrobial-impregnated central venous catheters on the risk for bloodstream infections in intensive care units, *Infect Control Hosp Epidemiol* 24:916, 2003.

A.S.P.E.N. Board of Directors and Clinical Guidelines Task Force: Guidelines for the use of parenteral and enteral nutrition in adults and pediatric patients, *J Parent Ent Nutr* 26(suppl):1SA, 2002.

Centers for Disease Control and Prevention: Guidelines for the prevention of intravascular catheter-related infections, *MMWR* 51(No. RR-10):1, 2002.

Davis A: Initiation, monitoring, and complications of pediatric parenteral nutrition. In Baker BB, Baker RD, Davis A, editors. *Pediatric parenteral nutrition*, New York, 1997, Chapman & Hall, pp. 212-237.

Koretz RL, Lipman TO, Klein S, American Gastroenterological Association: AGA technical review on parenteral nutrition, *Gastroenterology* 121:970, 2001.

Selected Bibliography

A.S.P.E.N. Board of Directors and Task Force on Standards for Specialized Nutrition Support for Hospitalized Adult Patients: Standards for specialized nutrition support: adult hospitalized patients, *Nutr Clin Prac* 17: 384, 2002.

Cowl CT et al: Complications and cost associated with parenteral nutrition delivered to hospitalized patients through either subclavian or peripherally-inserted central catheters, *Clin Nutr* 19:237-243, 2000.

Dominguez-Cherit G et al: Total parenteral nutrition, *Curr Opin Crit Care* 8:285-289, 2002.

Heyland DK et al: Total parenteral nutrition in the surgical patient: a meta-analysis, *Can J Surg* 44:102-111, 2001.

Irving SY et al: Nutrition for the critically ill child: enteral and parenteral support, *AACN Clinical Issues* 11:541, 2000.

Klein GL: Aluminum contamination of parenteral nutrition solutions and its impact on the pediatric patient, *Nutr Clin Prac* 18:302, 2003.

Kumpf VJ: Update on parenteral iron therapy, *Nutr Clin Prac* 18:318, 2003.

Rice H: *Fluid therapy for the pediatric surgery patient.* Updated June 13, 2003. Available at http://www.emedicine.com/ped/topic2954.htm. Accessed January 20, 2004.

Vanek V: The ins and outs of venous access: part I, *Nutr Clin Pract* 17:85, 2002.

MEDICAL NUTRITION THERAPY

III

Acute and chronic illnesses are treated in a variety of settings, including acute care hospitals, rehabilitation centers, extended care facilities, clinics, offices of private practitioners, and patients' homes. Whatever the setting, however, nutritional care is an essential part of treatment. In recognition of its importance, assessment, planning, and nutritional care of medical, surgical, and emotional conditions is often referred to as medical nutrition therapy.

Metabolic Stress: Critical Illness and Trauma

10

Critical illness and wound healing are stressors that result in **hypermetabolism,** or markedly increased energy expenditure. Nutritional care is a priority to minimize nutritional deficits during the period of hypermetabolism and to promote repair during convalescence.

The Stress Response
Pathophysiology

Injury and critical illness are accompanied by a stress response. The stress response is designed to perform two important tasks:

- *Produce adequate energy to meet increased metabolic needs from surgery and injury.* Increased secretion of glucagon, epinephrine, norepinephrine, and corticosteroids results in breakdown of glycogen, fat stores, and body proteins, especially in skeletal muscles. The net effect in severe injury is increased urinary nitrogen loss, muscle wasting, and weight loss.
- *Maintain the blood volume.* Antidiuretic hormone (ADH) secretion increases during the stress response, with decreased urine output and retention of fluid. In hypovolemia, increased aldosterone secretion occurs, and sodium and fluid are retained.

Impaired host defenses make the critically ill and injured person vulnerable to infection. Sepsis, the systemic response to infection, is believed to occur because of the release of inflammatory mediators such as cytokines, eicosanoids, and the hormones mentioned previously. The **systemic inflammatory response syndrome (SIRS)**, which includes sepsis, can occur in the absence of infection, when the presence of ischemic and necrotic tissue (e.g., trauma, burn, pancreatitis) stimulates a severe inflammatory response. Sepsis and SIRS result in hypermetabolism, insulin resistance and hyperglycemia, and increased protein catabolism and lipid release from the tissues. Lean body mass can be rapidly lost during severe inflammation.

Nutritional Care

The goal of nutritional care is to prevent or correct nutritional deficits that could impair healing. There is much ongoing research related to optimal nutritional support in trauma, sepsis, and burns. Investigators are exploring alternative energy sources (e.g., intravenous lipid emulsions with "structured" triglycerides that contain both medium- and long-chain fatty acids) and nutrients that potentially promote healing or enhance immune function (arginine, nucleotides, and omega-3 fatty acids). The optimal time frame for initiation of nutrition support is another question of considerable interest.

Assessment

Assessment is summarized in Table 10-1. A careful physical examination and nutritional history may be the most useful measures for determining nutritional risk in the ill or injured patient, because other parameters are unreliable in unstable patients. Changes in fluid balance in the acutely ill can alter anthropometric measurements. Moreover, serum protein concentrations are affected by many factors, including fluid balance, inflammation, the acute-phase response, and organ failure. In response to injury or infection, inflammatory mediators such as cytokines act to redirect liver protein metabolism from the synthesis of proteins such as albumin, transferrin, prealbumin (transthyretin), and retinol binding protein and toward the formation of the acute-phase reactants such as fibrinogen, C-reactive protein, complement-3, and haptoglobulin. Concentrations of serum albumin, transferrin, prealbumin, and retinol binding protein usually fall in the early period after injury or surgery (reverse acute-phase reaction), although decreased synthesis may not be the primary reason (especially for albumin, which

Table 10-1   Assessment in Metabolic Stress

Area of Concern	Significant Findings
Protein Energy Malnutrition (PEM)	*History* Increased needs caused by hypermetabolism from trauma, burns, surgery, fever, sepsis, pneumonia, or other infection; catabolic effects of corticosteroid therapy (head injury); weight loss before surgery, especially if >2% in 1 wk, >5% in 1 mo, >7.5% in 3 mo, or >10% in 6 mo; poor intake caused by anorexia, intestinal obstruction or ileus, nausea or vomiting, and alcoholism; increased losses caused by resection of small intestine, especially ileum, gastrectomy, fistula, burns (loss of serum proteins through damaged capillaries) *Physical Examination* Muscle wasting; triceps skinfold <5th percentile; edema; weight <10th percentile or BMI <18.5 *Laboratory Analysis* Not usually helpful in the early phase of care; after the acute phase, prealbumin and nitrogen balance can be used to evaluate efficacy of nutrition support
Altered Carbohydrate Metabolism	*History* Catabolism caused by trauma; corticosteroid therapy *Physical Examination* Muscle wasting *Laboratory Analysis* ↑ Serum glucose; glucosuria

Continued

Table 10-1 Assessment in Metabolic Stress—cont'd

Area of Concern	Significant Findings
Vitamin Deficiencies	
C	*History*
	Increased needs caused by trauma, burns, or major surgery; poor intake caused by anorexia
	Physical Examination
	Gingivitis; petechiae, ecchymoses; delayed wound healing
	Laboratory Analysis
	↓ Serum or leukocyte vitamin C
B complex	*History*
	Increased needs caused by fever or hypermetabolism; poor intake (same reasons as PEM)
	Physical Examination
	Glossitis; cheilosis; peripheral neuropathy; dermatitis
Mineral Deficiencies	
Iron (Fe)	*History*
	Blood loss, acute or chronic, as in stress ulcer, trauma, long-bone fracture; poor intake (same causes as PEM); impaired absorption, especially after gastrectomy
	Physical Examination
	Pallor; spoon-shaped nails; tachycardia
	Laboratory Analysis
	↓ Hct, Hgb, MCV; ↓ serum Fe and ferritin
Zinc (Zn)	*History*
	Increased losses from burns (loss of albumin to which Zn is bound), fistula drainage, diarrhea or steatorrhea; increased needs for healing of wounds; poor intake (same reason as PEM)

Table 10-1   Assessment in Metabolic Stress—cont'd

Area of Concern	Significant Findings
	Physical Examination Poor sense of taste, distorted taste; poor wound healing; alopecia; dermatitis
	Laboratory Analysis ↓ Serum Zn
Fluid and Electrolyte Imbalances Fluid deficit	*History* Increased losses from burns, persistent vomiting or diarrhea, gastric suction without adequate replacement, fever, tachypnea, fistula drainage, transient diabetes insipidus following head injury, use of radiant warmers or phototherapy (infants); poor intake caused by intestinal obstruction, coma, or confusion, causing failure to recognize or communicate thirst, use of tube feedings (especially in obtunded individual) without adequate fluid
	Physical Examination Poor skin turgor; acute weight loss (can be 5%-10% of usual weight within 3-7 days); oliguria (adult: <20 ml/hr; infant or child: <2-4 ml/kg/hr; infant <6 days: <1-3 ml/kg/hr); hypotension; dry skin and mucous membranes; sunken fontanel (infants)
	Laboratory Analysis Serum Na >150 mEq/L; ↑ serum osmolality, urine specific gravity, Hct, BUN

Continued

Table 10-1 Assessment in Metabolic Stress—cont'd

Area of Concern	Significant Findings
Potassium (K^+) excess	*History* Loss of K^+ from damaged cells into extracellular fluid caused by burns (early, usually within first 3 days) or crushing injuries
	Physical Examination Irritability; nausea, diarrhea; weakness
	Laboratory Analysis ↑ Serum K^+
K^+ deficit	*History* Increased losses caused by burns (after the fifth day), diarrhea, or vomiting
	Physical Examination Weakness; ↓ serum K^+
Phosphorus (P)	*History* Aggressive refeeding (especially high-carbohydrate feedings, as in TPN) in malnourished individuals; alcoholism; increased losses or impaired absorption caused by use of antacids (phosphate-binders) as prophylaxis/treatment for stress ulcer, severe diarrhea, or vomiting
	Physical Examination Tremor, ataxia; irritability progressing to stupor, coma, and death
	Laboratory Analysis ↓ Serum P; respiratory alkalosis (↑ blood pH, ↑ blood Pco_2)

has a long half-life). Hemodilution from fluid resuscitation and fluid retention may cause an apparent decrease in levels of these proteins, as does "capillary leak" of the proteins into the interstitial space. Thus the early decreases in the reverse acute-phase serum proteins are unrelated to nutrition status. Once the patient's clinical status has stabilized and adequate nutritional intake has been achieved, rising levels of prealbumin and retinol binding protein may be early signals of resolution of the acute-phase and the beginning of a response to nutritional therapy (Raguso et al., 2003).

Intervention and teaching

Nutrient needs

Fluids and electrolytes. Daily maintenance requirements for fluid and electrolytes are summarized in Table 8-3. Increased losses such as those from nasogastric suction, diaphoresis, and profuse diarrhea (short bowel syndrome) may substantially increase needs. Careful records of fluid output provide a guide to replacement. Fluid deficits in infants and small children can be estimated from changes in body weight: fluid deficit (liters) = usual weight – current weight, with weight in kg. For adults, fluid deficit can be estimated from serum sodium: fluid deficit (liters) = $0.6 \times$ body weight in kg – [(140/patient's sodium) $\times 0.6 \times$ body weight in kg], where sodium is in mEq/L or mmol/L, and 140 represents a normal serum sodium. Fluid resuscitation is a critical part of early burn care. Although standardized formulas are frequently used for estimating fluid resuscitation volumes, hemodynamic monitoring provides a more accurate assessment of the needs of the burn patient.

The syndrome of inappropriate antidiuretic hormone secretion (SIADHS) is especially likely to occur in individuals with closed head injury. In this condition, sodium is unusually low, usually less than 126 mEq/L. SIADHS does not result from sodium deficit but instead from fluid retention. It can be corrected by fluid restriction.

Energy. Energy needs of injured or postoperative individuals vary widely, and indirect calorimetry is the most accurate method for measuring energy needs. Where it is not available, estimates of energy expenditure in the initial period following injury may be made with a variety of formulas. Some examples include the following:

- The Harris-Benedict equations (see Box 2-5). If the Harris-Benedict equations are used, the results are often multiplied by "injury factors" that attempt to estimate total daily energy expenditure. Injury factors commonly range from 1.1 times the resting energy expenditure (REE), for each degree of fever consistently over 98.6° F (37° C), to 1.4 times REE for major trauma or head injury, and 1.5 to 2 times the REE for a major burn.

- The Ireton-Jones equations (see Box 2-5).
- The Curreri formula (for patients with greater than 20% to 30% body surface burned). Energy needs (kcal/day) = 25 kcal/kg + (40 kcal × % body surface burned). The Curreri formula overestimates energy expenditure in burned patients by 25% to 50% (EAST, 2003), which should be taken into account when using the formula.
- Estimates of initial energy needs of patients with trauma to the central nervous system (CNS) are as follows (EAST, 2003):
  - Severe head injury increases energy expenditure, at least partly because it stimulates a marked increase in the release of catecholamines, with a resulting increase in catabolism. Pharmacologic paralysis, frequently used in treatment of severe head injury, reduces oxygen demand and energy expenditure. For patients with severe closed head injury (Glasgow coma scale <8):
    a) Adult needs are approximately 140% of measured resting energy expenditure (~30 kcal/kg/day) if there is no pharmacologic paralysis.
    b) Energy needs with pharmacologic paralysis can be estimated as 100% of measured resting energy expenditure (~25 kcal/kg/day).
  - Energy needs of spinal cord injury patients decline because of the decrease in muscle energy use.
    a) Quadriplegia: 20 to 22 total kcal/kg/day (or 55% to 90% of predicted REE by Harris-Benedict equation).
    b) Paraplegia: 22 to 24 total kcal/kg/day (80% to 90% of predicted REE by Harris-Benedict equation).
  - For children with CNS injury, currently there are insufficient data available regarding needs, and the recommendation is to use weight-specific REE for children (e.g., Talbot, 1938), multiplied by the percentages given above for adults (Adelson et al., 2003).

Ongoing assessment is necessary to allow for adjustment of nutrition support as needed. Overfeeding of sick and injured patients contributes to increased morbidity—for example, hyperglycemia, infection, and prolonged need for ventilatory assistance and intensive care. In no case should carbohydrate be delivered at a higher rate than 5 mg/kg/min, and stressed patients may not tolerate delivery rates this high. Hyperglycemia is especially undesirable in perioperative patients because it appears to predispose patients to infection and prolonged hospital stays. The most effective measures to control hyperglycemia are avoiding overfeeding and using insulin if needed. Energy needs decline as healing takes place, and therefore needs should be reassessed repeatedly (as often as two times weekly), preferably with the use of indirect calorimetry, in order to adjust intake appropriately.

Protein. In adults, protein needs are estimated to be 1.25 to 2 g/kg daily in blunt or penetrating abdominal trauma, 1.5 to 2 g/kg/day in head injury, and 2 g/kg/day in burns (EAST, 2003). For children, protein needs are approximately 2 to 3 g/kg/day.

Vitamins and minerals. Needs for most vitamins and minerals increase in metabolic stress; however, energy needs are also high, and if energy needs are met, adequate amounts of most vitamins and minerals are usually provided. Vitamin C, vitamin A or beta-carotene, zinc, and iron intakes may need special attention, however.

Vitamin C, vitamin A (or retinoids), zinc, iron, and copper are all needed for collagen synthesis, an important part of wound healing. In addition to its role in collagen synthesis, vitamin A and other members of the retinoid family, such as beta-carotene, are involved in mediating the inflammatory response that initiates wound healing and regulating growth factors involved in healing, such as transforming growth factor (TGF)–β and insulin-like growth factor (IGF)–1. Zinc is required for DNA and protein synthesis, and zinc deficiency results in diminished wound strength and delayed epithelial coverage of the wound. Iron deficiency is relatively common in ill patients due to blood loss and inadequate intake, and very severe deficiency can impair both collagen synthesis and oxygen transport to wounds and damaged tissues. Although copper is necessary for collagen synthesis, deficiencies of copper are not as widespread as those of the other micronutrients.

In addition to their roles in healing, vitamin C, retinoids, and zinc play a role as antioxidants, along with selenium. Production of oxidants can be helpful, as in the killing of bacteria by white blood cells. However, metabolic stress is associated with increased release of "free radicals," which are especially reactive atoms with one or more unpaired electrons that can damage cells, proteins, and DNA by altering their chemical structures. Free radicals and other oxidants are believed to contribute to development of adult respiratory distress syndrome. An adequate intake of antioxidant nutrients may help to limit oxidant damage.

Although micronutrient needs in stressed patients are not well established, the following is a guide to doses used in supplementation.

- *Vitamin C:* 500 to 1000 mg daily (more than 5 to 10 times the Dietary Reference Intake, or DRI).
- *Vitamin A:* doses ranging from 1500 to 7500 μg daily (approximately 2 to 10 times the DRI) have been used. Excesses of preformed vitamin A may be toxic, however, and the higher doses should be used only with caution. Retinoids other than vitamin A have low toxicity.
- *Zinc:* commonly used zinc supplementation dosages are 6 mg/day IV during acute stress and 4 mg/day IV or 50 to 75 mg/day orally when stable. Unusually high small or large bowel output require zinc replacement; estimated zinc needs are 12 mg/L of small bowel drainage and 17 mg/kg of diarrheal stool or ileostomy drainage. Large doses of zinc provide no benefit unless deficiency or unusual losses are present.
- *Iron:* supplement with 25 to 50 mg elemental iron daily if low ferritin levels are present.

Nutrition support

Early enteral feeding (in comparison to either no artificial nutrition support or total parenteral nutrition [TPN]) has been shown to improve outcome in acutely ill patients. The beneficial effects of enteral feeding may result from better maintenance of the gastrointestinal (GI) tract integrity (because the GI tract uses a portion of the nutrients delivered enterally to meet its needs for energy and tissue synthesis) and/or reduction of the systemic stress response. The intact GI tract is a barrier to infection. In animal studies, lack of enteral nutrients causes GI mucosal atrophy and promotes translocation of microorganisms from the GI tract across the damaged gut and into the circulation. The importance of translocation in humans remains controversial. However, it is clear that the GI tract is an important component of the immune system and contains significant amounts of gut-associated lymphoid tissue (GALT). The beneficial effect of enteral feeding may be at least partly via improvement of the GI tract's immune function.

Delay in gastric emptying and gastric atony are common in acutely ill and injured patients, and this limits the amount of enteral formula that can be delivered intragastrically. Since feedings into the small bowel bypass the pyloric sphincter, it is possible to feed ill patients more aggressively via the small bowel as opposed to the stomach. However, patients with unstable hemodynamic status and those who require pressor therapy to maintain adequate blood pressure raise concerns about the possibility of ischemic bowel damage during feeding. Current recommendations are to use enteral feedings even in the acutely ill, starting at a low rate, once fluid resuscitation is complete and perfusion pressures are adequate. Guidelines for feeding patients at high risk for bowel ischemia have been suggested (McClave and Chang, 2003; Zaloga et al., 2003):

- *Enteral formula selection.* Isotonic, as opposed to hypertonic, formulas are likely to be best tolerated. Fiber-containing formulas should be avoided because they serve as a substrate for bacterial growth. Immune-enhancing formulas (enriched with arginine, nucleotides, omega-3 fatty acids, and antioxidants) have not proven to decrease mortality in general intensive care patients. However, they may have benefit in the sickest patients. In particular, they appear to enhance splanchnic (i.e., liver and bowel) blood flow in hemodynamically unstable patients and thus may improve feeding tolerance.

- *Monitoring gastrointestinal tolerance.* Patients should be monitored continually for evidence of ischemic bowel. Early indicators are those of feeding intolerance: nausea, diarrhea, bloating, and abdominal distension (repeated measurements taken at the umbilicus provide an objective indication of distension). Other signs and symptoms include crampy abdominal pain, ileus, and reduced passage of stool and flatus. These signs signal a need to reevaluate the patient, who may require a cessation of enteral feedings. Late signs, associated with significant injury, include high nasogastric output volumes, oliguria, metabolic acidosis, shock, and development of an acute abdomen. The abdominal radiographs may initially show dilated thickened loops of bowel; later there may be air in the wall of the intestine, the portal vein, or the peritoneal cavity.

- *Signs of need to stop enteral feedings.* In addition to increasing gastrointestinal intolerance, other indicators of a need to withhold enteral feeding are a sustained mean arterial blood pressure of 70 mm Hg or less, a need for increasing doses of pressor agents, or a requirement for increased ventilatory support.

Improved understanding of the nutrient needs in metabolic stress, as well as more objective tools for monitoring gut perfusion in acutely ill patients, will undoubtedly improve care of these patients in the future. TPN should be reserved for those patients that do not tolerate enteral feedings and are at high nutritional risk. Overfeeding should be avoided in all patients, whether nutrients are delivered enterally or parenterally, to reduce hyperglycemia, metabolic demands, and the risk of infection.

Organ Transplantation

Individuals undergoing organ transplantation (kidney, liver, heart, lung, small bowel, or pancreas) experience many of the same clinical problems as other critically ill and injured patients. However, the patient that experiences acute trauma or illness is likely to have been in good nutritional state prior to the illness or injury. In contrast, the organ transplant patient often has a variety of nutritional problems related to the underlying disease and its treatment (Box 10-1). Correction or control of these problems (to the extent possible) during the period of waiting for transplant improves graft survival and reduces morbidity and mortality.

Drug-Nutrient Interactions

After successful transplantation, most patients have improved quality of life, exercise tolerance, and nutritional status. However, they require long-term immunosuppressive therapy, which has significant drug-nutrient interactions (Table 10-2). Glucocorticoids may be used in the early postoperative period; their side effects include hyperglycemia and hyperlipidemia. The current practice is to wean corticosteroid dosages as rapidly as possible to reduce the metabolic side effects and risk of osteoporosis associated with this type of drug. Episodes of organ rejection may require increased drug dosages or additional drugs in the treatment regimen. Since many of the side effects of immunosuppressant drugs are dose related, this may have further impact on nutritional status.

Medical Nutrition Therapy after Transplant

- Protein intake of 1.2 to 2 g/kg per day for the first few weeks after surgery and 1 to 1.5 g/kg per day after the initial postoperative period is usually sufficient to allow for healing. This diet

Box 10-1   Factors Contributing to Malnutrition in Organ Transplant Candidates

All Solid Organs

Anorexia
Nausea, vomiting
Depression, fatigue
Hypermetabolism and chronic inflammation
Diet restrictions reducing palatability
Drug-nutrient interactions

Heart

Impaired absorption due to poor gastrointestinal circulation
↑ Cardiac and pulmonary energy expenditure
Poor nutrient delivery to tissues due to impaired circulation
Ascites and early satiety when hepatic congestion is present

Lung

↑ Work of breathing and resting energy expenditure
Complications related to cystic fibrosis: chronic infections, impaired absorption and steatorrhea, glucose intolerance and diabetes

Intestine

Complications of long-term TPN: cholestasis, cholelithiasis, hepatic dysfunction, portal hypertension, micronutrient deficiencies, metabolic bone disease

Liver

Protein intolerance
Fluid and electrolyte imbalances
Nutrient malabsorption and steatorrhea
Esophageal strictures and dysphasia
Mental alteration
Early satiety due to ascites
Impaired hepatic protein synthesis
Altered intermediary metabolism; ↑ use of amino acids for gluconeogenesis
Malabsorption due to ↓ bile salt concentrations
Small bowel dysfunction due to portal hypertension or lymphostasis

Continued

Box 10-1   Factors Contributing to Malnutrition in Organ
Transplant Candidates—cont'd

Glucose intolerance and diabetes
Essential fatty acid deficiency

Pancreas

Complications of diabetes: cardiovascular disease, nephropathy and albuminuria, gastroparesis

Kidney

Glucose intolerance
Hypertriglyceridemia and hypercholesterolemia
Abnormal metabolism of calcium, phosphorus, vitamin D
Anemia
Aluminum toxicity
↑ Protein degradation and protein loss

Adapted from Hasse JM, Roberts S: Transplantation. In Rombeau JL, Rolandelli
RH: *Clinical nutrition—parenteral nutrition*, ed 3, Philadelphia, 2001, Saunders.
Used with permission.

must be tailored to the patient's needs (e.g., reduced if renal failure develops).

- Hyperphagia stimulated by immunosuppressant drugs and by
  improved well-being, in conjunction with improved absorption,
  contributes to weight gain posttransplant. An increase in activity,
  behavioral measures to control eating behaviors, and instruction
  in healthy food choices are approaches to preventing or correcting unwanted weight gain. A modest reduction in energy intake is
  accomplished by limiting fried foods and high-fat foods such as
  pastries, whole milk and products made with whole milk, butter,
  margarine, oils, nuts, chips, and other snack foods. Limiting
  intake of meats to no more than 5 or 6 ounces daily also reduces
  fat and energy intake (see Chapter 7).
- If hypertriglyceridemia is present, avoid alcohol intake; restricting intake of simple sugars (sugar, candies, desserts) helps to control both hypertriglyceridemia and hyperglycemia.
- If low-density lipoprotein (LDL) cholesterol is elevated (>160
  mg/dl), limit cholesterol intake to 200 mg/day, total fat intake to
  less than 25% to 35% of total energy, and saturated fat to no

Table 10-2 Nutritional Impacts of Immunosuppressant Therapy

Drug	Gastrointestinal Side Effects	Electrolyte/Metabolic/ Serum Chemistry Alterations	Other
Azathioprine	Oral lesions, diarrhea, steatorrhea, nausea, vomiting, anorexia, ↓ taste acuity, pancreatitis (long-term therapy)	↓ Albumin	Antagonizes folic acid – anemia (long-term therapy); negative nitrogen balance
Basiliximab	Constipation, diarrhea, nausea, vomiting, abdominal pain, dyspepsis, oral moniliasis*	↓ or ↑ K, ↓ Ca, ↓ P, ↑cholesterol, ↑ glucose	Weight increase; peripheral edema
Daclizumab	Diarrhea, nausea, vomiting, abdominal pain, pyrosis, dyspepsia, abdominal distention, epigastric pain, flatulence		Peripheral edema
Muromonab-CD3	Diarrhea, vomiting, nausea		Peripheral edema
Mycophenolate mofetil	Diarrhea, constipation, nausea, vomiting, dyspepsia, oral moniliasis	↑ Cholesterol	Peripheral edema

Continued

Table 10-2   Nutritional Impacts of Immunosuppressant Therapy—cont'd

Drug	Gastrointestinal Side Effects	Electrolyte/Metabolic/Serum Chemistry Alterations	Other
Sirolimus	Diarrhea, constipation, nausea, vomiting, dyspepsia, abdominal pain, mouth ulceration or infection	↑ Cholesterol, ↑ triglycerides, ↓ K, anemia	Take consistently with or without food (food alters bioavailability of drug); avoid grapefruit juice
Tacrolimus	Diarrhea, constipation, nausea, vomiting, anorexia	↑ K	Take without food; grapefruit juice may raise drug concentrations

Ca, Calcium; *K,* potassium; *P,* phosphate.

*Infection with a fungus of the genus *Candida,* causing mouth pain and mucous membrane erosion.

more than 7% of energy intake. The same should be done if LDL cholesterol is borderline (>130 mg/dl but <160 mg/dl) and diabetes is present, or at least two other risk factors such as smoking, hypertension, or family history of premature cardiovascular disease are present. The Therapeutic Lifestyle Changes plan described in Chapter 14 can help to reduce cardiovascular risk.

▪ Supplements of vitamin D and calcium may help to prevent osteoporosis related to the disease state or corticosteroid therapy. Other measures to reduce osteoporosis include limiting alcohol intake, avoiding smoking, and increasing weight-bearing exercise.

REFERENCES

Adelson PD et al: Guidelines for the acute medical management of severe traumatic brain injury in infants, children, and adolescents. Chapter 18. Nutritional support, *Pediatr Crit Care Med* 4(suppl 3):S68, 2003.

EAST Practice Management Guidelines Workgroup: *Practice management guidelines for nutritional support of the trauma patient*, Allentown, Penn, 2003, Eastern Association for the Surgery of Trauma.

McClave SA, Chang WK: Feeding the hypotensive patient: does enteral feeding precipitate or protect against ischemic bowel? *Nutr Clin Prac* 18:279, 2003.

Raguso CA, Dupertuis YM, Pichard C: The role of visceral proteins in the nutritional assessment of intensive care unit patients, *Curr Opin Clin Nutr Metab Care* 6:211, 2003.

Talbot F: Basal metabolism standards for children, *J Dis Child* 55:455, 1938.

Zaloga GP, Roberts PR, Marik P: Feeding the hemodynamically unstable patient: a critical evaluation of the evidence, *Nutr Clin Prac* 18:285, 2003.

SELECTED BIBLIOGRAPHY

Campos ACL, Matias JEF, Coelho JCU: Nutritional aspects of liver transplantation, *Curr Opin Clin Nutr Metab Care* 5:297, 2002.

Flynn NE et al: The metabolic basis of arginine nutrition and pharmacotherapy, *Biomed Pharmacother* 56:427, 2002.

Hart DW et al: Effects of early excision and aggressive enteral feeding on hypermetabolism, catabolism, and sepsis after severe burn, *J Trauma* 54:755, 2003.

Hart DW et al: Persistence of muscle catabolism after severe burn, *Surgery* 128:312, 2000.

Lang JD et al: Oxidant-antioxidant balance in acute lung injury, *Chest* 122:314S, 2002.

Long CL et al: Ascorbic acid dynamics in the seriously ill and injured, *J Surg Res* 109:144, 2003.

Marino LV et al: To determine the effect of metoclopramide on gastric emptying in severe head injuries: a prospective, randomized, controlled clinical trial, *Br J Neurosurg* 17:24, 2003.

McCall M et al: Effect of neuromuscular blockade on energy expenditure in patients with severe head injury, *JPEN J Parenter Enteral Nutr* 27:27, 2003.

McKibbin B, Cresci G, Hawkins M: Nutrition support for the patient with an open abdomen after major abdominal trauma, *Nutrition* 19:56, 2003.

Montejo JC et al: Immunonutrition in the intensive care unit. A systematic review and consensus statement, *Clin Nutr* 22:221, 2003.

Williams JZ, Barbul A: Nutrition and wound healing, *Surg Clin North Am* 83:571, 2003.

Gastrointestinal Disorders

11

A variety of disorders that affect the gastrointestinal (GI) tract and its accessory organs—the liver, gallbladder, and pancreas—can impair nutritional status. Effects of these disorders include malabsorption, discomfort associated with eating, anorexia, impaired intake, and food intolerances. Disorders that often have an unfavorable impact on nutritional status and require medical nutrition therapy are discussed in this chapter.

Esophageal Disorders

Reflux, Obstruction, and Dysfunction

Pathophysiology

Among the problems that can interfere with normal esophageal function are gastroesophageal reflux, esophageal obstruction, and motor dysfunction. In **gastroesophageal reflux disease (GERD)**, reflux of stomach contents into the esophagus occurs, causing esophagitis and heartburn. Ulcer and stricture formation are two possible complications, and GERD is a major risk factor for development of Barrett's esophagus (a precancerous condition) and adenocarcinoma of the esophagus. Reduced lower esophageal sphincter (LES) pressure contributes to GERD. GERD is especially common in individuals with hiatal hernia, with the likelihood of reflux being related to the size of the herniation. Other contributing factors include impairments of gastric emptying or esophageal peristalsis.

Mechanical obstructions of the esophagus can result from strictures (e.g., from caustic injury caused by ingestion of lye or from GERD) or tumors. **Dysphagia** is a common symptom. Two motor disorders affecting the esophagus are **achalasia,** a complex neurologic condition that causes incomplete relaxation of the LES after swallowing, and *scleroderma,* a collagen-vascular disease causing proliferation of connective tissue and fibrosis in many organs. Achalasia obstructs the passage of food into the stomach, and dysphagia and regurgitation of food are common symptoms. Carcinoma of the esophagus is a potential long-term sequela. Scleroderma impairs peristalsis and LES closure; symptoms are the same as those of GERD.

Esophageal dysfunction places the patient at risk for pulmonary aspiration, dyspnea, and pneumonia.

Treatment

Antireflux measures include the following: elevation of the head of the bed; cessation of smoking, which reduces LES pressure; avoidance of medications that reduce LES pressure (e.g., anticholinergics, α-adrenergic antagonists, β-adrenergic agonists, calcium channel blockers, opiates, progesterone, and theophylline) if possible; use of antacids; and dietary modification (see the following discussion on nutritional care). Medications to reduce gastric acidity include histamine H_2-receptor antagonists (e.g., cimetidine and ranitidine) and proton pump inhibitors (e.g., omeprazole). Prokinetic medications such as metoclopramide increase LES pressure and promote gastric emptying. Antireflux surgery is a consideration for the patient who does not benefit from medical therapy.

Mechanical dilation may be used in treatment of strictures and achalasia, and surgery, or a combination of surgery and radiation therapy, is usually used in the treatment of esophageal tumors.

Nutritional Care

Assessment

Assessment is summarized in Table 11-1.

Intervention and teaching

Preventing or reducing reflux. To reduce the possibility of reflux, follow these guidelines:

- Reduce weight if overweight or obese.
- Consume small, frequent meals.

Table 11-1   Assessment in Gastrointestinal Disorders

Area of Concern	Significant Findings
Protein-Energy Malnutrition (PEM)	*History* Decreased food intake caused by pain associated with eating (e.g., gastroesophageal reflux [GER], gastric ulcer, cholecystitis, pancreatitis), alcohol abuse, nausea and vomiting, anorexia. Dysphagia, anticipation of dumping syndrome; increased losses (malabsorption) related to severe diarrhea or steatorrhea (stool greasy or difficult to flush away), pancreatic insufficiency (pancreatitis, cystic fibrosis), short-bowel syndrome, dumping syndrome; increased energy/protein needs in healing, infection, fever; increased work of breathing (cystic fibrosis); catabolism resulting from corticosteroids *Physical Examination* Muscle wasting; edema; triceps skinfold <5th percentile; weight <90% of that expected for height or BMI <18.5; failure to follow individual established pattern on growth charts (children) *Laboratory Analysis* ↓ Serum albumin, transferrin, or prealbumin; ↓ creatinine-height index
Fluid Deficit	*History* Excessive losses caused by severe vomiting or diarrhea (especially short-bowel syndrome and dumping syndrome)*

Continued

Table 11-1   Assessment in Gastrointestinal Disorders—cont'd

Area of Concern	Significant Findings
	Physical Examination Poor skin turgor; dry, sticky mucous membranes; feeling of thirst; acute loss of >3%-5% of body weight; hypotension
	Laboratory Analysis ↑ BUN; ↑ Hct; ↑ serum Na
Vitamin Deficiencies	
A	*History* Decreased absorption as a result of steatorrhea or pancreatic insufficiency
	Physical Examination Drying of skin and cornea; popular eruption around hair follicles (follicular hyperkeratosis)
	Laboratory Analysis ↓ Serum retinol; ↓ retinol-binding protein (indicating PEM, with inadequate protein to manufacture carrier for vitamin A)
E	*History* Decreased absorption as a result of steatorrhea or pancreatic insufficiency
	Physical Examination Neuromuscular dysfunction (causing extreme weakness)
	Laboratory Analysis ↓ Serum tocopherol; hemolysis
K	*History* Decreased absorption as a result of steatorrhea or pancreatic insufficiency; decreased production caused by destruction of intestinal bacteria by antibiotic usage (e.g., in hepatic encephalopathy or cystic fibrosis)

Table 11-1   Assessment in Gastrointestinal Disorders—cont'd

Area of Concern	Significant Findings
	Physical Examination Petechiae, ecchymoses
	Laboratory Analysis Prolonged prothrombin time (PT)
B_{12}	*History* Decreased absorption as a result of gastrectomy (loss of intrinsic factor necessary for absorption), distal ileal disease (e.g., Crohn's disease), or resection (loss of absorptive sites); bacterial overgrowth in the bowel competing for vitamin B_{12} (seen in short-bowel syndrome or gastric resection)
	Physical Examination Pallor; sore, inflamed tongue; neuropathy
	Laboratory Analysis $\downarrow$ Serum vitamin B_{12}; $\downarrow$ Hct, $\downarrow$ MCV
Mineral/Electolyte Deficiencies Calcium (Ca)	*History* Decreased intake of milk products caused by lactose intolerance; increased losses as a result of steatorrhea or corticosteroid use; hip or vertebrae fractures related to osteoporosis
	Physical Examination Tingling of fingers; muscular tetany and cramps, carpopedal spasm; convulsion
	Laboratory Analysis $\downarrow$ Serum Ca (severe deficits only); $\downarrow$ bone mineral density (chronic Ca deficit)

Continued

Table 11-1   Assessment in Gastrointestinal Disorders—cont'd

Area of Concern	Significant Findings
Magnesium (Mg)	*History* Inadequate intake as a result of alcoholism; increased losses as a result of steatorrhea or diarrhea, vomiting, loss of small bowel fluid (e.g., short-bowel syndrome, fistula) *Physical Examination* Tremor, hyperactive deep reflexes; convulsions *Laboratory Analysis* ↓ Serum Mg
Iron (Fe)	*History* Blood loss; impaired absorption caused by decreased acid within upper GI tract, resulting from gastrectomy or chronic antacid or cimetidine use; decreased intake (e.g., restriction of protein foods in liver disease) *Physical Examination* Spoon-shaped nails; pallor, blue sclerae; fatigue *Laboratory Analysis* ↓ Hct, Hgb, MCV; ↓ serum Fe and ferritin
Zinc (Zn)	*History* Increased losses as a result of diarrhea/steatorrhea, loss of intestinal fluid (e.g., short-bowel syndrome, high output ileostomy, fistula drainage); decreased intake caused by protein restriction; delayed growth in children

Table 11-1   Assessment in Gastrointestinal Disorders—cont'd

Area of Concern	Significant Findings
	Physical Examination Anorexia; poor sense of taste, distorted taste; alopecia; poor wound healing; diarrhea; dermatitis
	Laboratory Analysis ↓ Serum Zn
Potassium (K^+)	*History* Increased losses caused by diarrhea
	Physical Examination Muscle weakness, ileus; diminished reflexes
	Laboratory Analysis ↓ Serum K^+; inverted T wave on ECG
Nutrient Excess of Iron (Fe)	*History* Family history of hemochromatosis
	Physical Examination No abnormalities if diagnosed early; later: bronze skin (in areas not exposed to sun)
	Laboratory Analysis ↑ Serum Fe, ↑ ferritin, ↑ transferrin saturation

*When diarrhea is severe, stools should be weighed or measured to determine output accurately.

- Alcohol, mint, chocolate, chili, and onions reduce LES pressure and may contribute to reflux. Limit these in the diet.
- Do not lie down within 2 hours of a meal. Eat the last meal of the day several hours before bedtime, and avoid late-night snacking.
- Keep the head of the bed elevated at least 15 cm (6 in).
- Avoid smoking, because nicotine reduces LES pressure.

Coping with dysphagia. Solid foods and thin liquids usually cause the most difficulty. Foods that create a semisolid bolus when chewed are generally best tolerated.

- Liquids can be thickened with dry infant cereals, mashed potatoes or potato flakes, cornstarch, or yogurt.
- Commercial supplements designed for use in dysphagia are available; these have the consistency of nectars, honey, or even thicker consistencies, depending on the needs of the individual.
- Try fluids in frozen form (e.g., sherbet or fruit ices).
- Consult with a speech therapist, who may be able to assist dysphagic individuals in improving their swallowing techniques.

Wait until dilation or surgical therapy has been performed before trying to increase oral intake in the person with achalasia; the risk of pulmonary aspiration is high before treatment.

Providing nutritional support as needed. Where esophageal obstruction exists or reflux or dysphagia is severe, impairing intake so much that weight loss occurs or placing the individual at high risk of pulmonary aspiration, tube feedings (via gastrostomy or jejunostomy if esophageal obstruction is present) may be needed. Special care must be taken to reduce the risk of pulmonary aspiration (e.g., elevation of the head of the bed). Nasoenteric feedings are generally not used before definitive therapy for achalasia has been provided.

Gastric Disorders

Gastrectomy

Pathophysiology

Partial or total resection of the stomach is sometimes required for treatment of peptic ulcer or gastric cancer. Two problems are likely after gastrectomy: fat malabsorption and dumping syndrome. Fat malabsorption results from the bypass of the duodenum by the Roux-en-Y esophagojejunostomy and other common gastrectomy procedures. Bacteria multiply within the bypassed duodenum, and the bacteria deconjugate bile salts, making micelle formation and fat absorption inadequate (see p. 234 for a discussion of fat absorption). Dumping syndrome results from the rapid passage of foods into the small bowel, caused by the loss or bypass of the pyloric sphincter. Rapid hydrolysis (digestion) of nutrients increases the osmolality (concentrations of solutes) within the upper small bowel. Fluid from the plasma and extracellular space is drawn into the bowel to dilute the hypertonic intestinal contents. Symptoms include nausea, abdominal pain, weakness, diaphoresis (sweating), diarrhea, and weight loss.

Nutritional Care

Assessment

Assessment is summarized in Table 11-1.

Intervention and teaching

Dietary modifications and their rationale. To maintain a stable body weight, select a high-protein, high-energy diet. Fat absorption may be improved if fat intake is not excessive (no more than 30% of total energy intake). To achieve these goals, follow these guidelines:

- Use skinned poultry, lean meats, skim or low-fat milk, and dairy products made from skim or low-fat milk.
- Use plant proteins such as dried beans and peas regularly.
- Limit fried or fatty foods.

Reduce the likelihood of dumping syndrome with the following measures:

- Eat small meals and snacks often; six meals a day may be needed.
- Avoid beverages at mealtime. Drink fluids at least 1 hour before or after meals.
- Avoid concentrated sweets (e.g., candy, cookies, pies, cakes, jam, jelly, soft drinks, sugared beverages or foods). Although they are high in simple carbohydrates, fresh fruits are often well-tolerated because of their soluble fiber (pectin) content. They can be used as desserts and snacks.
- Maintain nonstressful eating practices. Eat slowly in a relaxed setting. Lying down for about 1 hour after meals can also help prevent dumping syndrome.
- Pectin or guar gum taken with meals and snacks may delay gastric emptying and carbohydrate absorption, reducing the risk of dumping syndrome.

Supplementation. Calcium and iron may be poorly absorbed postoperatively because these minerals are absorbed best in an acidic environment. Normally, much of their absorption takes place in the duodenum, because that segment of the small intestine is acidified by the entry of the stomach contents, and the GI contents have not yet been alkalinized by the pancreatic secretions. Secretion of gastric acid is greatly reduced postoperatively, which makes the duodenum less acidic. Supplements of calcium and iron help to reduce the risk of osteoporosis and iron-deficiency anemia.

Intrinsic factor and hydrochloric acid, both produced in the stomach, are required for absorption of vitamin B_{12}. Therefore, supplemental vitamin B_{12} (regular injections or high-dose oral supplements) is usually required for the remainder of the person's life.

Intestinal Disorders

Nutrients are absorbed at specific sites in the small intestine (see Figure 1-5); therefore, the location and the extent of small intestinal disease or resection determine which nutrients will be affected. Generally, the proximal small intestine is more effective in increasing its absorptive capacity following resection of the distal bowel than the distal bowel is in adapting to the loss of the proximal intestine. However, the proximal small intestine cannot take on the absorption of vitamin B_{12}.

Osteoporosis is especially common among individuals with diseases causing malabsorption. The etiology and nutritional treatment of osteoporosis is summarized in Box 11-1.

Short-Bowel Syndrome
Pathophysiology

Massive resection of the small bowel, creating **short-bowel syndrome,** severely reduces the area available for the absorption of nutrients. This procedure is sometimes required in Crohn's disease, necrotizing enterocolitis (see Chapter 20), congenital atresias, acute volvulus, strangulated hernias, mesenteric artery occlusion, and similar disorders. Malabsorption and diarrhea are greater if (1) more than 80% of the small bowel is resected, (2) the ileum is resected, (3) the ileocecal valve is removed, or (4) the unresected bowel is damaged. For at least the first 2 years after massive bowel resection, adaptation occurs via bowel hyperplasia and hypertrophy. This response takes place in phases:

Phase 1: In the immediate postoperative period there are enormous losses of fluids, electrolytes, magnesium, calcium, zinc, and

Box 11-1 Osteoporosis Related to Gastrointestinal Disorders

Possible Etiologies

- Malabsorption of vitamin D and calcium due to steatorrhea
- Impaired absorption of calcium due to decreased acidity in proximal small intestine (e.g., gastrectomy)
- Chronic (3 months or longer) or repeated treatment with corticosteroids
- Inflammatory processes (bone resorption is stimulated by the inflammatory cytokines)
- Lactose intolerance
- Alcohol abuse (increased excretion of calcium, possibly poor dietary intake)

Nutrition and Lifestyle Measures to Reduce the Risk of Osteoporosis

- Adequate calcium intake: at least 1000 mg daily in young men and premenopausal women and 1200 mg daily for men over 50 years and postmenopausal women; individuals with malabsorption may need increased amounts.

   Section 1.01   Dietary sources include milk and milk products, calcium fortified juices, sardines and other canned fish, and most dark green leafy vegetables.

   Section 1.02   Supplements of calcium carbonate (40% calcium) or calcium citrate (24% calcium) may be needed to achieve adequate intakes. Calcium citrate has higher bioavailability and may cause less bloating and constipation.

   Section 1.03   If renal calcium loss is high, kidney stones may occur. Urine calcium should be measured; individuals excreting more than 4 mg/kg/day are at risk of stone formation. Thiazide diuretics can be used to decrease calcium.

- Adequate vitamin D intake: healthy adults need 5 to 10 µg/day (200 to 400 IU/day), and those with malabsorption may need several times more.

   Section 1.04   Vitamin D may cause toxicity, including hypercalcemia and hypercalciuria, at high doses, and therefore vitamin D intake should be carefully evaluated.

- Avoid smoking.
- Avoid excessive alcohol intake.
- Obtain weight-bearing exercise most days of the week.

amino acids. In addition to the loss of absorptive area, temporary gastric hypersecretion contributes to fluid and electrolyte losses.

Phase 2: Diarrhea diminishes, along with fluid and electrolyte problems.

Phase 3: The individual achieves a stable weight determined by the amount of bowel remaining.

Treatment

Antidiarrheal and anticholinergic drugs, such as codeine, loperamide (Imodium), diphenoxylate with atropine (Lomotil), or glycopyrrolate (Robinul), may be helpful in controlling diarrhea during phases 1 and 2. If the ileum is removed, large amounts of bile salts may enter the colon and cause diarrhea by stimulating colonic water secretion. At least 100 cm of ileum is required for complete absorption of bile salts. Cholestyramine is sometimes used to bind the bile salts and reduce diarrhea. Some patients with short-bowel syndrome have undergone small bowel transplantation, which may become much more common in the future. In preliminary studies, glucagon-like peptide 2 enhanced mucosal growth and improved absorption (Drucker, 2002).

Nutritional Care

Assessment

Assessment is summarized in Table 11-1. Massive small bowel resection can be expected to affect absorption of almost every nutrient and to have great potential for causing malnutrition.

Intervention and teaching

Replacing losses and preventing malnutrition

Phase 1: Intravenous (IV) support is essential to replace fluids, electrolytes, and other nutrient losses. Most individuals require total parenteral nutrition (TPN) for at least a few weeks after surgery. It is especially important to replace zinc losses (12 to 17 mg of zinc is lost per kilogram of feces or ileostomy drainage) because wound healing is impaired without zinc, and standard TPN solutions do not contain enough zinc to replace diarrheal losses.

Phase 2: The presence of nutrients within the GI tract is necessary for bowel adaptation to occur. Enteral feedings are often started as soon as the volume of fecal losses decreases to less than

1 L/day. Typically, TPN continues as continuous tube feedings are begun. Small oral feedings may also be started. They are generally low in fat (less than 10 g/day) and fiber and high in starch. White rice, enriched white bread and toast, noodles, macaroni, and peeled boiled or baked potato (all without added milk, cheese, margarine, butter, or other fat) are examples of possible foods.

Phase 3: Oral feedings can be advanced. They should be small and frequent. Fat intake can be increased unless **steatorrhea** worsens. Concentrated sugars, excessive fat, or alcohol consumption may worsen malabsorption. Medium-chain triglycerides (MCTs) may be used for caloric supplementation, but excessive amounts often worsen diarrhea. MCTs can be used in cooking or added to juice or applesauce to increase caloric intake. TPN will continue to be required if the individual is unable to maintain adequate nutriture with oral or oral plus enteral tube feedings.

The individual will need instruction in a high-energy diet with small, frequent feedings. The need for a low-fat diet (Table 11-2) is determined on an individual basis; individuals with severe steatorrhea are often more comfortable when they restrict fat intake. Fat restriction appears to be most effective in individuals who still have the colon. Lactose intolerance is common, but yogurt, hard cheeses, milk accompanied by intake of lactase enzyme, and calcium-fortified juices provide well-tolerated calcium sources. Osteoporosis is common in individuals with short-bowel syndrome, and adequate vitamin D and calcium are needed to replace fecal losses (see Box 11-1).

Patients with a high jejunostomy should not drink plain water, but instead should use electrolyte-containing drinks. Fluid and electrolyte losses are so great that plain water results in more losses than it replaces.

Hyperoxaluria (excessive urinary excretion of oxalates), which may result in formation of urinary stones, occurs in some individuals with steatorrhea because they fail to absorb adequate calcium as a result of formation of calcium soaps with fat in the stool. Normally, calcium binds oxalate in the gut to inhibit oxalate absorption, but excessive fecal calcium losses allow increased amounts of oxalate to be absorbed. A calcium supplement can reduce oxalate absorption. A low-oxalate diet can be used if the calcium supplement does not correct the hyperoxaluria. Foods high in oxalate are

Table 11-2   Fat-Restricted Diet

Type of Food	Foods to Include	Foods to Avoid
Milk products	Milk products made with skim milk	Milk products made with 2% or whole milk
Meat and meat substitutes	Lean meat, fish (water packed, if canned), poultry without skin, egg whites	Fried meats, sausage, frankfurters, poultry skins, duck, goose, salt pork, luncheon meats, peanut butter, egg yolk except as allowed*
Breads and cereals	Plain pasta, cereals, whole-grain or enriched bread or rolls	Biscuits, doughnuts, pancakes, sweet rolls, waffles, muffins, high-fat rolls such as croissants
Fruits	All except avocado	Avocado except as allowed*
Vegetables	All if plainly prepared	Fried, au gratin, creamed, or buttered
Dessert	Sherbet made with skim milk, angel food cake, gelatin, pudding made with skim milk, fruit ice	Cake, pie, pastry, ice cream (except fat-free or light, as allowed*), or any dessert containing fat or chocolate
Sweets	Jelly, jam, syrup, sugar, hard sugar candies, jelly beans, gum drops	Any candy made with chocolate, nuts, butter, or cream

*The following contain 5 g of fat per serving and must be used only in limited amounts. Usually no more than 5 to 6 of these fat servings per day are included in a low-fat diet: 1 tsp butter, margarine, oil, shortening, or mayonnaise; 1 tbsp salad dressing or heavy cream; 1 strip crisp bacon; ⅛ avocado; 6 small nuts; 10 peanuts; 5 small olives; ½ cup "light" ice cream; 1 egg yolk or whole egg.

nuts; coffee; chocolate; green beans; green, leafy vegetables; beets; rhubarb; eggplant; celery; carrots; artichokes; plums; blackberries; and whole wheat.

Supplementation

Individuals not receiving TPN: Daily supplements are often necessary, particularly in water-miscible forms of vitamins A, D, E, and K; iron; calcium; magnesium; and zinc.

Severe steatorrhea: Water-miscible forms of vitamins A, D, E, and K may be better absorbed than standard fat-soluble forms. Hypomagnesemia and hypocalcemia are common; a low-fat diet combined with supplements of these minerals helps to correct deficiencies. Zinc supplements may also be needed.

Absence of the terminal ileum: Vitamin B_{12} supplements are needed, usually in regularly scheduled injections. Some patients may absorb enough B_{12} if they take large oral doses (1000 μg) daily.

Emotional support. The effects of massive bowel resection are catastrophic and are likely to be permanent. The individual and family need encouragement and reinforcement, particularly if home TPN or tube feedings are required.

Home nutritional support. Some individuals will need instruction in home TPN or tube feedings because these may need to continue at least until maximal adaptation occurs (see Chapters 8 and 9).

Celiac Disease (Nontropical Sprue or Gluten-Sensitive Enteropathy)

Pathophysiology

Celiac disease is a genetic disorder that results from an immune reaction to the **gliadin** portion of **gluten** (a protein found in wheat) and to closely related proteins in rye and barley. The immune response brings about a marked decrease in the length of the villi and in the surface area of the bowel, and disaccharidase and peptidase activity is low because these enzymes, which digest carbohydrates and proteins, are found in the intestinal mucosal cells. Diarrhea, steatorrhea, impaired absorption of all macronutrients (carbohydrate, protein, and fat), muscle wasting, weight loss or failure to gain weight (in children), and anemia are common signs and symptoms. Dermatitis herpetiformis is a severe itchy, blistering skin disease caused by gluten intolerance. While it is a separate disease, individuals with dermatitis herpetiformis are likely to have intestinal damage similar to those with celiac disease.

A small bowel biopsy to look for microscopic evidence of blunting of the villi is currently the definitive diagnosis. As antibody testing (for antiendomysial or tissue transglutaminase antibody titers, which rise in celiac disease) becomes easier, more widespread, and more sensitive, this may replace the biopsy. Improvement of symptoms in response to a trial of a gluten-restricted diet (and relapse when gluten consumption is restarted) is further evidence of celiac disease.

Nutritional Care

Assessment

Assessment is summarized in Table 11-1.

Intervention and teaching

Gluten-free diet. Permanent removal of gliadin and related proteins from the diet is the only treatment for celiac disease. Following the diet is especially important because GI lymphoma appears to be more common in individuals who fail to do so. This diet is difficult to follow because grain products are so widely used in processed foods. The individual and family need extensive encouragement and reinforcement.

Recommendations for restricting gluten include the following:

- Avoid wheat, barley, rye, and all products made with these grains. Table 11-3 lists foods to include and to avoid in gluten sensitivity. Alternative names for wheat products, such as graham (whole wheat), durum, and semolina, are frequently used on food packaging.
- The use of oats in celiac disease is controversial. Some evidence suggests that oats (at least up to 60 g daily) may be tolerated by most adults with celiac disease, but data regarding the safety of oats in celiac disease is not yet conclusive. If oats are included in the diet, it is necessary to be sure that they come from a source where there is no chance of contamination with wheat, barley, and rye during harvesting, storage, or processing.
- Buckwheat is a grass not related to wheat, and it is acceptable for use.

Table 11-3   Diet for Gluten Intolerance

Type of Food	Foods to Include	Foods to Avoid
Milk products	All except those with gluten additives	Malted milk, some milk drinks, and some flavored or frozen yogurt
Meat, poultry, fish, eggs, dry beans and peas, and nuts	All fresh, unprocessed meat, poultry, and fish; dried beans and peas; soybeans; nuts; peanut butter; cold cuts, frankfurters, and sausage without fillers	Breaded products; some sausages, frankfurters, luncheon meats, and sandwich spreads (with fillers); self-basting turkey; and some egg substitutes
Cheeses	All natural cheeses	Any cheese containing oat gum* and some pasteurized process cheese
Breads and starches	Potatoes, potato flour, rice, rice flour, wild rice, corn, cornstarch, hominy, grits, buckwheat, amaranth, bean or pea flour, quinoa, flax, sago, teff, tapioca, sago, arrowroot, soy flour, millet, sorghum, and special gluten-free pasta and breads	All products containing wheat, rye, oats,* barley, triticale (wheat-rye hybrid), wheat starch, wheat bran, wheat germ, graham or durum flour, bulgur, farina, spelt, kamut, wheat-based semolina, cereals with malt flavoring or extracts
Vegetables	All plain fresh, frozen, or canned	Creamed, au gratin, or breaded (unless made with gluten-free starch); canned baked beans; and some French fries

Continued

Table 11-3   Diet for Gluten Intolerance—cont'd

Type of Food	Foods to Include	Foods to Avoid
Fruits	All fresh, frozen, or canned	Some commercial fruit pie fillings
Beverages	Pure instant and ground coffee, tea, carbonated drinks, wine made in the United States, and rum	Flavored instant coffee, hot cocoa mixes, herbal tea, alcohol distilled from cereal grains (e.g., whiskey, gin, beer, ale), and malted beverages
Miscellaneous	Most seasonings and flavorings; sauces, soups and condiments prepared with allowed ingredients; butter, margarine, and oils; sugar, honey, plain chocolate, coconut, molasses, meringue, and marshmallows; and xanthan and guar gums	Some nondairy creamers; commercial salad dressings; prepared soups; condiments, sauces, and seasonings prepared with grains that are not allowed; and licorice

*Evidence suggests that oats may be acceptable for a gluten-free diet, but this remains under study.

- Read labels carefully because gluten and gluten-containing grains are added to many products. When it is unclear whether a product contains gluten, contact the manufacturer or distributor (whose address must appear on the food label) or consult their website to obtain further information.
- In restaurants, ask whether unfamiliar foods contain restricted grains.
- Cornmeal; cornstarch; flour made from rice, peas, beans, or potatoes; amaranth; and tapioca are examples of products that can be used instead of wheat flour for thickening foods and preparing breads.

Celiac disease support groups can provide recipes, practical information, and support for the affected individual and the family. Local groups can be located via the national Celiac Sprue Association (see Appendix I).

Supplementation. At the time of diagnosis, a complete blood count and measurement of serum ferritin, folate, and vitamin B_{12} should be obtained (American Gastroenterological Association [AGA], 2001).

- Supplements of iron, folic acid, and vitamin B_{12} may be needed if deficiency is indicated, although levels of these nutrients often normalize as the person follows the gluten-free diet and absorption improves.
- Severe hypokalemia and hypomagnesemia may be present due to losses in steatorrhea. Immediate correction of these deficits should be carried out; as the patient responds to the change in diet, these problems will not recur.
- Osteoporosis is common among individuals with celiac disease, and some may require calcium supplementation. See Box 11-1 for other nutritional interventions.

Inflammatory Bowel Disease (Crohn's Disease and Ulcerative Colitis)
Pathophysiology

Inflammatory bowel disease (IBD) can affect individuals of all ages. In **Crohn's disease** (regional ileitis), inflammation extends through all layers of the bowel wall. It can affect any part of the GI tract but most often affects the terminal ileum. In acute exacerbations, abdominal pain, fever, nausea, and diarrhea occur. In chronic disease, weight loss, anorexia, anemia, and steatorrhea are common.

In **ulcerative colitis,** congestion, edema, and ulcerations affect the mucosal and submucosal layers of the bowel. It usually involves the rectum and colon and sometimes extends to the ileum. Bloody diarrhea, abdominal and rectal pain, weight loss, and anorexia are common.

Diagnosis is made by barium enema, endoscopy (sigmoidoscopy, colonoscopy, or esophagoscopy), and intestinal biopsy.

Treatment

Drugs that are often used include corticosteroids to decrease inflammation; antidiarrheals, such as diphenoxylate (Lomotil); and antispasmodics, such as tincture of belladonna, to decrease discomfort. Sulfasalazine is used in ulcerative colitis for its antiinflammatory and antimicrobial effects. Infliximab reduces inflammation in Crohn's disease by blocking the effects of tumor necrosis factor–α. (See Appendix H for drug-nutrient interactions.) Surgery may be necessary if fistulas, hemorrhage, perforation, or intestinal obstruction occurs. Resection of the colon is often performed after several acute exacerbations of ulcerative colitis because of the risk of developing colon cancer.

Nutritional Care

Assessment

Assessment is summarized in Table 11-1.

Intervention and teaching

Diet and other lifestyle modifications

Acute disease: Supportive therapy with intravenous (IV) fluids and a clear liquid diet is often provided. In severe disease, or when a fistula is present, TPN without any oral intake may be used for several weeks in an effort to rest the bowel and promote healing. Evidence suggests that enteral tube feedings of an elemental diet may be as effective as TPN in promoting healing.

Chronic disease: A low-fat diet (see Table 11-2) may be prescribed to decrease steatorrhea, which is common with ileal involvement. A high-protein diet (1.5 to 2 g/kg/day) helps promote bowel regeneration and replace losses.

If areas of intestinal stenosis are present, then a restricted-fiber diet that eliminates berries, raw fruits except banana and avocado, raw vegetables, whole grains, and dried beans or peas is often recommended to reduce the potential for bowel obstruction.

Lactose intolerance is common in Crohn's disease. Some lactose-intolerant individuals can tolerate yogurt, buttermilk, and hard cheeses. Lactase enzyme can be consumed with milk to hydrolyze the lactose.

Stress can exacerbate inflammatory bowel disease (IBD). Furthermore, chronic disease imposes its own stresses. Development of coping and stress-reduction skills improves quality of life.

Supplementation. The following supplements may be needed:

- Iron if blood loss is sufficient to cause anemia.
- Vitamins A, D, and E; calcium; magnesium; and zinc if steatorrhea is present. Osteoporosis is common among individuals with IBD. See Box 11-1 for nutrition intervention to reduce the risk of osteoporosis.
- Vitamin B_{12} if the terminal ileum is involved.

Pancreatic Dysfunction

Pancreatitis (Acute or Chronic)

Pathophysiology

Pancreatitis refers to inflammation, edema, and necrosis of the pancreas as a result of digestion of the pancreas by enzymes normally secreted by the pancreas. Alcoholism, biliary tract disease, trauma, obstruction of the pancreatic duct, peptic ulcer disease, hyperlipidemia, and the use of certain drugs (glucocorticoids, sulfonamides, chlorothiazides, and azathioprine) may cause pancreatitis. Symptoms include pain in the epigastric region, persistent vomiting, abdominal rigidity, and elevated serum amylase. Malabsorption and decreased glucose tolerance are common in chronic pancreatitis.

Treatment

Anticholinergic agents, such as atropine, may be used to decrease pancreatic secretion. Meperidine is used for pain relief. Use of pancreatic enzymes with food intake can reduce the stimulus for the pancreas to release enzymes and therefore reduce pancreatic damage and pain.

Nutritional care

Assessment

Assessment is summarized in Table 11-1.

Intervention and teaching

Acute pancreatitis. The goal of treatment is to avoid pain and reduce inflammation caused by pancreatic stimulation.

- All oral feedings may be withheld during severe attacks. IV fluids and electrolytes are given to replace the massive losses that occur during inflammation. In the past, TPN has often been recommended for individuals with pancreatitis, because it causes little or no stimulation of pancreatic secretion, thus promoting healing. However, jejunal feedings of a low-fat-defined formula diet stimulate pancreatic secretion very little and are well-tolerated by most patients with acute pancreatitis.
- Once pain has subsided, clear liquids by mouth are usually introduced, and the diet is progressed as tolerated. A low-fat (<20% of total energy intake), high-carbohydrate diet usually causes less pain than an unrestricted diet. MCTs can be added if needed for adequate energy intake. The diet is gradually liberalized as the patient tolerates it.
- Alcohol is contraindicated because it increases pancreatic damage and pain.

Chronic pancreatitis. The goal of treatment is to promote healing and compensate for the decrease in pancreatic secretion.

- A high-protein, high-carbohydrate diet with as much fat as can be tolerated promotes healing. Skinned, baked, or broiled poultry; lean meats; low-fat cheeses; and vegetable proteins, such as dried beans and peas, provide protein with a low to moderate fat intake.
- The individual may need to limit fat in the diet if it causes steatorrhea or pain (see Table 11-2). If additional food energy is needed, MCT oil can be used to replace the usual dietary fats in cooking, combined into a shake with milk and ice milk, or served in juice.
- Pancreatic enzyme replacement may be administered with each meal to improve digestion.

- Alcohol intake is contraindicated.
- Insulin secretion is likely to be impaired. If glucose intolerance is present, then the patient is treated as a diabetic (see Chapter 17).

Supplementation. If fat malabsorption is severe, water-miscible forms of vitamins A and E, as well as supplements of zinc and calcium, may be needed.

Cystic Fibrosis

Pathophysiology

Cystic fibrosis (CF) results from a genetic defect in a cell membrane protein, the cystic fibrosis transmembrane conductance regulator (CFTR), that regulates the passage of chloride out of cells. Indirectly, this defect disrupts the sodium and water balance across cell membranes. The respiratory system is especially vulnerable to the effects of this disruption because there is not enough water on the airway surface to maintain normal, well-hydrated mucus secretions. Instead, viscous mucus collects in the respiratory tract, which can obstruct the airways and provide a favorable environment for growth of microorganisms. Other areas that are likely to be obstructed by thickened secretions include the pancreatic duct, through which the pancreatic digestive enzymes enter the duodenum, the common bile duct, and the vas deferens of the male reproductive tract. Involvement of the pancreas (and, to a lesser extent, the common bile duct) results in malabsorption, with fat being the nutrient most affected. Consequently, stools tend to be large and bulky and growth failure is common unless aggressive nutritional intervention is initiated. In contrast to most of the body cells, which normally secrete chloride, the sweat glands reabsorb it. The defect in the CFTR results in increased losses of chloride in sweat and provides a key tool for diagnosis of CF. Sweat chloride concentrations greater than 60 mmol/L are indicative of CF.

Treatment

Prevention of atelectasis and respiratory infections is a primary goal of treatment. Daily chest physiotherapy, including percussion and postural drainage, is especially effective. Antibiotics are given as necessary to treat or prevent pneumonia. Inhalation of human recombinant DNase has been effective in improving pulmonary function in clinical trials. Lung transplantation has been performed in some patients with end-stage pulmonary disease. A variety of experimental treatments are under study, including new mucolytics and hydrating agents to liquefy secretions and gene therapy to insert normal CFTR in the respiratory tract.

As many as 85% of individuals with CF have pancreatic insufficiency and require pancreatic enzyme replacement with all meals and snacks to correct malabsorption.

Nutritional Care

Assessment

Assessment is summarized in Table 11-1.

Intervention and teaching

Promoting optimum growth and preventing malnutrition. Adequate energy intake is needed to compensate for malabsorption, increased work of breathing, and increased needs imposed by infection. Each day, healthy children need about 1000 kcal plus 100 kcal per year of life. Depending on the extent of their disease, children with CF may grow well on this number of kcal or may need 120% to 150% of this amount and 2 to 2.5 g of protein per day.

A high-protein, moderate- to high-fat diet (30% to 40% of total energy) should be encouraged. Some individuals experience abdominal pain and severe steatorrhea with unrestricted fat intake. Adjustment of their pancreatic enzyme dosages usually improves their fat tolerance. MCT oil may be used to increase caloric intake when steatorrhea is severe. If oral intake is inadequate to prevent or correct malnutrition, then enteral tube feedings to supplement oral intake have been found to be beneficial in improving nutritional status. Nasal polyps are common in CF, and therefore nasogastric and nasointestinal tubes may be poorly tolerated. Gastrostomy feedings are an alternative.

Supplementation. Zinc, magnesium, and calcium supplements and water-miscible forms of vitamins A, D, E, and K may be necessary in individuals with steatorrhea. Food should be generously salted, especially in hot weather, to replace abnormal electrolyte losses in sweat.

Emotional support. Cystic fibrosis is a chronic, incurable disease. The affected person and family need much support to cope with the illness. The disease can be mild to severe, making it difficult to foresee exactly what the individual's functional level and length of survival will be. The median age of survival is continually increasing with improved treatment. Individuals should be encouraged to participate in all activities compatible with their functional abilities. Support groups may be of great help to the individuals and their families.

Hepatic Diseases

Hepatitis

Pathophysiology

Hepatitis is an inflammation of the liver caused by a virus, toxin, obstruction, parasite, or drug (alcohol, chloroform, or carbon tetrachloride). Symptoms include jaundice, abdominal pain, hepatomegaly, nausea, vomiting, and anorexia. Elevated serum levels of bilirubin, aspartate aminotransferase (AST, or SGOT), alanine aminotransferase (ALT, or SGPT), and lactic dehydrogenase (LDH) are commonly present.

Treatment

If the cause of hepatitis is known, then it should be removed. Rest and nutritional therapy are the primary treatments.

Nutritional Care

Assessment

Assessment is summarized in Table 11-1.

Intervention and teaching

Promotion of liver regeneration. A high-energy, high-protein (70 to 100 g), moderate-fat diet promotes healing. Lean meats, poultry, legumes, and cheese or cottage cheese made with skim or low-fat milk are good protein sources that are low to moderate in fat. Starches, such as pasta, rice, potatoes, cereals, and breads, are good energy sources. Frequent, small feedings are better tolerated than large feedings. Alcohol is toxic to the liver and should be avoided during convalescence. Individuals with hepatitis C should be especially careful to abstain from alcohol intake, because of the likelihood of the disease progressing to cirrhosis.

Supplementation. If steatorrhea is present, then supplemental water-miscible vitamins A, D, and E; calcium; and zinc may be needed.

Nonalcoholic Fatty Liver Disease

Pathophysiology

Nonalcoholic fatty liver disease (NAFLD) is an increasingly common cause of liver dysfunction. Liver function tests are elevated in NAFLD, as in hepatitis, and prothombin time may be prolonged. After ruling out other causes of liver disease (e.g., consumption of more than 20 to 30 g [1 to 2 drinks] of alcohol per day), NAFLD may be diagnosed by liver biopsy. Fatty infiltration of the liver (steatosis) is present, and there may be necrosis of the hepatocytes and fibrosis, a form of NAFLD referred to as nonalcoholic steatohepatitis (NASH). The disorder may progress to cirrhosis and liver failure. NAFLD is present in all age groups, with the prevalence rising among the obese. The disorder is often associated with the metabolic syndrome (described in Chapter 15), which includes abdominal obesity, insulin resistance, diabetes, hypertriglyceridemia, and hypertension. The cause of NAFLD is not well understood.

Treatment

There is no specific drug therapy for NAFLD. Hepatoprotective agents such as betaine, vitamin E, vitamin C, and ursodeoxycholic acid (a bile acid) have been used in small clinical trials and have shown some promise. Good control of disorders associated with NASH, such as diabetes and hyperlipidemia, is recommended.

Nutritional Care

Assessment

Assessment is summarized in Table 11-1.

Intervention and teaching

Weight control. Weight loss is recommended for individuals with NAFLD who have a BMI greater than 25, with the initial goal being a loss of 10% of body weight, at a rate of 0.5 to 1 kg (1 to 2 lb) per week. Lifestyle changes to bring about gradual weight loss are described in Chapter 7. Rapid weight loss should be avoided, because it may worsen steatohepatitis and contribute to liver failure. The risk of gallstone formation is also markedly increased with losses of more than 1.5 kg/week. Surgery for weight reduction is a consideration for morbidly obese individuals (BMI of 35 or greater), but these patients must be carefully evaluated to ensure that rapid weight loss is unlikely to precipitate hepatic failure (AGA, 2002).

Cirrhosis and Hepatic Encephalopathy or Coma

Pathophysiology

Cirrhosis occurs following hepatic damage. Causes of damage include alcoholism, biliary tract obstruction, and viral infection. Although the liver is able to regenerate much of the damaged tissue, some fibrous tissue develops, impairing the normal flow of blood, bile, and hepatic metabolites. Portal vein hypertension occurs, with esophageal and gastric varices, GI bleeding, hypoalbuminemia, ascites, and jaundice. Severe liver dysfunction results in intolerance to protein and **hepatic encephalopathy.** Signs of encephalopathy include confusion, increased serum ammonia levels (worsened by high-protein intake), and a flapping hand tremor, with progression to somnolence and coma. Aromatic amino acids (phenylalanine and tyrosine) and methionine appear to contribute to the problem, perhaps by formation of false neurotransmitters in the central nervous system. Intestinal bacteria digest blood in the GI tract, and ammonia released by this process is absorbed into the body, worsening hepatic encephalopathy.

Treatment

Drug therapy includes use of lactulose, which reduces absorption of ammonia from the GI tract, and poorly absorbed antibiotics such as neomycin, which are given orally to destroy intestinal bacteria that produce ammonia.

Nutritional Care

Assessment

Assessment is summarized in Table 11-1.

Intervention and teaching

Dietary modifications. The goal is to avoid inducing encephalopathy or worsening symptoms, while providing as nutritious a diet as possible.

- Alcohol intake must be eliminated because it increases liver damage.

- A high-energy diet (45 to 50 kcal/kg) prevents breakdown of body tissues to meet energy needs (which releases ammonia and other wastes that worsen encephalopathy). Carbohydrates provide most of the energy. Moderate fat (30% of total energy intake) can be provided unless steatorrhea is present. If steatorrhea occurs, then fat can be reduced. MCTs can be used to increase energy intake where steatorrhea is present.
- Protein intake is usually limited to 1 to 1.5 g/kg desirable weight per day unless hepatic encephalopathy is impending. In encephalopathy, protein is often limited to 0.5 g/kg or less. With improvement, intake can be gradually liberalized, with the eventual goal being 1 g/kg/day. Vegetable protein appears to be better tolerated than meat protein by some patients with chronic hepatic encephalopathy. There is some evidence that increased intakes of branched-chain amino acids (BCAAs) are beneficial for selected patients with encephalopathy. Enteral formulas high in BCAAs (Hepatic-Aid II and NutriHep [Nestle]) can be taken orally or delivered by tube. BCAA-enriched amino acid solutions are available for use in TPN.
- Restriction of sodium intake to 500 to 1500 mg (20 to 65 mEq) per day of sodium helps to control fluid retention and ascites. (See Box 14-3 for sodium-restricted diets.)
- Small, frequent feedings are better tolerated than larger, less frequent ones. Soft foods that are low in fiber help prevent bleeding from esophageal varices, which may result in elevated ammonia levels as the blood proteins are absorbed or in shock if severe acute bleeding occurs.

Supplementation. Supplements providing at least two to three times the RDA of B complex vitamins, especially folic acid, are often used. Many individuals with cirrhosis are alcoholics and have followed poor diets; they have poor tissue stores of vitamins.

Hemochromatosis
Pathophysiology

Hemochromatosis is a genetic disorder in which excessive iron is stored in various organs, especially the liver, pancreas, heart, gonads, skin, and joints, disrupting organ function. Cirrhosis of the liver, bronzing of the skin, and diabetes are likely to occur if the disorder is left untreated. The laboratory evidence of hemochromatosis includes elevated serum iron and ferritin concentrations, saturated iron-binding capacity, and excessive parenchymal iron in liver biopsy tissue.

Treatment

Regular phlebotomy is used to remove excessive iron stores, with the goal being to maintain serum ferritin at 50 µg/L or less.

Nutritional Care

Assessment

Assessment is summarized in Table 11-1.

Intervention and teaching

Limit dietary iron and its absorption.   To limit dietary iron, follow these guidelines:

- Avoid medicinal iron and iron-containing mineral supplements, breakfast cereals, and other foods highly fortified with iron, and use of iron cookware.
- Avoid consuming vitamin C supplements or food sources rich in vitamin C with meals, and avoid supplements with excessive amounts of vitamin C, which can increase iron absorption.
- Choose foods rich in fiber and drink tea, coffee, or milk with meals, to reduce the absorption of iron from the meal.
- Avoid alcohol intake or consume alcohol in very limited amounts. Alcohol potentiates liver damage from hemachromatosis and increases the likelihood of cirrhosis and death.

REFERENCES

American Gastroenterological Association medical position statement: celiac sprue, *Gastroenterology* 120:1522, 2001.

American Gastroenterological Association medical position statement: nonalcoholic fatty liver disease, *Gastroenterology* 123:1702, 2002.

Drucker DJ: Gut adaptation and the glucagon-like peptides, *Gut* 50:428, 2002.

SELECTED BIBLIOGRAPHY

Aldhous MC, Meister D, Ghosh S: Modification of enteral diets in inflammatory bowel disease, *Proc Nutr Soc* 60:457, 2001.

Al-Omran M, Groof A, Wilke D: Enteral versus parenteral nutrition for acute pancreatitis, *Cochrane Database Syst Rev*: CD002837, 2003.

Arteel G et al. Advances in alcoholic liver disease, *Best Pract Res Clin Gastroenterol* 17:625, 2003.

Balistreri WF et al: Acute and chronic hepatitis: Working Group Report of the First World Congress of Pediatric Gastroenterology, Hepatology, and Nutrition, *J Pediatr Gastroenterol Nutr* 35(suppl 2):S62, 2002.

Bernstein C, Leslie W, Leboff M: AGA technical review on osteoporosis in gastrointestinal diseases, *Gastroenterology* 124:795, 2003.

Cabre E, Gassull MA: Nutritional aspects of liver disease and transplantation, *Curr Opin Clin Nutr Metab Care* 4:581, 2001.

Dolbey CH: Hemochromatosis: a review, *Clin J Oncol Nurs* 5:257, 2001.

Gassull MA: Nutrition and inflammatory bowel disease: its relation to pathophysiology, outcome and therapy, *Dig Dis* 21:220, 2003.

Kastin DA, Buchman AL: Malnutrition and gastrointestinal disease, *Curr Opin Clin Nutr Metab Care* 5:699, 2002.

Katz PO: Optimizing medical therapy for gastroesophageal reflux disease: state of the art, *Rev Gastroenterol Disord* 3:59, 2003.

Li SD et al: Nutrition support for individuals with liver failure, *Nutr Rev* 58:242, 2000.

Lord LM et al: Management of the patient with short bowel syndrome, *AACN Clin Issues* 11:604, 2000.

Petersen JM, Forsmark CE: Chronic pancreatitis and maldigestion, *Semin Gastrointest Dis* 13:191, 2002.

Song Z et al: Treatment of alcoholic liver disease, *Curr Gastroenterol Rep* 6:71, 2004.

Thompson T: Oats and the gluten-free diet, *J Am Dietet Assoc* 103:376, 2003.

Cancer

12

Cancer and nutrition are closely related. Evidence suggests that nutritional factors have a role in development of many types of tumors. Once cancer has developed, it can have severe adverse effects on nutritional status. Not only does the cancerous tumor draw nutrients from the host, but also the treatment modalities and the psychologic impact of cancer can interfere with maintenance of adequate nutrition.

Cancer Prevention

At least one third of all cancers in western countries are estimated to be nutrition and diet related, and thus dietary changes are an important area for primary prevention. Chapter 1 describes in more detail the recommendations for a diet likely to be low in cancer risk, which can be summarized as follows:

- *Maintain a desirable body weight.* Obesity is linked to numerous types of cancer and appears to establish a hormonal climate suitable to cancer development. Fat cells release numerous hormones and metabolic effectors, some of which have stimulatory effects on tumor growth. Obesity is frequently associated with insulin resistance, a condition in which there are high circulating insulin levels. Insulin's actions can include growth-stimulating effects on tumor cells.
- *Eat a varied diet.* Foods not only contain a variety of nutrients with anticarcinogenic properties, such as antioxidants, but they also provide nonnutritive substances such as isoflavones, flavonoids, allylic sulfides (garlic), capsaicin, indoles, and protease inhibitors with anticarcinogenic activity. It is especially important to include a variety of fruits and vegetables daily and to include fiber-containing foods such as whole grains, legumes,

fruits, and vegetables. In one large study, lung cancer rates were inversely related to the number of fruit servings consumed daily (Miller et al., 2004).

▪ *Limit total fat intake.* Unlike heart disease, where saturated fat is the primary form of fat contributing to elevated LDL-cholesterol and cardiovascular risk, all types of fat are associated with increased prevalence of cancer.

▪ *Limit intake of alcoholic beverages, if consumed at all.* For example, one drink a day raises a woman's risk of breast cancer by 7%.

▪ *Limit consumption of salt-cured, smoked, nitrite-preserved, and charbroiled food.* Gastric cancers, in particular, are more common among individuals with diets high in these types of food.

Future work may make it possible to understand the complex interactions between an individual's genetic make-up, environment, and diet that contribute to carcinogenesis. Individualized recommendations regarding nutrient needs to alter gene transcription and susceptibility to cancer may become possible.

Pathophysiology of Cancer's Nutritional Effects

Cancerous tumors differ according to their site, size, cellular types, and metabolic effects. Some cancers can have very serious impacts on nutritional status, but these impacts are not strongly correlated with tumor size. **Cancer cachexia** is a severe form of malnutrition associated with a poor prognosis and characterized by anorexia, early satiety, weight loss, anemia, weakness, and muscle wasting. Metabolic alterations—including futile metabolic cycles, insulin resistance causing glucose intolerance, increased lipolysis or fat breakdown, and increased tissue protein turnover—contribute to the nutritional problems of people with cancer. The inflammatory actions of tumor necrosis factor and other cytokines are involved in these metabolic changes, as well as the fatigue and anorexia many patients experience. Appetite may be impaired by altered neurotransmitter (serotonin) levels in the central nervous system or elevated levels of lactate produced by anaerobic metabolism, a method of metabolism favored by tumors. Other factors that can inhibit intake include psychologic stress and dysgeusia (distorted taste) or aversions to specific foods. About 70% of individuals with cancer experience food aversions, either because of the effects of the tumor itself or because of the effects of chemotherapy. Mucositis, impaired salivation, nausea, vomiting, loss of the senses of taste and smell, and diarrhea resulting from cancer therapies are all factors in reduced food intake.

Cancer Treatment—Interaction with Nutrition

Surgery, radiation therapy, and chemotherapy are used alone or in combination in cancer treatment. Table 12-1 demonstrates some of the nutritional effects of cancer therapies. Poor nutritional status can interfere with cancer treatment. For example, it may be necessary to reduce the chemotherapy dosages for a malnourished person. A poorly nourished surgical patient is more likely to develop pneumonia, wound dehiscence, or other postoperative complications.

Nutritional Care

The goals of nutritional care are to identify and prevent or correct nutritional deficiencies resulting from cancer or its therapies, and to maintain or improve functional capacity and quality of life.

Assessment

Assessment is summarized in Table 12-2.

Intervention and Teaching
Nutritional Needs
Energy and protein

Encourage a high-energy, high-protein intake to maintain or increase weight and tissue stores. Adults with good nutritional status may need no more than 25 to 30 kcal/kg/day to maintain their weight. Undernourished individuals may need 35 kcal/kg/day or more to promote weight gain. Children need adequate energy intake to promote continued growth, generally no less than 1000 kcal plus 100 kcal/year of life. Individuals with anorexia may consume more if small amounts of food are given frequently. Sweets and sugar are rich in energy, but the person with cancer may have little appetite for sweets. *Glucose oligosaccharides*, *glucose polymers*, and *corn syrup solids* are terms that refer to short chains of glucose molecules; they are less sweet than sugar and are not objectionable to most individuals. They can be added to beverages (except carbonated beverages); shakes; and foods such as cereals, pudding, and

Text continued on p. 345

Table 12-1   Nutritional Effects of Cancer Therapy

Site of Restriction	Surgery — Effect on Nutrition
Tongue, mouth, jaw	Oral intake precluded (temporary)
Esophagus	Oral intake precluded (temporary); gastric stasis and fat malabsorption as a result of vagotomy
Stomach	Dumping syndrome; impaired absorption of vitamin B_{12} and iron
Pancreas (pancreatoduodenectomy)	Diabetes mellitus; impaired absorption of fat and fat-soluble vitamins, calcium, zinc, magnesium, and protein
Small bowel	Depends on extent of resection and portion of bowel involved (see Figure 1-5); lactose intolerance possible; ileal resection: impaired absorption of fat and fat-soluble vitamins, calcium, zinc, magnesium, and vitamin B_{12}; impaired absorption of bile salts with resulting diarrhea and loss of fluid and electrolytes; with massive resection, loss of all nutrients, weight loss, and dehydration occur unless adequate nutritional support is given promptly
Colon	Impaired absorption of water and electrolytes

Radiation Therapy

Site of Restriction	Acute Effect	Long Term Effect*
Central nervous system	Anorexia, nausea, vomiting (occasionally)	
Head and neck	Xerostomia (dry mouth), mucositis, anorexia, hypogeusia ("mouth blindness")	Xerostomia, bony necrosis, dental caries, altered taste
Esophagus, lung	Dysphagia, sore throat	Esophageal stenosis
Upper abdomen	Anorexia; nausea, vomiting	Gastrointestinal (GI) ulcer
Whole abdomen	Nausea, vomiting; diarrhea; cramping	GI ulcer; diarrhea, malabsorption; chronic enteritis or colitis
Pelvis	Diarrhea	Diarrhea; chronic enteritis or colitis

Chemotherapy

Chemotherapeutic Agent	Effect on Nutrition
Anastrozole, bleomycin, bortezomib, carboplatin, carmustine, cisplatin, cyclophosphamide, cytarabine, dacarbazine, doxorubicin, epirubicin, estramustine, etoposide, floxuridine, fluorouracil, fulvestrant, gemcitabine, ifoxfamide, imatinib, lomustine, mechlorethamine, mesna, methotrexate, mitotane, mitoxantrone, octreotide, oxaliplatin, paclitaxel, procarbazine, thiotepa, topotecan, trastuzumab, vinblastine, vincristine, vinorelbine	Anorexia, nausea, vomiting

Continued

Table 12-1   Nutritional Effects of Cancer Therapy—cont'd

Chemotherapy	
Chemotherapeutic Agent	Effect on Nutrition
Bleomycin, cytarabine, docetaxel, doxorubicin, epirubicin, floxuridine, fluorouracil, gemcitabine, methotrexate, mitoxantrone, paclitaxel, oxaliplatin, vinblastine, vincristine	Mucositis (stomatitis, esophagitis, intestinal ulcerations)
Bortezomib, capecitabine, cytarabine, estramustine, fluorouracil, gefitinib, gemcitabine, imatinib, mesna, methotrexate, mitotane, mitoxantrone, octreotide, paclitaxel, topotecan, trastuzumab, vinblastine	Diarrhea
Gemcitabine, topotecan, vinblastine, vincristine	Constipation/paralytic ileus
Asparaginase, megestrol acetate, streptozocin	Hyperglycemia
Megestrol acetate	Unwanted weight gain/increased appetite

*Long-term effects may occur within a few months of therapy or may appear years later.

Table 12-2   Assessment in Cancer

Area of Concern	Significant Findings
Protein-Energy Malnutrition (PEM)	*History* Poor intake of protein and energy as a result of food aversions, anorexia, nausea, vomiting, bad taste in mouth, difficulty chewing or swallowing (especially meats), inadequate financial resources; increased needs as a result of infection, abscess or fistula; glucocorticoid treatment; impaired absorption caused by dumping syndrome, ileal or pancreatic resection, or lactose intolerance; weight loss, especially if >2% in 1 wk, >5% in 1 mo, >7.5% in 3 mo, >10% in 6 mo *Physical Examination* Muscle wasting; edema; delayed wound healing; diarrhea (↓ oncotic pressure in the gut); triceps skinfold <5th percentile; weight <90% standard for height or BMI <18.5, or decline of weight and/or height growth pattern by 10% or more (children) (see Appendix D) *Laboratory Analysis* ↓ Serum albumin, transferrin, or prealbumin; ↓ creatinine-height index
Vitamin Deficiencies A	*History* Poor intake (same reasons as listed for PCM); steatorrhea; ileal or pancreatic resection *Physical Examination* Dry, scaly skin; dry cornea; ↓ night vision

Continued

Table 12-2   Assessment in Cancer—cont'd

Area of Concern	Significant Findings
K	*Laboratory Analysis* ↓ Serum retinol *History* Antibiotic usage *Physical Examination* Petechiae, ecchymoses *Laboratory Analysis* ↓ Prothrombin time
C	*History* Poor intake of citrus and other fruits as a result of stomatitis, esophagitis, or anorexia *Physical Examination* Petechiae, ecchymoses; delayed wound healing *Laboratory Analysis* ↓ Serum or lymphocyte ascorbic acid
Folate	*History* Poor intake of fruits, vegetables, and fortified foods caused by anorexia, nausea, vomiting, stomatitis, or esophagitis; methotrexate (a folic acid antagonist) treatment; alcohol abuse

Mineral/Electrolyte Deficiencies	
Iron (Fe)	*Physical Examination* Pallor, glossitis *Laboratory Analysis* ↓ Hgb, ↑ MCV, ↓ serum or red blood cell folate
	History Poor intake as a result of aversions to or difficulty chewing/swallowing meats, poultry, or fish; anorexia; nausea; vomiting; dysgeusia; increased losses from acute or chronic blood loss; decreased absorption caused by gastric resection *Physical Examination* Pallor, blue sclerae; spoon-shaped nails *Laboratory Analysis* ↓ Hgb, Hct, MCV, ↓ serum Fe and ferritin
Zinc (Zn)	*History* Poor intake caused by same factors as listed for Fe; increased losses caused by diarrhea or fistula drainage; impaired absorption as a result of pancreatic or small bowel resection *Physical Examination* Poor sense of taste, distorted taste; alopecia; delayed wound healing; dermatitis *Laboratory Analysis* ↓ Serum Zn

Continued

Table 12-2   Assessment in Cancer—cont'd

Area of Concern	Significant Findings
Potassium (K⁺)	*History* Increased losses from vomiting or diarrhea *Physical Examination* Malaise, weakness *Laboratory Analysis* ↓ Serum K⁺
Magnesium (Mg)	*History* Poor intake as a result of alcoholism; increased losses/decreased absorption caused by prolonged vomiting, diarrhea, steatorrhea, fistula drainage, pancreatic or small bowel resection *Physical Examination* Tremor, hyperactive deep reflexes; disorientation *Laboratory Anaylsis* ↓ Serum Mg

applesauce to increase the energy content. Box 12-1 provides suggestions for improving energy intake.

Intake of 1.2 to 2 g of protein per kg/day usually provides adequate amino acids for tissue synthesis, if carbohydrate and fat intake is sufficient to meet energy needs. Snacking on foods such as nuts or seeds, soy nuts, boiled or deviled eggs, hummus, cheese, and yogurt is a good way to increase both protein and energy intake. Where regular foods are inadequate to meet nutritional needs, commercial supplements may be beneficial. See Tables 8-1 and 8-2 for examples.

Iron

Iron-deficiency anemia can result from blood loss or aversions to iron-containing foods. Poultry and fish may be acceptable to the individual with aversion to red meat, and green, leafy vegetables and whole-grain or enriched breads and cereals provide additional iron. In addition, cast iron cookware increases the iron content of food prepared in it. If an iron supplement is needed, milk, tea, or coffee should not be consumed with it because they impair iron absorption. Foods containing vitamin C improve iron absorption. Iron supplements often cause some gastrointestinal distress. Taking them with meals or just before bedtime may improve tolerance. If ferrous sulfate, a commonly used form of iron supplementation, is poorly tolerated, then ferrous gluconate or another form of iron may be better accepted. Supplementation continues until concentrations of serum ferritin, a storage form of iron, rise to normal. Supplementation may continue to be needed for maintenance of adequate stores if intake is poor.

Some anemia in cancer patients is not related to iron deficiency—at least not in the early stages of the anemia. The anemia of myelosuppression can be treated with recombinant forms of the hormone erythropoietin (i.e., epoetin alfa). Adequate iron stores are needed in order to respond effectively to these drugs, and patients who require chronic treatment almost always require iron supplementation. Anemia of chronic disease occurs in patients with some malignancies, as well as those with renal failure and other chronic illnesses. In this type of anemia, the bone marrow fails to produce adequate red blood cells, but iron stores may be normal. The anemia is often normocytic (normal-sized cells), rather than microcytic, as in iron deficiency (see Chapter 2). Iron therapy does not correct anemia of chronic disease. Serum ferritin

Box 12-1   Suggestions for Increasing Energy Intake

Use Fat Liberally Because It Is an Especially Concentrated Source of Energy*

- Salad dressings, cooking oils, mayonnaise, nuts, cream, sour cream, sauces, and gravies should be used as often as possible.
- Butter or margarine provides 35 kcal/tsp. Add them to hot foods such as soup, vegetables, mashed potatoes, cooked cereals, and rice. Serve hot bread because more butter is used when it melts into the bread.
- Peanut butter is high in fat, providing 90 kcal/tbsp. It can be served on bread or crackers, apple or pear slices, bananas, or celery.

Serve Small Meals Frequently

Keep Snacks Available at All Times

Nuts, hummus, dried fruits, bagels or muffins, cookies, crackers and cheese, granola, ice cream or sherbet, yogurt or frozen yogurt, milkshakes made with ice cream, and puddings are good energy sources.

Prepare Foods in a Manner That Will Make Them as Energy-Dense as Possible

- Soups, hot cereals, cocoa from a mix, and instant puddings can be prepared with whole milk or half and half, rather than water.
- Sauces can be added to cooked vegetables and pastas. Alfredo sauce, prepared with cream, contains more energy than tomato-based pasta sauces.

Do Not Allow Foods of Low Energy Density to Displace More Concentrated Energy Sources

- Beverage consumption is best delayed until after, rather than before or during, meals. Low-calorie or no-calorie beverages (artificially sweetened drinks, unsweetened tea or coffee, water) should be avoided as much as possible. Glucose oligosaccharides (also called *corn syrup solids* and glucose *polymers*) can be added to tea, coffee, or juices (see Table 8-2).

Box 12-1   Suggestions for Increasing Energy
Intake—cont'd

- Raw vegetables and salads should be served only at the end
  of the meal, or energy-dense foods (cheese, egg, poultry,
  meat, beans, salad dressing) should be added liberally.

---

*Individuals with malabsorption and steatorrhea may not tolerate increased fat
intake. MCT oil (see Chapter 8) is one potential source of energy.

levels help to distinguish between anemia of chronic disease and
iron-deficiency anemia because serum ferritin is low in iron deficiency but may be high or in the high-normal range in anemia of
chronic disease. If ferritin measurements do not provide clear-cut
separation between the two anemias (e.g., ferritin is low-normal),
then measurement of iron stores in a bone marrow aspirate will distinguish between them.

Calcium

Lactase deficiency is a common result of the intestinal damage
caused by radiation or chemotherapy, since this enzyme is located
in the intestinal mucosa. Lactose intake can cause cramping, bloating, and diarrhea in lactase-deficient individuals. Calcium intake is
likely to be low if dairy products are avoided. Lactose-intolerant
individuals often tolerate yogurt, cheese, cottage cheese, or buttermilk, as well as small amounts of milk. Milk treated with lactase
enzyme is commercially available, as are lactase enzyme tablets
to be taken with milk. Other reliable calcium sources include
calcium-fortified juices, tortillas, and foods prepared with milk,
such as pancakes (see Figure 3-1). A supplement of 800 to 1200
mg of calcium per day, in the form of salts such as calcium carbonate,calcium citrate, or calcium gluconate, can be used to replace
milk products.

Zinc

Zinc is found in many of the same foods as iron, and food aversions
can limit intake. Zinc needs during healing and anabolism (tissue
building) are high. A supplement (15 to 30 mg of elemental zinc)
may be needed.

Nutritional Problems Associated with Cancer Therapy

Box 12-2 summarizes problems often encountered during cancer therapy and approaches that may help alleviate them.

Nausea and vomiting are especially common during chemotherapy and can accompany radiation therapy. Medications to relieve nausea and vomiting promote comfort and help make adequate nutritional intake possible if they are given on a regularly scheduled basis or before mealtime.

Mucositis can affect any area of the GI tract, but involvement of the mouth and esophagus is especially troublesome during chemotherapy and radiation of the head and neck. Mouth pain greatly inhibits nutritional intake, and the ulcerations are susceptible to infection. Frequent rinsing of the mouth with saline has been shown to be as effective as antiseptic solutions (dilute hydrogen peroxide) in treating stomatitis. Viscous lidocaine is an effective anesthetic, but the patient must be very careful when using it to avoid inadvertently biting the numbed tissues or burning them with hot food. Magnesium hydroxide (milk of magnesia) rinses are soothing but can dry the mucosa. Other treatments that have been used to promote healing include sucralfate application, hydroxypropyl cellulose films used to form a barrier over lesions, and vitamin E. Cryotherapy (holding ice chips in the mouth) at the time of chemotherapy administration causes vasoconstriction and reduces oral damage. Capsaicin, from chili peppers, has had some success in both relief of pain and stimulation of the regrowth of the oral mucosa.

Food aversions can develop as a conditioned response in individuals suffering from nausea and vomiting caused by radiation or chemotherapy. For example, aversions to red gelatin have occurred in individuals receiving doxorubicin (Adriamycin), a red drug. Individualization of the diet through a process of trial and error appears to be the most successful way of dealing with food aversions.

Complementary and Alternative Medical (CAM) Therapies

CAM therapies are believed to be widely used among patients with cancer, although the exact percentages of patients using CAM therapies remain unclear. All patients with cancer should be asked about their use of CAM therapies—for example, herbs, special diets, manipulation, immune therapies, medicinal teas, and any other therapies not

Box 12-2   **Common Nutritional Problems and Dietary Suggestions for Individuals with Cancer**

Nausea and Vomiting

Diet: Liquids and soft foods served cold: juices, carbonated beverages, gelatin, fruits; dry, bland foods: toast, crackers, plain bagels; tart foods and fluids: lemonade; serve small amounts frequently.

Supplements:[*] Glucose oligosaccharides, clear liquids such as Resource Fruit Drink (Novartis).

Suggestions: Keep environment cool, well ventilated, free of cooking odors; dry starchy foods (crackers, toast) before rising can help prevent vomiting; liquids should be sipped slowly; distraction, imagery, and relaxation techniques may help; premedicate with antiemetics if appropriate; plan the medication schedule so that drugs with high emetic potential are not given close to mealtime, if possible; avoid serving favorite foods during nausea to reduce the risk of developing aversions to them; avoid coaxing or pressure to increase intake.

Problem foods: Hot foods, fatty foods, foods with strong odors, spicy foods.

Anorexia

Diet: Regular foods served attractively, with variety in texture and color; small frequent feedings.

Supplements: Glucose oligosaccharides and other modular products; complete liquid supplements (allow the individual to taste several and select the one[s] preferred); milk powder added to liquid milk, cereals, mashed potatoes (if lactose tolerance not a problem); Resource Benecalorie (Novartis); tube feedings if necessary.

Suggestions: Avoid offering beverages until individual has finished eating, since fluids can be filling; encourage physical activity; children may eat more if they are involved in food preparation or if foods are decorated (e.g., sandwiches cut with cookie cutters).

Problem foods: Large meals can overwhelm the person and suppress appetite.

Continued

Box 12-2   Common Nutritional Problems and Dietary
Suggestions for Individuals with Cancer—cont'd

Mucositis (Stomatitis, Esophagitis)

Diet: Nonabrasive, soft foods served cold or at room temperature: sherbet; canned or soft, fresh, low-acid fruits; fruit ices; popsicles; custard; gelatin, ice cream; yogurt; cottage cheese; puddings; canned or cooked vegetables; eggs; sandwiches; cooked cereals (warm, not hot).

Supplements: Glucose oligosaccharides, complete liquid supplements.

Suggestions: Rinse mouth often with saline, plain water, sodium bicarbonate solution (1 tsp baking soda/500 ml water), or hydrogen peroxide diluted to one sixth strength; viscous lidocaine provides topical analgesia, but the patient must be careful in eating after using it because numbed tissues may inadvertently be bitten or burned by hot foods or beverages.

Problem foods: Acidic fruits and juices such as citrus (evaluate vitamin C intake when citrus fruits are avoided); salty or spicy foods; hard or abrasive foods such as chips, pretzels, nuts, seeds; foods served hot.

Dysphagia

Diet: Emphasize foods that form a semisolid bolus in the mouth (e.g., macaroni and cheese).

Supplements: Carbohydrate or protein modules added to foods, thickened liquid supplements (see Suggestions); pudding-type supplements; commercial thickened foods and thickeners to be added to foods and beverages.[†]

Suggestions: Thicken liquids with dry infant cereals, mashed potatoes, potato flakes, or cornstarch; use gravies and sauces to moisten meats and vegetables; if dysphagia is severe, consider tube feedings.

Problem foods: Thin liquids such as water, tea, coffee; foods that are not uniform in consistency such as stews; dry foods such as overcooked meats, hard rolls, nuts; foods that stick to the palate, such as peanut butter and white bread; slippery foods such as gelatin.

Box 12-2   **Common Nutritional Problems and Dietary Suggestions for Individuals with Cancer—cont'd**

Xerostomia (Reduced Saliva Production)

Diet: Regular, moist foods: casseroles, gravies, sauces; encourage fluids, including popsicles, fruit ices, sherbet, gelatin, soups.

Suggestions: Use good oral hygiene because dental caries is common when saliva production is insufficient to buffer acids produced by mouth bacteria; rinse mouth often with saline or mouthwash; use sugar-free candies and gum between meals to promote saliva flow; use artificial saliva if problem is severe.

Problem foods: Breads, dry foods, sweet sticky foods, sugars in gum or candy.

Hypogeusia ("Mouth Blindness")

Diet: Regular foods with strong flavors or seasonings and interesting textures.

Supplements: Complete liquid supplements with added flavors if necessary.

Problem foods: Bland foods.

Dysgeusia (Altered Taste)

Diet: Regular foods; use trial and error to determine the most suitable foods.

Supplements: Fruit-flavored supplements, glucose oligosaccharides.

Problem foods: Coffee, chocolate, red meats, others (varies with the individual).

Diarrhea

Diet: Low-lactose, low-fat; increase fluids; emphasize starches.

Supplements: Glucose oligosaccharides, lactose-free liquid supplements; live lactobacillus supplements.

Problem foods: Milk, cream soups, ice cream, fatty or fried foods.

Constipation

Diet: High-fiber; at least 50 ml fluid per kg/day.

Supplements: Bran, 2 tbsp/day.

Continued

Box 12-2   Common Nutritional Problems and Dietary
Suggestions for Individuals with Cancer—cont'd

Neutropenia with Potential for Infection

Diet: Regular.

Suggestions: Cook eggs, meats, poultry, and fish well; thoroughly wash fruits and vegetables to be eaten raw (after bone marrow transplant and in severe neutropenia, it is sometimes necessary to avoid raw foods altogether); avoid cross-contamination (e.g., carefully clean cutting boards used for trimming raw meat before using them to prepare raw vegetables); refrigerate cooked foods immediately after meal; discard any leftovers within 3 days.[‡]

Supplements: Glucose oligosaccharides, canned supplements.

Problem foods: Raw or undercooked eggs, meats, poultry, fish, shellfish (e.g., shrimp, lobster) rare meats, sushi, homemade mayonnaise, raw oysters, key lime pie, and "royal" icing or other decorative icings and glazes unless they are known not to contain raw eggs.

---

[*]See Tables 8-1 and 8-2 for listings of supplements.
[†]Examples include Resource Thicken-Up and Resource Thickened Coffee, Juice and Water (Novartis) or Thick & Easy products (Hormel Health Labs).
[‡]For further food safety information, see Appendix K.

---

prescribed by their conventional health care provider. CAM therapies used by cancer patients range from treatments for symptom control (i.e., antinausea and pain treatments) to those aimed at cancer suppression. Box 12-3 lists selected therapies used by cancer patients. A summary of available information about other therapies and links to additional resources are available at the websites of the National Cancer Institute (http://www.cancer.gov/cancerinfo/treatment/cam/) and the Office of Cancer Complementary and Alternative Therapy (http://www3.cancer.gov/occam/).

The health provider should discuss these topics with the patient considering use of CAM therapies (National Cancer Institute, National Center for Complementary and Alternative Medicine, 2003):

■ What benefits can be expected from this therapy?
■ What are the risks associated with this therapy?

Box 12-3   Complementary and Alternative Medical Therapies Used by Some Cancer Patients

Cartilage (Shark, Bovine [Cow], AE-941/Neovastat [Aqueous Extract of Shark Cartilage])

Use: Inhibition of angiogenesis.

Adverse effects: Shark—nausea, vomiting, abdominal cramping and/or bloating, constipation, hypotension, hyperglycemia, generalized weakness, and hypercalcemia; bovine—dysgeusia (unpleasant taste), fatigue, nausea, fever, and dizziness; AE-941/Neovastat—nausea, vomiting, and dyspepsia.

Comments: AE-941/Neovastat is undergoing clinical trials.

Essiac and Flor-Essence (Herbal Tea Mixtures)

Use: Stengthen immune system and shrink tumor.

Adverse effects: Mild, including nausea, vomiting, and increased stools.

Comments: No human trials have ever been reported. Some of the individual herbs in the tea have cytotoxic effects.

Mistletoe Extract (Viscum Species)

Use: Immune enhancement, direct cytotoxic effects on target cells, and improved quality of life.

Adverse effects: Minimal, including soreness at the injection site, fever, headache, and chills. (Also, mistletoe berries and leaves are poisonous and have caused seizures and death)

Comments: Clinical trials have not shown conclusive evidence of any benefit.

Laetrile/amygdalin (from Fruit Pits)

Use: Cytotoxic effects.

Adverse effects: Symptoms of cyanide poisoning, including nausea, vomiting, dizziness, cyanosis, hypotension, ataxia, confusion, coma, and death. Toxicity is potentiated by high doses of vitamin C and by taking laetrile with raw almonds, celery, peaches, carrots, or bean sprouts. Can be taken orally or by injection; toxicity is higher with oral doses.

Comments: Clinical trials did not warrant further study of laetrile in cancer cases.

Continued

Box 12-3   Complementary and Alternative Therapies Used by Some Cancer Patients—cont'd

Ginger

Use: Reduces duration and severity of nausea after chemotherapy.

Adverse effects: Irritation or a bad taste in the mouth, heartburn, belching, bloating, and nausea.

Comments: Intake should be limited to 4 g daily. There is no evidence of ginger's safety or efficacy in children. It is available in many forms, including fresh or dried root, powder, and tea.

Mushroom (*Coriolus versicolor* [Turkey Tail Mushroom] and its extracts polysaccharide K and Polysaccharide-Peptide)

Use: Antimicrobial, antiviral, and antitumor properties when used as a supplement with chemotherapy and/or radiotherapy.

Adverse effects: Uncommon.

Comments: Patients should not attempt to identify these mushrooms on their own due to the risk of selecting a poisonous variety.

Echinacea (American Coneflower)

Use: Immune enhancement.

Adverse effects: Mild, including stomach discomfort, nausea, sore throat, rash, and a low white blood cell count (with chronic use).

Comments: There is no evidence of effectiveness against cancer, though it may shorten the duration of colds.

Aloe Vera

Use: Oral—adjuvant to other cancer therapies through stimulation and modulation of immune function; topical—care of the skin during radiation therapy.

Adverse effects: Oral—purgative; topical—dermatitis; four deaths have been linked to injection of aloe vera (which is illegal in the United States).

Comments: There is no conclusive evidence regarding efficacy.

- Do the known benefits outweigh the risks?
- What side effects can be expected?
- Will the therapy interfere with conventional treatment?
- Is this therapy part of a clinical trial? If so, who is sponsoring the trial?
- Will the therapy be covered by health insurance?

Among the most common CAM therapies are vitamin and mineral supplements. In particular, patients are likely to take supplements of antioxidant nutrients such as vitamins C and E, beta-carotene, and selenium. The overall effects of this are not known. Some research has shown beneficial effects of antioxidants, either alone or together. Vitamin E appears to reduce chemotherapy-induced stomatitis and cancer pain. Both selenium and vitamin E have shown some promise as adjunctive therapy in improving response to standard chemotherapy. Balanced against this is the fact that one theory of the way that both chemotherapy and radiation therapy kill tumor cells is by stimulating oxidative processes, which might be inhibited by high antioxidant intakes. In four large studies in smokers, beta-carotene had no benefit in preventing cancer, and two of the studies actually found an increase in the rates of lung cancer and overall mortality. Also, at very high doses, nutrients that normally have an antioxidant effect can become pro-oxidants. Selenium, in particular, is toxic in large doses (more than 1 mg, about 15 times the DRI), causing irritation of the respiratory system, rhinitis, pulmonary edema, bronchopneumonia, and a metallic taste in the mouth; large doses of selenium dioxide have resulted in skin necrosis. For these reasons, and because foods may have beneficial effects beyond their vitamin and mineral content, a diet rich in fruits and vegetables (5 to 10 servings daily) is the preferred way of ensuring adequate antioxidant intake. A daily multivitamin-mineral supplement providing the DRI can be recommended for patients receiving conventional cancer therapies. However, there is little evidence of benefit from doses larger than the DRI (reviewed in Norman et al., 2003).

Nutrition Support

Oral feedings

- *Indications:* Method of choice whenever feasible; requires bowel motility and ability to ingest food orally.

- *Example of use:* Mild to moderate anorexia related to any type of tumor.
- *Comments:* Supplements (modular components or complete formulas) can be used where regular foods are insufficient. See Tables 8-1 and 8-2 for suitable supplements. Oral intake is often insufficient for children and adults receiving intensive chemotherapy or abdominal radiation.

Enteral tube feedings

Enteral tube feedings are given via nasogastric (NG), nasoduodenal or nasojejunal (ND/NJ), gastrostomy, or jejunostomy tubes.

- *Indications:* Inadequate oral intake, impaired digestion or absorption requiring an elemental diet, ND/NJ feedings are useful if delayed gastric emptying is present; requires adequate bowel motility, unobstructed lower gastrointestinal (GI) tract.
- *Example of use:* Severe anorexia, oral or upper GI tumor preventing oral intake, short-bowel syndrome, pancreatic resection.
- *Comments:* ND/NJ feedings may be tolerated by the nauseated patient who cannot tolerate feedings into the stomach, but the tubes are unlikely to stay in place during active vomiting.

Total parenteral nutrition (TPN)

- *Indications:* GI obstruction preventing tube feeding; severely impaired digestion or absorption that prevents adequate enteral intake or causes dehydration, uncontrollable vomiting.
- *Example of use:* Severe short-bowel syndrome; jejunal or ileal obstruction; high-output enterocutaneous fistula, where bowel rest may promote healing.
- *Comments:* TPN is generally reserved for malnourished individuals, or those likely to become malnourished as a result of treatment, for whom an effective cancer therapy is available. Those individuals who are terminally ill and for whom no further treatment is contemplated do not receive much benefit from TPN.

Home Care

The patient and/or caregivers must have a basic understanding of the patient's dietary needs and the nutritional contributions of foods in the diet. The patient may need to keep daily records of intake as a basis for evaluating the diet and developing strategies for improving it. The patient and/or caregivers must also monitor nutritional status regularly. In particular, the patient should weigh at least weekly while at home, and progressive weight loss should be reported to the health care team so that appropriate interventions can be planned.

Many individuals find it impossible to maintain their weight and nutritional status without aggressive nutrition support. Home tube feeding or TPN is often appropriate for those receiving long-term therapy. Chapters 8 and 9 describe procedures for safe delivery of nutrition support.

REFERENCES

Miller AB et al: Fruits and vegetables and lung cancer: Findings from the European Prospective Investigation into Cancer and Nutrition, *Int J Cancer* 108:269, 2004.

National Cancer Institute, National Center for Complementary and Alternative Medicine: *Complementary and alternative medicine in cancer treatment: questions and answers.* Available at http://cis.nci.nih.gov/fact/9_14.htm, Updated August 12, 2003. Accessed December 20, 2003.

Norman H et al: The role of dietary supplements during cancer therapy, *J Nutr* 133(11 suppl 1):3794S, 2003.

SELECTED BIBLIOGRAPHY

Brown JK: A systematic review of the evidence on symptom management of cancer-related anorexia and cachexia, *Oncology Nursing Forum* 29:517, 2002.

Go VLW et al: Diet, nutrition, and cancer prevention: the postgenomic era, *J Nutr* 133(11 suppl 1):3830S, 2003.

Guenter PJ et al: Understanding tumor-induced weight loss, *MEDSURG Nurs* 11:215, 2002.

Strasser F: Eating-related disorders in patients with advanced cancer, *Support Care Cancer* 11:11, 2003.

Ravasco P et al: Nutritional deterioration in cancer: the role of disease and diet, *Clin Oncol (R Coll Radiol)* 15:443, 2003.

Worthington HV, Clarkson JE: Prevention of oral mucositis and oral candidiasis for patients with cancer treated with chemotherapy: Cochrane systematic review, *J Dent Educ* 66:903, 2002.

HIV Infection 13

Individuals infected with the human immunodeficiency virus (HIV) display a variety of responses, ranging from asymptomatic infection to acquired immunodeficiency syndrome (AIDS).

Pathophysiology

The retrovirus HIV selectively targets lymphocytes bearing the CD4 cell marker. Using the DNA from the host CD4 cell and the reverse transcriptase enzyme, HIV is able to replicate itself and create an inactive provirus. The provirus is activated by protease in the cell nucleus, and the resulting mature, infectious virus is able to bud from the CD4 cell into the plasma, where it can infect other CD4 cells.

The infected individual is susceptible to opportunistic infections and cancers such as Kaposi's sarcoma and non-Hodgkin's lymphoma. Weight loss and malnutrition are common, even in the early stages of the infection, and 80% or more of individuals with AIDS report unintentional weight loss. Malnutrition can decrease functional capacity, contribute to immune dysfunction, and increase the morbidity associated with the disease. Multiple factors are responsible for the nutritional impairments associated with HIV infection. Respiratory infections, such as *Pneumocystis carinii* pneumonia, cause anorexia; dyspnea; fever; and increased needs for protein, energy, and vitamins. Diarrhea is a common finding, occurring as a result of gastrointestinal (GI) pathogens, including fungi, viruses, bacteria, and protozoans; medications used; or enteropathy caused by HIV itself. Central nervous system (CNS) infections caused by HIV or by opportunistic organisms cause confusion, dementia, and impaired coordination, which interfere with food intake. Medications may impair food intake or absorption, and depression can result in anorexia. Finally, some investigations, but not all, have found resting energy expenditure (and thus energy needs) to be increased in stable individuals infected with HIV.

Treatment

Three types of antiretroviral agents have been approved by the U.S. Food and Drug Administration (FDA) for HIV treatment: (1) nucleotide reverse transcriptase inhibitors (abacavir, zidovudine, didanosine, zalcitabine, stavudine, tenofovir, and lamivudine), (2) nonnucleotide reverse transcriptase inhibitors (efavirenz, nevirapine, and delavirdine), and (3) protease inhibitors (amprenavir, saquinavir, ritonavir, indinavir, and nelfinavir). Combination therapy (highly active antiretroviral therapy, or HAART) is common, making the patient vulnerable to a variety of medication side effects and drug-nutrient or drug-drug interactions. Secondary infections require the use of appropriate antibiotic agents, and, when applicable, patients also receive cancer therapy (see Chapter 12). The side effects of commonly used medications include anorexia, nausea and vomiting, mucosal lesions, and diarrhea (Table 13-1).

Nutritional Care

Nutritional care of the person with HIV infection focuses on identifying and correcting, if possible, nutritional deficits that might weaken the individual, exacerbate immune dysfunctions, or impair quality of life.

Several pharmacologic agents to improve nutritional status are in clinical use or are undergoing experimental evaluation. Dronabinol, a marijuana derivative, and megestrol acetate, a progesterone-like drug, are approved for treatment of anorexia. These agents have been successful in promoting weight gain in some HIV-infected individuals. In some studies, however, it appears that much of the weight gained by adults has been fat rather than lean body tissue. Children have been found to gain weight without growing in height when taking megesterol acetate. Human growth factor, insulin-like growth factor–1, and the anabolic steroid oxandrolone have been used experimentally and have shown promise in increasing lean body mass.

Serum levels of several micronutrients have been reported to be low in individuals with HIV infection. These include zinc; magnesium; total carotenes; folate; and vitamins B_{12}, B_6, A, and E.

Table 13-1 Nutritional Impacts of Medications Commonly Prescribed for Persons with HIV Infection

Drug	Side Effect					
	Nausea/ Vomiting	Diarrhea	Sore Mouth/ Abdominal Pain	Dry Mouth/ Throat*	Unpleasant Taste	Anorexia
AIDS Chemotherapeutic Agents						
Abacavir	X	X				
Amprenavir	X	X	X		X	X
Delaverdine	X	X		X	X	X
Didanosine		X*				
Efavirenz	X	X	X			X
Indinavir	X	X				
Lamivudine	X	X	X			X
Nelfinavir	X	X	X	X		
Nevirapine	X	X	X	X		
Ritonavir		X		X	X	
Saquinavir	X	X	X	X		
Stavudine	X	X		X		X
Tenofovir	X	X				
Zalcitabine	X	X	X'	X	X	
Zidovudine	X	X	X			X

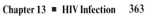

Antifungal Agents						
Amphotericin B	X	X	X	X			X
Caspofungin	X						
Fluconazole	X	X	X				
Flucytosine	X	X	X				
Itraconazole	X	X	X				X
Ketoconazole	X	X	X				
Nystatin	X	X	X				
Terbinafine	X	X	X				
Voriconazole	X	X	X				
Antiviral Agents						
Acyclovir	X	X	X				X
Cidofovir	X	X	X	X	X		X
Famciclovir	X	X	X				X
Fomivirsen	X	X	X		X	X	X
Foscarnet	X	X	X	X			X
Ganciclovir	X	X	X				X
Interferon Alfa-2a	X	X	X				
Interferon Alfa-2b	X	X	X				
Valacyclovir	X	X					X

Continued

Table 13-1 Nutritional Impacts of Medications Commonly Prescribed for Persons with HIV Infection—cont'd

	Side Effect					
Drug	Nausea/ Vomiting	Diarrhea	Sore Mouth/ Abdominal Pain	Dry Mouth/ Throat*	Unpleasant Taste	Anorexia
Valganciclovir	X	X	X			
Vidarabine	X	X	X			
Antiprotozoal Agents						
Atavaquone	X	X	X			X
Metronidazole	X	X	X	X	X	
Pentamidine						
IV or IM	X					
Inhalable	X		X	X	X	X

*Diarrhea most likely with the oral suspension; consider use of the chewable tablet form for a patient with diarrhea.

Assessment

Nutrition assessment is summarized in Table 13-2.

Intervention and Teaching

Principles of a healthful diet

Optimal nutrition will help to maintain functional capacity, improve quality of life, and improve tolerance of treatment. Many individuals infected with HIV are extremely interested in nutrition and its potential benefits in controlling disease, and it is possible to build on this interest in teaching about diet. The DASH diet (see Chapters 1 and 14) provides a healthful eating pattern that can be used as a teaching tool.

Weight loss and undernutrition

Weight loss is more common in individuals with the highest viral loads, and it is associated with higher rates of morbidity and mortality. Nutrition counseling with frequent follow-up, use of supplements as appropriate, and use of oxandrolone, a synthetic androgen, has been effective in stabilizing or increasing weight and lean body mass in some instances. Energy needs can be estimated (see Box 2-5) if indirect calorimetry is not available to measure them. A high-protein diet (>1.5 g/kg/day) provides the amino acids needed for tissue synthesis. Issues to consider include the following:

- Diarrhea may improve if a low-fat, high-starch diet is followed. Medium-chain triglycerides can be added to the diet if additional energy is needed.
- Modular ingredients (see Table 8-2) may be added to foods and beverages to increase the protein and energy content.
- Lactose intolerance is common in individuals with HIV infection and can cause diarrhea, cramping, and bloating. Yogurt and hard cheeses are usually better tolerated than liquid milk in lactose intolerance. Milk treated with lactase enzyme is available commercially, or lactase capsules can be taken along with milk. Lactose-free products should be chosen if oral supplements or enteral tube feedings are used (see Table 8-1).
- Appetite stimulants (dronabinol, megestrol acetate, or cyproheptadine) may be effective in increasing intake. If they are prescribed, the patient should take them about 30 minutes before meals (usually twice daily).

Table 13-2   Nutrition Assessment of the HIV-Infected Individual

Area of Concern	Significant Findings
Protein-Energy Malnutrition (PEM)	*History* Nutrient losses caused by diarrhea, malabsorption (from AIDS enteropathy, GI infections, medications), vomiting; increased needs because of infection and fever; poor intake caused by anorexia (related to respiratory or other infections, depression, medications), oral and esophageal pain (e.g., *Candida* or herpes esophagitis, endotracheal Kaposi's sarcoma), dyspnea, dysphagia, distorted sense of taste, related to medication use of zinc deficiency, dementia, or CNS infections *Physical Examination* Recent weight loss; weight <90% of desirable or BMI <18.5, or decline in percentiles for height or weight on growth chart for children; wasting of muscle and subcutaneous tissue; triceps skinfold <5th percentile *Laboratory Analysis* ↓ Serum albumin, transferrin, or prealbumin; negative nitrogen balance; ↓ creatinine-height index
Mineral Deficiencies Iron (Fe)	*History* Poor intake (same causes as PEM); increased losses or impaired utilization caused by medications such as pentamidine, amphotericin B, foscarnet *Physical Examination* Pallor, spoon-shaped nails, fatigue, tachycardia

Table 13-2 Nutrition Assessment of the HIV-Infected
Individual—cont'd

Area of Concern	Significant Findings
Zinc (Zn)	*Laboratory Analysis* ↓ Hct, Hgb, MCV, serum ferritin *History* Poor intake (same reasons as PEM); impaired absorption in diarrhea *Physical Examination* Poor sense of taste, distorted taste, delayed wound healing, alopecia, dermatitis, diarrhea *Laboratory Analysis* ↓ Serum Zn
Vitamin Deficiencies A	*History* Decreased absorption as a result of diarrhea; poor intake because of anorexia, nausea, vomiting *Physical Examination* Drying of skin and cornea; papular eruption around hair follicles *Laboratory Analysis* ↓ Serum retinol; ↓ retinol-binding protein (indicating PEM, with inadequate protein to manufacture carrier for vitamin A)
B_{12}	*History* Poor intake because of poverty, difficulty chewing protein foods, vegetarian diet, anorexia; impaired absorption; diarrhea *Physical Examination* Pallor, glossitis, fatigue, paresthesias *Laboratory Analysis* ↓ Hct; ↑ MCV; ↓ serum vitamin B_{12}

Continued

Table 13-2   Nutrition Assessment of the HIV-Infected
Individual—cont'd

Area of Concern	Significant Findings
Folate	*History* Poor intake of fruits and vegetables because of mouth soreness, unconventional diet, poverty, anorexia; impaired absorption because of trimethoprim-sulfamethoxazole or pentamidine use *Physical Examination* Pallor, glossitis, fatigue *Laboratory Analysis* ↓ Hct; ↑ MCV; ↓ serum or RBC folate
Dyslipidemia	*History* Highly active antiretroviral therapy, especially protease inhibitor therapy *Physical Examination* Fat loss in the extremities with truncal fat accumulation *Laboratory Analysis* ↑ Triglycerides, ↓ HDL cholesterol
Glucose Intolerance	*History* Highly active antiretroviral therapy, especially protease inhibitor therapy *Physical Examination* Fat loss in the extremities with truncal fat accumulation *Laboratory Analysis* ↑ Fasting and postprandial plasma glucose

- Acute episodes of diarrhea may be better controlled if antidiarrheals are administered on a routine schedule rather than after diarrhea occurs.
- Antiemetic medications (if ordered) should be scheduled to be taken before mealtimes.

- Small, frequent meals are usually best tolerated if dyspnea is present, and foods of high energy density (cheese, meats, muffins, vegetables with sauces, etc.) are preferable to foods with low energy density (raw green leafy vegetables, no- or low-calorie beverages, etc.). If oxygen is needed, use of a nasal cannula during meals often improves eating ability.

- Individuals with dementia or neurologic dysfunction may need to be reminded and encouraged to eat. Occupational therapists can assist in evaluating patients with motor problems and selecting special eating utensils that can improve their ability to feed themselves. Those who cannot feed themselves should be fed in a calm, unhurried manner, with family members or friends being involved whenever possible.

- A daily multivitamin and mineral supplement that supplies 100% of the DRI is commonly recommended. Some treatment centers also recommend increased supplementation with vitamins C, B_{12}, B_6, and E, as well as zinc, selenium, and beta-carotene, either because they may be poorly absorbed or because needs (especially of antioxidant nutrients) may be increased. The impact of potential drug-nutrient interactions (see below and Appendix H) must be considered, especially if the individual is taking several drugs, and the supplementation regimens must be adjusted accordingly.

Specialized nutrition support

A variety of oral nutritional supplements (see Table 8-1) are available for patients with difficulty consuming an adequate diet from regular food. HAART involves numerous doses of medication daily. Taking oral medications with an oral nutritional supplement (unless the medication should be taken without food [see Drug-Nutrient Interactions in the following text]) offers several opportunities daily to obtain extra nutrients.

For patients who cannot consume or absorb enough nutrients administered orally, enteral or parenteral (TPN) feedings may be necessary. The enteral route is preferred whenever possible because it is less likely to be associated with sepsis, more economical, and possibly more effective in maintaining normal GI mucosa and immune function, an important barrier to infection. TPN may be necessary if the GI tract is nonfunctional or the energy requirements are so high that they cannot be met entirely via the enteral route. Careful attention to infection control measures is important during both enteral and parenteral feedings (as is the case in all patients, not just those with HIV infection; see Chapters 8 and 9).

Individuals with malabsorption usually tolerate enteral tube feedings better if they are given continuously or slowly delivered intermittently rather than as bolus feedings. Formulas that are low in total fat or those in which a substantial portion of the fat is in the form of medium-chain triglycerides (MCTs) are likely to be better absorbed than formulas that are rich in long-chain triglycerides (see Table 8-1). Where oral or esophageal infections are present, the patient may be unable to tolerate a nasogastric, nasoduodenal, or nasojejunal tube. Gastrostomy or jejunostomy feedings may be more appropriate.

Complications of the infection and therapy

Many of the disease- and drug-related symptoms (anorexia, nausea and vomiting, stomatitis and esophagitis, dysphagia, neutropenia, diarrhea) are similar to those in the person with cancer. Interventions for these problems are summarized in Box 12-2.

Drug-nutrient interactions

In addition to the general side effects of the antiretroviral drugs, some of the drugs are associated with specific drug-nutrient interactions. These include the following:

- *Indinavir:* Increases the risk of renal *lithiasis* (stones). Adults taking this drug must consume a minimum of 1500 ml fluid daily to reduce the risk.
- *Didanosine powder:* Supplies 1380 mg sodium per single dose packet (100, 167, or 250 mg). The tablet form may be preferable for the patient needing a sodium-restricted diet.
- *Didanosine tablets:* Contain 36.5 mg phenylalanine/200 mg tablet, and this must be considered if the individual has phenylketonuria (PKU; inability to metabolize phenylalanine).
- *Amprenavir:* Contains several times the DRI for vitamin E. The total amount of vitamin E in the recommended daily adult dose of amprenavir is 1167 mg (compared with an adult DRI of approximately 15 mg); 1 ml of the oral suspension (used for small children) contains approximately 5 times the DRI for this age group. Patients should be cautioned not to take supplemental vitamin E if taking this drug.

Taking antiretroviral agents with food, or with specific dietary components, may alter absorption and metabolism of the drugs. Patients receiving these drugs need to be aware of the following drug and food relationships:

- *Amprenavir:* Do not take with a high-fat meal, which reduces absorption.
- *Didanosine:* Do not take with food, which can reduce absorption as much as 50%.
- *Indinavir:* Take on an empty stomach or after a small meal. A meal high in energy, fat, and protein may significantly decrease absorption of the drug. Do not take with grapefruit, which alters drug metabolism.
- *Ritonavir:* Take with food, which increases drug absorption.
- *Stavudine:* Take at least 2 hours before a meal; a high-fat meal can reduce absorption.
- *Tenofovir:* Take with a meal, which increases the bioavailability of the drug.
- *Zalcitabine:* Avoid taking with food, which reduces absorption.
- *Zidovudine:* Avoid taking with a high-fat meal, which reduces absorption.

Lipodystrophy

With more successful combination therapy, many individuals with HIV infection are experiencing weight gain rather than rapid weight loss during therapy. Unfortunately this weight may not reflect an increase in lean body mass but instead may represent an increase in fat. Protease inhibitors have been associated with **lipodystrophy syndrome** (redistribution of body fat, particularly accumulation of fat in the truncal region, accompanied by wasting of fat in the extremities). This creates body image disturbances for some patients and may cause them to discontinue the medication. Unfortunately, lipodystrophy is associated with elevated triglyceride levels, insulin resistance, and diabetes. Hyperglycemia and diabetes is especially common with use of abacavir, amprenavir, and delaverdine; hypertriglyceridemia is most frequently found during use of abacavir, delaverdine, and ritonavir. Patients taking protease inhibitors must be regularly screened for lipid abnormalities and hyperglycemia. Nutrition and lifestyle modifications are summarized briefly in the following text and described more fully in Chapters 14 and 17.

- Both hypertriglyceridemia and insulin resistance/diabetes
  - Be moderately physically active, as tolerated, daily or almost every day. (See Chapter 5 for estimates of energy expenditure during physical activity; try to increase activity enough to use at least an additional 200 kcal daily.)
  - Choose a diet rich in both soluble (viscous) and insoluble fiber, and add psyllium or other fiber supplements if needed to make a total of at least 25 to 30 g of fiber daily.
  - Limit high-fat and high-energy foods that are low in nutritional value (e.g., snack foods, pastries, doughnuts, cakes).
  - Choose a diet adequate in protein. Vegetable protein sources (e.g., legumes; vegetable burgers, sausages, and ground meat substitutes) are especially beneficial because they tend to be good sources of fiber, as well as relatively low in fat.
  - Consume at least five to 10 servings of fruits and vegetables daily.
  - Determine energy needs (e.g., estimate with calculations in Box 2-5). Monitor weight frequently and adjust energy intake as needed to maintain or achieve a desirable BMI (inside back cover).
- Insulin resistance/diabetes
  - Use carbohydrate counting to individualize dietary intake, consuming an energy intake calculated to maintain or achieve desirable weight.
  - Divide dietary carbohydrate into three or more meals or snacks and spread it throughout the day rather than consuming it in one or two large meals.
- Hypertriglyceridemia
  - Limit intake of carbohydrates, particularly sugars and sweets.
  - Avoid alcohol. If this is not acceptable to the patient, alcohol use should be infrequent and low in volume (never more than one drink daily for women or two drinks for men).
  - Increase intake of monounsaturated fat (e.g., olive, canola, and high oleic forms of sunflower and safflower oils; almonds; hazelnuts; and avocados) if the reduction in carbohydrate intake makes energy intake too low.

Complementary and alternative medical (CAM) therapies

Use of **complementary** and **alternative medical (CAM) therapies** is very common among individuals with HIV. Health care providers need to familiarize themselves with the types of therapies being used in order to evaluate them and give informed advice. Many CAM treatments have not been evaluated in large-scale trials, and therefore their risks and benefits are not fully known. Brief descriptions of some popular CAM therapies follow (see also Box 12-3):

- *Vitamin and/or other micronutrient supplements:* Most studies have been short-term and have shown no effect on lymphocyte markers. However, in a long-term study of HIV-infected individuals, being in the quartile with the highest intakes of B vitamins and carotene was a predictor of survival. Chronic vitamin A intakes >50,000 IU/day can be toxic and should be avoided.
- *Exercise:* Some short-term studies have found a trend toward an increase in natural killer activity and CD4 counts with regular exercise. Exercise may also stabilize or increase lean body mass. Weight training, or a combination of aerobic exercise and weight training, appears to be more effective than aerobics alone.
- *Massage:* Massage does not appear to have any consistent benefit on markers of disease progression, but it has been effective in stress relief.
- *Chinese herbs and acupuncture:* Several Chinese herbs are used, with or without acupuncture. These therapies have afforded symptom relief to some patients. Ginseng is undergoing further study for possible immune-enhancing effects. Ephedra-containing compounds, including the popular product "ma huang," are banned in the United States because of instances of toxicity (hypertension, stroke, seizures, and death).
- *Other herbal treatments:* Echinacea (coneflower) is reported to enhance immune function. Thus far, it has shown little benefit in prevention of respiratory infections, but it may shorten the duration of colds.

In one large-scale survey, 50% of individuals with HIV were using one or more forms of CAM, and 26% of patients using these therapies had not told their health care providers about their CAM use (Hsiao et al., 2003). Nearly 30% of CAM usage involved herbal therapies or megadoses of vitamins. These are of concern because of possible toxicity and also because of potential interactions with conventional retroviral therapy (e.g., St. John's wort, an herbal treatment for depression, decreases blood levels of indinavir). The health care provider should question each patient in detail about use of CAM therapies.

Safe handling practices for food

Infection with food-borne organisms is 20 to 300 times more common in individuals with HIV than in the general population, and these infections are more likely to lead to sepsis and other severe complications in HIV-infected patients. Individuals with HIV and their caregivers need instruction in choosing, preparing, and storing foods carefully. Appendix K summarizes important food safety guidelines. Food safety information specifically prepared for the individual with AIDS is also available from the FDA Center for Food Safety and Nutrition website (http://www.cfsan.fda.gov) and the food information hotline (800-FDA-4010).

Summary

HIV treatment is a complicated process requiring numerous therapeutic agents taken one or more times daily. Optimal antiviral therapy may conflict with the nutrition care plan. For example, the dyspneic individual may be able to eat more if he/she consumes small amounts frequently, but many of the antiretroviral agents are better absorbed if not taken when there is food in the stomach. Individualization of the therapeutic regimen is vital to maximize quality of life and response to therapy.

References

Hsiao AF et al: Complementary and alternative medicine use and substitution for conventional therapy by HIV-infected patients, *J Acquir Immune Defic Syndr* 33:157, 2003.

Selected Bibliography

Batterham MJ, Garsia R, Greenop P: Prevalence and predictors of HIV-associated weight loss in the era of highly active antiretroviral therapy, *Int J STD AIDS* 13:744, 2002.

Chen D, Misra A, Garg A: Clinical review 153: Lipodystrophy in human immunodeficiency virus-infected patients, *J Clin Endocrinol Metab* 87: 4845, 2002.

Earthman CP et al: Body cell mass repletion and improved quality of life in HIV-infected individuals receiving oxandrolone, *J Parenter Enteral Nutr* 26:357, 2002.

Fawzi WW et al: Randomized trial of vitamin supplements in relation to transmission of HIV-1 through breastfeeding and early child mortality, *AIDS* 16:1935, 2002.

Hendricks KM et al: High-fiber diet in HIV-positive men is associated with lower risk of developing fat deposition, *Am J Clin Nutr* 78:790, 2003.

Knox TA et al: Assessment of nutritional status, body composition, and human immunodeficiency virus-associated morphologic changes, *Clin Infect Dis* 36:S63, 2003.

Nerad J et al: General nutrition management in patients infected with human immunodeficiency virus, *Clin Infect Dis* 36:S52, 2003.

Risa KJ et al: Alternative therapy use in HIV-infected patients receiving highly active antiretroviral therapy, *Int J STD AIDS* 13:706, 2002.

Tang AM et al: Weight loss and survival in HIV-positive patients in the era of highly active antiretroviral therapy, *J Acquir Immune Defic Syndr* 31:230-236, 2002.

Heart Disease 14

Heart disease, the leading cause of death in the United States, encompasses a variety of conditions, including coronary heart disease, hypertension, and congestive heart failure.

Coronary Heart Disease

Pathophysiology

Coronary heart disease (CHD) occurs when plaques containing lipoproteins, cholesterol, tissue debris, and calcium form on the intima, or interior surface of blood vessels. The plaques roughen the intima, and platelets are attracted to the roughened areas, forming clots. When the plaques enlarge sufficiently to occlude the blood flow, tissues distal to the occlusion are deprived of oxygen and nutrients, creating an area of infarct. CHD is manifested when a myocardial infarction (MI) occurs or when myocardial ischemia is present, causing the painful disorder known as *angina pectoris*.

Serum cholesterol is carried by several **lipoproteins** classified by their density. In order of increasing density, the lipoproteins are **chylomicrons**, **very-low-density lipoproteins (VLDLs)**, **low-density lipoproteins (LDLs)**, and **high-density lipoproteins (HDLs)**. LDLs carry the most cholesterol and are the most closely correlated with CHD. HDLs reduce the risk from CHD by transporting cholesterol from the tissues to the liver, where it is metabolized and excreted. Total cholesterol levels <200 mg/dl are desirable, with levels between 200 and 239 mg/dl being borderline high and levels of 240 mg/dl or greater being high. However, the LDL cholesterol level is a more specific indicator of CHD risk than total cholesterol is. LDL cholesterol levels can be categorized as follows: *optimal*, <100 mg/dl; *near optimal* or *above* *optimal*, 100 to 129 mg/dl; *borderline high*, 130 to 159 mg/dl; *high*, 160 to 189 mg/dl; and *very high*, ≥190 mg/dl. LDL cholesterol is directly related to risk of CHD, but the Adult Treatment Panel III of the National Cholesterol Education Program (ATP III [*Third Report of the National Cholesterol Education Program (NCEP) Expert Panel on Detection, Evaluation, and Treatment of High Blood Cholesterol in Adults (Adult Treatment Panel III)*, 2002]) recognizes other factors that increase risk. These include the presence of known CHD or a CHD risk equivalent (e.g., peripheral vascular disease). Diabetes is classified as a CHD risk equivalent. Other risk factors include: (1) cigarette smoking, (2) hypertension (blood pressure ≥140/90 mm Hg or use of an antihypertensive medication), (3) low HDL cholesterol (<40 mg/dl for males or <50 mg/dl for females), (4) family history of premature CHD (CHD in male first-degree relative before age 55; CHD in female first-degree relative before age 65), (5) age (≥45 years in men and ≥55 years in women. On the other hand, if high HDL-cholesterol (≥60 mg/dl) is present, then one risk factor can be deducted from the individual's total count. Goals for therapy are determined based on the presence or absence of risk factors, as shown in Table 14-1.

Prevention and Treatment

An elevated LDL cholesterol level is the primary target of therapy. The initial approach to elevated LDL cholesterol involves **therapeutic lifestyle changes** (TLC). These changes are described in more detail below. If the goal for LDL cholesterol has not been achieved after an appropriate trial of TLC (~3 months), drug therapy may be initiated. Drugs used include the HMG CoA reductase inhibitors (statins) that inhibit cholesterol synthesis; the bile acid sequestrants cholestyramine and colestipol; nicotinic acid, which lowers total and LDL cholesterol, as well as triglycerides; and fibric acid derivatives such as gemfibrozil and clofibrate, which reduce triglycerides and raise HDL cholesterol. Additionally, the presence of the metabolic syndrome, defined as three or more of the following findings—abdominal obesity (waist circumference >40 inches in men or >35 inches in women), glucose intolerance (fasting glucose >110 mg/dl), BP >130/85 mm Hg, high triglycerides (>150 mg/dl), or low HDL (<40 mg/dl in men or <50 mg/dl in women)—increases the degree of risk. More aggressive weight control measures and

Table 14-1   LDL Cholesterol Goals for Risk Levels

Risk Level	LDL Cholesterol Goal
CHD or CHD risk equivalent	<100 mg/dl
Multiple (2+) risk factors*	<130 mg/dl†
0-1 risk factors*	<160 mg/dl

From Adult Treatment Panel (ATP) III. *Third Report of the National Cholesterol Education Program (NCEP) Expert Panel on Detection, Evaluation, and Treatment of High Blood Cholesterol in Adults (Adult Treatment Panel III),* Washington, 2002, National Institutes of Health, National Heart, Lung and Blood Institute.
CHD, Coronary heart disease; *LDL,* low-density lipoprotein.

*When HDL cholesterol is ≥60 mg/dl, deduct 1 risk factor.
†When the risk of "hard" CHD (myocardial infarction or death from CHD) within 10 years is >20%, the LDL cholesterol goal is <100 mg/dl. The 10-year risk is determined by the number and type of risk factors. An online/downloadable version of the risk calculator is available at *http://nhlbi.nih.gov/health/prof/heart/index.htm.*

increases in physical activity may be needed to combat the metabolic syndrome.

Nutritional Care

LDL cholesterol is the primary target, and therefore the primary goal of care is to achieve LDL cholesterol levels associated with low risk (see Table 14-1). An elevated triglyceride level is an independent risk factor for CHD, as is the presence of the metabolic syndrome. Therefore, if they are present, they are also a target of therapy.

Assessment

Assessment is summarized in Table 14-2. The MEDFICTS (Meats, Eggs, Dairy, Frying foods, In baked goods, Convenience foods, Table fats, Snacks) assessment tool (Box 14-1) has been developed by the ATP III to provide a score indicating how closely an individual's diet approximates the TLC diet and identifying areas needing change.

Intervention and teaching

Therapeutic lifestyle changes

The therapeutic lifestyle changes (TLC), developed by the ATP III (2002), provide a plan for lowering cardiovascular risk. The TLC

Text continued on p. 385

Table 14-2   Assessment in Heart Disease

Area of Concern	Significant Findings
Overweight/ obesity	*History* Excessive energy intake; sedentary lifestyle *Physical Examination* Wt >120% of desirable or BMI >25; triceps skinfold >95th percentile for age and sex
Underweight (seen primarily in congestive heart failure)	*History* Poor intake because of dyspnea or fatigue; impaired absorption because of inadequate bowel perfusion; increased energy needs if dyspneic or suffering from concomitant infection *Physical Examination* Wt <90% of desirable or BMI <18.5 or BMI height, or weight <5th percentile for age (children); triceps skinfold <5th percentile for age and sex
Elevated serum lipid levels	*History* Daily use of foods high in saturated fat and cholesterol; sedentary lifestyle; family history of hyperlipidemia; diabetes *Physical Examination* Xanthomas, or yellowish plaques deposited on the skin Laboratory Analysis ↑ Total serum cholesterol; HDL <40 mg/dl; LDL >130 mg/dl
Elevated blood pressure	*History* Daily use of high-sodium (processed) foods and salt at the table; psychosocial stress; family history of hypertension; obesity; excessive alcohol intake; diabetes *Physical Examination* Edema; elevated blood pressure

Box 14-1   MEDFICTS Dietary Assessment Questionnaire

In each food category for both Group 1 and Group 2 foods, check one box from the "Weekly Consumption" column (number of servings eaten per week) and then check one box from the "Serving Size" column. If you check Rarely/Never, do not check a serving size box. See p. 386 for score.

| Food Category | Weekly Consumption | | | Serving Size | | | Score |
	Rarely/ never	3 or less	4 or more	Small <5 oz/d 1 pt	Average 5 oz/d 2 pts	Large >5 oz/d 3 pts	
Meats ▪ Recommended amount per day: ≤5 oz (equal in size to 2 decks of playing cards). ▪ Base your estimate on the food you consume most often. ▪ Beef and lamb selections are trimmed to ⅛" fat.							
Group 1. 10 g or more total fat in 3 oz cooked portion **Beef** – Ground beef, ribs, steak (T-bone, flank, porterhouse,	☐	☐ 3 pts	☐ 7 pts ×	☐ 1 pt	☐ 2 pts	☐ 3 pts	————

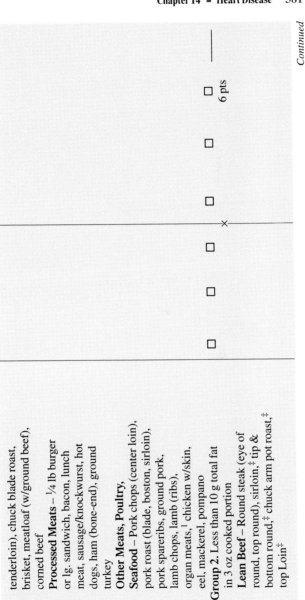

tenderloin), chuck blade roast, brisket, meatloaf (w/ground beef), corned beef

Processed Meats – ¼ lb burger or lg. sandwich, bacon, lunch meat, sausage/knockwurst, hot dogs, ham (bone-end), ground turkey

Other Meats, Poultry, Seafood – Pork chops (center loin), pork roast (blade, boston, sirloin), pork spareribs, ground pork, lamb chops, lamb (ribs), organ meats,¹ chicken w/skin, eel, mackerel, pompano

Group 2. Less than 10 g total fat in 3 oz cooked portion

Lean Beef – Round steak (eye of round, top round), sirloin,‡ tip & bottom round,‡ chuck arm pot roast,‡ top Loin‡

6 pts

Continued

Box 14-1   MEDFICTS Dietary Assessment Questionnaire—cont'd

Low-Fat Processed Meats—Low-fat lunch meat, Canadian bacon, "lean" fast food sandwich, boneless ham

Other Meats, Poultry,

Seafood—Chicken, turkey (w/o skin),[§] most seafood,[†] lamb leg shank, pork tenderloin, sirloin top loin, veal cutlets, sirloin, shoulder, ground veal, venison, veal chops and ribs,[†] lamb (whole leg, loin, fore-shank, sirloin)[‡]

Eggs—Weekly consumption is the number of times you eat eggs each week. Check the number of eggs eaten each time.

						≤1	2	≥3	Score
Group 1. Whole eggs, yolks	☐	☐ 3 pts	☐	☐ 7 pts	×	☐ 1 pt	☐ 2 pts	☐ 3 pts	___
Group 2. Egg whites, egg substitutes (½ cup)	☐		☐						___

Dairy

Milk—Average serving 1 cup

						≤1	2	≥3	Score
Group 1. Whole milk, 2% milk, 2% buttermilk, yogurt (whole milk)	☐	☐ 3 pts	☐	☐ 7 pt	×	☐ 1 pt	☐ 2 pts	☐ 3 pts	___

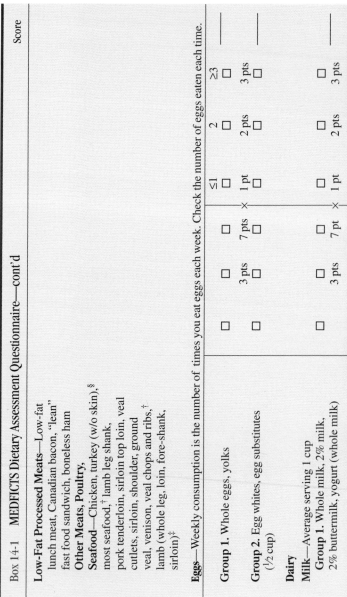

Food					×			
Group 2. Fat-free milk, 1% milk, fat-free buttermilk, yogurt (Fat-free, 1% low fat)	☐	☐	☐	☐		☐	☐	☐
Cheese—Average serving 1 oz								
Group 1. Cream cheese, Cheddar, Monterey Jack, colby, Swiss, American processed, blue cheese, regular cottage cheese (½ cup), and ricotta (¼ cup)	☐	☐	☐ 3 pts	☐ 7 pts	×	☐ 1 pt	☐ 2 pts	☐ 3 pts
Group 2. Low-fat & fat-free cheeses, Fat-free milk mozzarella, string cheese, low-fat, fat-free milk & fat-free cottagecheese (½ cup) and ricotta (¼ cup)	☐	☐	☐	☐	×	☐	☐	☐
Frozen Desserts—Average serving ½ cup								
Group 1. Ice cream, milk shakes	☐	☐	☐ 3 pts	☐ 7 pts	×	☐ 1 pt	☐ 2 pts	☐ 3 pts
Group 2. Low-fat ice cream, frozen yogurt	☐	☐						
Frying Foods—Average servings: see below. This section refers to method of preparation for vegetables and meal.								
Group 1. French fries, fried vegetables (½ cup), fried chicken, fish, meat (3 oz)	☐	☐	☐ 3 pts	☐ 7 pts	×	☐ 1 pt	☐ 2 pts	☐ 3 pts

Continued

Box 14-1   MEDFICTS Dietary Assessment Questionnaire—cont'd

							Score
Group 2. Vegetables, not deep fried (½ cup), meat, poultry, or fish—prepared by baking, broiling, grilling, poaching, roasting, stewing: (3 oz)	☐	☐	☐	☐	☐	☐	—
In Baked Goods—1 Average serving							
Group 1. Doughnuts, biscuits, butter rolls, muffins, croissants, sweet rolls, Danish, cakes, pies, coffee cakes, cookies	☐	☐ 3 pts	☐ 7 pts ×	☐ 1 pt	☐ 2 pts	☐ 3 pts	—
Group 2. Fruit bars, low-fat cookies/cakes/ pastries, angel food cake, homemade baked goods with vegetable oils, breads, bagels	☐	☐	☐	☐	☐	☐	—
Convenience Foods							
Group 1. Canned, packaged, or frozen dinners; e.g., pizza (1 slice), macaroni & cheese (1 cup), pot pie (1), cream soups (1 cup), potato, rice & pasta dishes with cream/cheese sauces (½ cup)	☐	☐ 3 pts	☐ 7 pts ×	☐ 1 pt	☐ 2 pts	☐ 3 pts	—

	☐	☐	×	☐	☐	☐
Group 2. Diet/reduced calorie or reduced fat dinners (1), potato, rice & pasta dishes without cream/cheese sauces (½ cup)	☐	☐		☐	☐	☐
Table Fats—Average serving: 1 Tbsp						
Group 1. Butter, stick margarine, regular salad dressing, mayonnaise, sour cream (2 Tbsp)	☐ 3 pts	☐ 7 pts	×	☐ 1 pt	☐ 2 pts	☐ 3 pts
Group 2. Diet and tub margarine, low-fat & fat-free salad dressing, low-fat & fat-free mayonnaise	☐	☐		☐	☐	☐
Snacks						
Group 1. Chips (potato, corn, taco), cheese puffs, snack mix, nuts (1 oz), regular crackers (½ oz), candy (milk chocolate, caramel, coconut) (about 1½ oz), regular popcorn (3 cups)	☐ 3 pts	☐ 7 pts	×	☐ 1 pt	☐ 2 pts	☐ 3 pts

Continued

Box 14-1 MEDFICTS Dietary Assessment Questionnaire—cont'd						Score
Group 2. Pretzels, fat-free chips (1 oz), low-fat crackers (½ oz), fruit, fruit rolls, licorice, hard candy (1 med piece), bread sticks (1-2 pcs), air-popped or low-fat popcorn (3 cups)	☐	☐	☐	☐	☐	——
					Final score ——

From *Third Report of the National Cholesterol Program (NCEP) Expert Panel on Detection, Evaluation, and Treatment of High Blood Cholesterol in Adults (ATP III).* Washington, DC: 2002, NIH, NHLBI.

† Organ meats, shrimp, abalone, and squid are low in fat but high in cholesterol.
‡ Only lean cuts with all visible fat trimmed. If not trimmed of all visible fat, score as if in Group 1.
‡ Score 6 pts if this box is checked.
§ All parts not listed in group 1 have <10 g total fat.

To Score: For each food category, multiply points in weekly consumption box by points in serving size box and record total in score column. If Group 2 foods checked, no points are scored (except for Group 2 meats, large serving = 6 pts).

Example:

☐	☑	×	☐	☐	☑		21 pts
3 pts	7 pts		1 pt	2 pts	3 pts	21 pts	——

Add all scores to get final score.

Key:
≥70 Need to make some dietary changes
40-70 Heart-healthy diet
<40 TLC diet

dietary changes require individualized counseling. A registered dietitian is the professional best prepared to provide the detailed diet counseling needed, although physicians and nurses working with individuals with CHD or risk for CHD should thoroughly understand the diet principles. The components of the TLC are as follows:

- Macronutrient intakes
  - Dietary fat: 25% to 35% of total energy intake
    - This moderate level of fat intake is recommended because very-low-fat diets usually require increases in carbohydrate intake that may worsen hypertriglyceridemia.
    - Monounsaturated fats supply up to 20% of total energy intake. Good sources are olive oil, canola (rapeseed) oil, and the high oleic forms of safflower and sunflower oil; almonds; hazelnuts; pecans; peanuts; and peanut butter. (The ingredient labels of safflower and sunflower oils usually state "high oleic" if the oil is that type.) Avocado is a fair source of monounsaturated fat.
    - Polyunsaturated fats supply up to 10% of total energy intake. Good sources are sunflower, soybean, cottonseed, and corn oils; walnuts and walnut oil; pecans; and fish oils.
    - Omega-3 (n-3) fatty acids from fish should be consumed frequently. The TLC does not specify a level of omega-3 intake, but the American Heart Association (AHA) recommends that individuals with CHD consume ~1 g/day of omega-3 fatty acids, preferably from oily fish (Table 14-3). Because this amount may be difficult for many individuals to consume in their diets, the AHA suggests that fish oil supplements providing eicosapentanenoic acid (EPA) and docosahexaenoic acid (DHA) be considered in consultation with the physician (Kris-Etherton et al., 2002). Most commercially prepared fried fish (in restaurants and frozen convenience items) is low in omega-3 fatty acids. Certain vegetable oils (e.g., canola, walnut, flaxseed [linseed], and soybean) are also sources of omega-3 fatty acids, and they can be encouraged. However, the omega-3 fatty acids they contain are not EPA and DHA, and it is not known if the benefits from these oils are the same as those from fish.

Table 14-3   Omega-3 (n-3) Fatty Acids in Fish

Type of Fish	Omega-3 (EPA and DHA), in g
Salmon, Atlantic	2.1
Herring, Atlantic	2.1
Salmon, pink, canned	1.7
Tuna, bluefin	1.3
Mackerel, Atlantic	1.3
Trout, rainbow	1.1
Sardines, oil-canned	1.0
Tuna, water-canned, white	0.9
Bass, freshwater	0.8
Halibut	0.6
Sole/flounder	0.5
Crab, Alaskan king	0.4
Shrimp	0.3
Catfish, farmed	0.2
Tuna, water-canned, light	0.2

Data are derived from the USDA National Nutrient Database, SR 15. Accessed May 15, 2003 at *www.nutrition.gov.*

Values are for 100 g (~3 oz) servings of broiled, steamed, or baked fish (except where canned is specified).

- The combination of saturated and *trans* fat provide no more than 7% of total energy. Dietary cholesterol should be no more than 200 mg/day. Table 14-4 describes the foods to choose more often and those to choose less often to comply with these guidelines. Partially hydrogenated fats (stick margarines and shortening) contain *trans* forms of fatty acids, rather than the *cis* forms more common in nature (see Figure 1-1). *Trans*–fatty acids raise LDL cholesterol even more than saturated fats do. Liquid vegetable oil, soft (tub) margarine, and *trans*–fatty acid–free margarine are preferable to butter, stick margarine, and shortening.
- The American Heart Association recommends that all Americans *without* CHD, diabetes, or high LDL cholesterol concentrations consume a diet providing no more than 10% of energy as saturated and *trans* fats and no more than 300 mg of cholesterol per day, in order to reduce the risk of developing CHD at a later date.

Table 14-4 Guide to Therapeutic Lifestyle Changes (TLC)

	Healthy Lifestyle Recommendations for a Healthy Heart		
Food Items to Choose More Often	Food Items to Choose Less Often	Recommendations for Weight Reduction	Recommendations for Increased Physical Activity
Breads and Cereals ≥6 servings per day, adjusted to caloric needs Breads, cereals, especially whole grain; pasta; rice; potatoes; dry beans and peas; low fat crackers and cookies **Vegetables** 3-5 servings per day fresh, frozen, or canned, without added fat, sauce, or salt **Fruits** 2-4 servings per day fresh, frozen, canned, dried	**Breads and Cereals** Many bakery products, including doughnuts, biscuits, butter rolls, muffins, croissants, sweet rolls, Danish, cakes, pies, coffee cakes, cookies Many grain-based snacks, including chips, cheese puffs, snack mix, regular crackers, buttered popcorn **Vegetables** Vegetables fried or	**Weigh Regularly** Record weight, BMI, & waist circumference **Lose Weight Gradually** Goal: lose 10% of body weight in 6 months. Lose ½ to 1 lb per week **Develop Healthy Eating Patterns** ■ Choose healthy foods (see Column 1) ■ Reduce intake of foods in Column 2 ■ Limit number of eating	**Make Physical Activity Part of Daily Routines** ■ Reduce sedentary time ■ Walk, wheel, or bike-ride more, or drive less; take the stairs instead of an elevator; get off the bus a few stops early and walk the remaining distance; mow the lawn with a push mower; rake leaves; garden; push a stroller; clean the house; do exercises or pedal a stationary bike

Continued

Table 14-4   Guide to Therapeutic Lifestyle Changes (TLC)—cont'd

	Healthy Lifestyle Recommendations for a Healthy Heart		
Food Items to Choose More Often	Food Items to Choose Less Often	Recommendations for Weight Reduction	Recommendations for Increased Physical Activity
Dairy Products 2–3 servings per day Fat-free, 1/2%, 1% milk, buttermilk, yogurt, cottage cheese; fat-free & low-fat cheese **Eggs** ≤2 egg yolks per week Egg whites or egg substitute **Meat, Poultry, Fish** ≤5 oz per day Lean cuts: loin, leg, round; extra lean hamburger; cold cuts made with lean meat or soy protein; skinless poultry; fish	prepared with butter, cheese, or cream sauce **Fruits** Fruits fried or served with butter or cream **Dairy Products** Whole milk/2% milk, whole-milk yogurt, ice cream, cream, cheese **Eggs** Egg yolks, whole eggs **Meat, Poultry, Fish** Higher fat meat cuts; ribs, T-bone steak, regular hamburger,	occasions ■ Select sensible portion sizes ■ Avoid second helpings ■ Identify and reduce hidden fat by reading food labels to choose products lower in saturated fat and calories, and ask about ingredients in ready-to-eat foods prepared away from home ■ Identify and reduce sources of excess carbohydrates such as	while watching television; play actively with children; take a brisk 10-minute walk or wheel before work, during your work break, and after dinner **Make Physical Activity Part of Exercise or Recreational Activities** ■ Walk, wheel, or jog; bicycle or use an arm pedal bicycle; swim or do water aerobics; play basketball; Join a

Fats and Oils Amount adjusted to caloric level: unsaturated oils; soft or liquid margarines and vegetable oil spreads, salad dressings, seeds, and nuts **TLC Diet Options** Stanol/sterol-containing margarines; viscous fiber food sources: barley, oats, psyllium, apples, bananas, berries, citrus fruits, nectarines, peaches, pears, plums, prunes, broccoli, brussels sprouts, carrots, dry beans, peas, soy products (tofu, miso)	bacon, sausage; cold cuts; salami, bologna, hot dogs; organ meats; liver, brains, sweetbreads; poultry with skin; fried meat; fried poultry; fried fish **Fats and Oils** Butter, shortening, stick margarine, chocolate, coconut	fat-free and regular crackers; cookies and other desserts; snacks; and sugar-containing beverages	sports team; play wheelchair sports; golf (pull cart or carry clubs); canoe; cross-country ski; dance; take part in an exercise program at work, home, school, or gym

From *Third Report of the National Cholesterol Program (NCEP) Expert Panel on Detection Evaluation, and Treatment of High Blood Cholesterol in Adults (ATP III)*. Washington, 2002, NIH, NHLBI

- Carbohydrate: 50% to 60% of total energy intake
    - Whole grains, fruits, and vegetables are the most important sources of carbohydrate.
    - An intake of 20 to 30 g of dietary fiber daily is recommended.
- Protein: approximately 15% of total energy intake
    - Soy protein, along with the isoflavones and other phytochemicals naturally associated with it, has an LDL-cholesterol-lowering effect. Isoflavone supplements alone have not been found to be as effective. Therefore, the AHA recommends consumption of ≥25 g/day of soy protein (Erdman, 2000). One soy burger or sausage (~70 g) or 3 oz (85 g) of soy meat substitute (e.g., steak-style strips or ground beef substitute) provide ~11 to 13 g of soy protein. Soy milk and soy flour are other good sources of soy protein.
- The so-called Mediterranean diet, modeled after the traditional diet of Mediterranean countries, has been found in one large prospective study to reduce recurrence of myocardial infarction (MI) in patients that had had one MI (Kris-Etherton et al., 2001). The Mediterranean diet emphasizes fruits; vegetables; breads and other grains; potatoes, beans, nuts, and seeds. Olive oil, which is rich in monounsaturated fat, is an important component. Dairy products, fish, and poultry are included in low to moderate amounts, eggs are consumed zero to four times weekly, and there is little red meat. Wine is consumed in low to moderate amounts. Overall, fiber intake is higher than that in the traditional American diet, and saturated fat and cholesterol intakes are lower. This diet is similar to the TLC diet and the dietary guidelines of the American Heart Association. Research continues into the benefits offered by the Mediterranean diet pattern.
- Therapeutic options for LDL lowering. Motivated individuals or those requiring extra measures to lower their cholesterol to the target range may try these options.
    - Special margarines containing esters formed from plant *sterols* or *stanols* have been shown to reduce LDL cholesterol by decreasing the absorption of cholesterol. The esters are included in margarines because they require lipid to be soluble. Margarines that contain plant sterol/stanol esters are labeled with the amount. People who use these products

must be cautioned to adjust their intake of energy from other sources to compensate for the energy provided by the margarine. The recommended amount of sterols and stanols is approximately 2 g/day (ATP III, 2002; Lichtenstein & Deckelbaum, 2001). Gelcaps containing plant sterols are also available.

- Sterol/stanol esters reduce absorption of carotenoids, and people using them need to consume five or more servings daily of fruits and vegetables, including good sources of carotenoids (e.g., orange vegetables such as winter squash, pumpkin, and carrots; deep green leafy vegetables; peppers; tomatoes; and orange fruits such as cantaloupe, orange, tangerine, and papaya).
- Viscous, or soluble, fiber (10 to 25 g/day [ATP III, 2002]) has a cholesterol-lowering effect. Good sources of viscous fiber are listed in Box 14-2.

- Body weight goals
  - The patient should maintain a desirable body weight, gradually reduce weight, or prevent weight gain, as applicable. Figure 7-1 provides an algorithm for determining the appropriate weight control strategy, based on BMI.
  - BMI should be determined at every visit. Times when weight gain is likely (e.g., perimenopausal period, times of high life stress, smoking cessation) should be anticipated, and the patient should be counseled in advance regarding prevention of weight gain, and follow-up visits should be scheduled to evaluate success of weight control strategies.
  - Patients who are overweight need counseling regarding the benefits of a modest (10%) weight reduction. Lifestyle patterns that promote weight loss, portion control, and ways to obtain daily physical activity are part of teaching (see Chapter 7). Follow-up visits should be scheduled to evaluate weight and BMI and to discuss barriers to adherence to the plan. Weight reduction is an important part of lipid-lowering therapy, but emphasis on it may be delayed to avoid overwhelming the patient with too many lifestyle changes at once.
    - Once LDL-cholesterol-lowering measures are being implemented, an intensified focus on weight reduction and physical activity is warranted to reduce the features of the metabolic syndrome. Both weight reduction and physical activity improve insulin action. Moreover, weight control

---

Box 14-2   Good Dietary Sources of Viscous (Soluble) Fiber

3 or More g/Serving*

Psyllium seeds, ground, 1 tbsp
Lima or kidney beans, ½ cup
Brussels sprouts, ½ cup

1.5 to 2 g/Serving*

Citrus fruit (orange, grapefruit), 1 medium
Pears, 1 medium
Black, navy, or pinto beans, ½ cup
Northern beans, ½ cup
Prunes, ¼ cup

1 g/Serving

Barley, oatmeal, or oat bran, cooked, ½ cup
Apple, banana, or plum, 1 medium
Blackberries, ½ cup
Nectarine or peach, 1 medium
Lentils, chickpeas, black-eyed peas, ½ cup
Broccoli, ½ cup
Carrots, ½ cup

---

*Within these categories, foods with the highest viscous fiber content are listed first.

measures have been found to be effective in reducing abdominal fat stores, associated with the metabolic syndrome and **hepatic steatosis (nonalcoholic fatty liver disease).**
- Moderate physical activity sufficient to use at least 200 kcal (837 kJ) daily (see Table 5-3)
    - At least 30 minutes of moderate activity daily decreases cardiovascular risk.
    - The patient needs help in identifying ways to integrate physical activity into his/her lifestyle.
    - At follow-up visits, assess level of activity and discuss barriers to daily physical activity and ways to overcome these barriers.
- Other dietary measures that may reduce risk for CHD
    - Vitamin supplementation (folic acid and vitamins B_6 and B_{12})

- High plasma homocysteine concentrations have been associated with CHD risk in many, but not all, studies. Supplementation with folic acid and vitamins B_6 and B_{12} have been shown to lower homocysteine levels. Whether or not this reduces CHD is still under study, but certainly consuming the DRI for these vitamins daily can be recommended.
- Antioxidants
  - Oxidation of LDL appears to be involved in atherogenesis, but studies to date have not shown that supplementation with antioxidants is protective against CHD. Consuming the DRI for vitamins C and E is recommended.
  - Vitamin C needs of smokers are increased. The CHD risk from smoking is so great that every effort should be made to stop smoking. For those individuals who do smoke, a daily supplement providing the DRI of vitamin C is advisable, along with a diet rich in vitamin C sources (see Appendix A).
- Moderate intake of alcohol
  - Numerous studies indicate that there is reduced CHD risk in men over 45 years of age and women over 55 years of age with moderate alcohol intake. The type of alcohol consumed does not alter the results.
  - Advice to use alcohol should be given only after weighing the advantages and disadvantages. Alcohol abuse is common in the United States, and excessive intakes pose numerous health risks, including elevated blood pressure, dysrhythmia, acute pancreatitis, hypertriglyceridemia, and increased risk of breast cancer in women. Only middle-aged and older adults benefit from use of alcohol, and people who do not drink should not be encouraged to start in order to reduce CHD risk.
  - If alcohol is consumed, intakes should be no more than 1 drink daily for women and 2 for men. One drink is 5 oz (150 ml) of wine, 12 oz (360 ml) of beer, or 1.5 oz (45 ml) of 80-proof alcohol.
- Hypertriglyceridemia, in particular, is an independent risk factor for CHD. In addition to weight loss and increased activity, the following measures are recommended to reduce triglyceride concentrations:
  - Avoid alcohol intake. If this is not acceptable to the patient, intake should be limited as much as possible.

- Maintain a fat intake of ~30 to 35 g/day, emphasizing mono-unsaturated fats.
- Consume 3 g or more of omega-3 fatty acids daily. This level almost always requires supplementation.
- Avoid simple sugars; carbohydrates should be primarily complex (starches and fiber).

In a short-term trial, a diet low in saturated fat and supplemented with viscous fiber, plant sterols, and almonds was effective in lowering LDL-cholesterol and the inflammatory marker C-reactive protein (which is elevated in those at high risk for heart disease) as much as statin treatment, with none of the side effects that might be experienced with drug therapy (Jenkins et al., 2003). This underscores the potential for risk factor reduction with appropriate diet and lifestyle practices. Changes in diet and lifestyle may seem less overwhelming if people are counseled to make them gradually. For example, the transition from whole milk to skim milk may be easier if the individual first changes to 2% milk, and later to skim milk. Changes do not have to result in a restrictive or unpalatable diet (Table 14-5). Tasty, attractive meals can be prepared within the guidelines.

Eating away from home is likely to pose challenges for the person trying to follow the TLC diet. Some suggestions to make the experience easier include the following:

- Ask service personnel in restaurants about preparation methods and fat content of foods if this information is not clear from the menu.
- Avoid fried foods and large portions of red meats. Salads (with as few high-fat ingredients such as meat, cheese, or bacon bits as possible) or grilled items are preferable.
- Order foods without sauces, butter, and sour cream.
- Ask that salad dressings be served on the side, and use limited amounts, or request low-fat dressings.
- Choose small amounts of sunflower seeds and olives over high-saturated fat toppings such as bacon, chopped eggs, and cheese.
- Avoid eating everything if portions are large. Share with a companion, or plan to take some food home for another meal.
- Move away from buffet tables or other areas where food is available at parties.

Table 14-5   Dietary Changes to Reduce Risk of Heart Disease

Previous Intake	Revised Intake
Breakfast	*Breakfast*
Doughnut	Shredded wheat with sliced
Orange juice	banana (Fi, SF)*
Coffee	Grapefruit half (Fi)
Nondairy creamer	Coffee
	Skim milk (SF)
Lunch	*Lunch*
Quarter-pound	Grilled chicken sandwich
hamburger	(SF)
French fries, salted	Side salad with low-fat
Soft drink	dressing (Fi, SF, Na)
Fried fruit pie	Soft drink
	Dried fruit snack pack (SF,
	Fi, Na)
Snack	*Snack*
Chocolate bar	Trail mix with chocolate
	chips, unsalted nuts, and
	seeds (SF, Fi)
Dinner	*Dinner*
Prime rib	Herbed chicken (SF)
Baked potato with	Brown rice pilaf (SF, Fi, C)
sour cream	Green beans cooked with
Green beans cooked	thyme (Na)
with salt	Mixed greens with raspberry
Mixed greens with	vinaigrette (SF)
blue cheese dressing	Iced tea
Iced tea	
Snack	*Snack*
Fudge cake with icing	Blueberry-oatmeal crisp
Whole milk	(SF, Fi)
	Skim milk (SF, C)

*Abbreviations refer to reductions in cholesterol (C), saturated fat (SF), and sodium (Na) and an increase in fiber (Fi) intake.

Hypertension

Hypertension—defined as systolic blood pressure greater than 140 mm Hg or diastolic pressure greater than 90 mm Hg—affects approximately 50 million individuals in the United States. Systolic blood pressure between 120 and 139 mm Hg or diastolic blood pressure between 80 and 89 mm Hg is regarded as prehypertension and is a signal that the person is at risk for developing hypertension.

Pathophysiology

Increases in blood volume, heart rate, and peripheral vascular resistance can lead to hypertension, but a large percentage of cases are essential hypertension—that is, no cause is known. Nevertheless, it is clear that there is a close association of hypertension with cardiovascular disease (CVD). For each increment of 20 mm Hg in systolic blood pressure or 10 mm Hg in diastolic blood pressure, the risk of heart attack, heart failure, stroke, or kidney disease is doubled (National High Blood Pressure Education Program, 2003).

Treatment

Nutrition and lifestyle changes are key components in treatment of hypertension, as are an extensive list of pharmacologic agents. Drugs used in treatment of hypertension include diuretics, aldosterone receptor blockers, beta-adrenergic blocking agents, calcium channel blockers, angiotensin-converting enzyme (ACE) inhibitors, and angiotensin II antagonists. Commonly two or more drugs are used in treatment of hypertension, increasing the risk of drug-drug and drug-nutrient interactions.

Nutritional Care

The goal is to reduce blood pressure to normal if possible. Even if complete normalization is not achieved, every 2 mm Hg reduction in systolic blood pressure decreases the risk of heart disease by 5% and decreases the risk of stroke by 8%. Lifestyle changes, including diet modifications, can reduce blood pressure, enhance the response to drug therapy, and reduce CVD risk.

Assessment

Assessment is summarized in Table 14-2.

Intervention and teaching

Lifestyle changes to reduce blood pressure

The National High Blood Pressure Education Program (2003) states that specific lifestyle changes can reduce blood pressure; the program has provided the following estimates of the reduction in systolic blood pressure for each change:

- Weight reduction for individuals who are overweight or obese, 5 to 20 mm Hg decrease per 10 kg (22 lb) loss
- Adhering to the Dietary Approaches to Stop Hypertension (DASH) eating plan described below, 8 to 14 mm Hg
- Reducing sodium intake to no more than 100 mmol (2.4 g, equivalent to 6 g of sodium chloride) daily, 2 to 8 mm Hg
- Engaging in regular aerobic activity at least 30 minutes on most days of the week, 4 to 9 mm Hg
- Moderation of alcohol intake to no more than 2 drinks/day in men and 1 drink/day in women or small men, 2 to 4 mm Hg

Weight reduction. Overweight and insulin resistance are linked with hypertension in the metabolic syndrome. Although the obese individual may not achieve ideal body weight, even a 10 kg weight loss (or approximately 10%) can improve hypertension significantly. Chapter 7 provides more information about weight loss measures.

The DASH eating plan. The DASH plan is rich in fruits, vegetables, and low-fat dairy products and low in saturated fats and cholesterol. Red meats, sweets, and sugar-containing beverages are limited, with fish, poultry, nuts, and whole grains being encouraged. The resulting diet is high in calcium, magnesium, potassium, and fiber. Supplements of these nutrients alone, outside of the DASH diet, have not been found to be as successful at lowering blood pressure as the DASH diet itself. Table 14-6 shows the food choices encouraged in the DASH eating plan. The table shows an eating plan providing 2000 kcal/day, but the diet can easily be adapted to fewer or greater numbers of kcal by altering the numbers of servings. Gradual changes may be more successful than sudden, radical changes. In implementing the DASH diet, for instance, if the individual currently eats only one serving of vegetables daily, encourage him/her to add one serving at lunch and one at dinner. Once that habit has been established, progressively make other needed dietary changes.

Sodium restriction. The DASH diet itself is not a low-sodium diet, although the fruits, vegetables, and whole grains encouraged by the eating plan provide healthful, low-sodium food choices. Most of the

Table 14-6   DASH Eating Plan

The DASH eating plan shown here is based on 2000 calories a day. The number of daily servings in a food group may vary from those listed, depending on caloric needs.

Food Group	Daily Servings (Except as Noted)	Serving Sizes	Examples and Notes	Significance of Each Food Group to the DASH Eating Plan
Grains and grain products	7-8	1 slice bread 1 oz dry cereal* ½ cup cooked rice, pasta, or cereal	Whole wheat bread, English muffin, pita bread, bagel, cereals, grits, oatmeal, crackers, unsalted pretzels and popcorn	Major sources of energy and fiber
Vegetables	4-5	1 cup raw leafy vegetable ½ cup cooked vegetable 6 oz vegetable juice	Tomatoes, potatoes, carrots, green peas, squash, broccoli, turnip greens, collards, kale, spinach, artichokes, green beans, lima beans, sweet potatoes	Rich sources of potassium, magnesium, and fiber
Fruits	4-5	6 oz fruit juice 1 medium fruit	Apricots, bananas, dates, grapes, oranges, orange juice,	Important sources of potassium,

			magnesium, and fiber
Lowfat or fat free dairy foods	2-3	8 oz milk 1 cup yogurt 1½ oz cheese	Fat free (skim) or lowfat (1%) milk, fat free or lowfat buttermilk, fat free or lowfat regular or frozen yogurt, lowfat and fat free cheese	Major sources of calcium and protein
Meats, poultry, and fish	2 or less	3 oz cooked meats, poultry, or fish	Select only lean; trim away visible fats; broil, roast, or boil, instead of frying; remove skin from poultry	Rich sources of protein and magnesium
Nuts, seeds, and dry beans	4-5 per week	½ cup or 1½ oz nuts 2 Tbsp or ½ oz seeds ½ cup cooked dry beans, peas	Almonds, filberts, mixed nuts, peanuts, walnuts, sunflower seeds, kidney beans, lentils	Rich sources of energy, magnesium, potassium, protein, and fiber
Fats and oils[†]	2-3	1 tsp soft margarine	Soft margarine, lowfat mayonnaise, light salad	DASH has 27%

Continued

Table 14-6   DASH Eating Plan—cont'd

The DASH eating plan shown here is based on 2000 calories a day. The number of daily servings in a food group may vary from those listed, depending on caloric needs.

Food Group	Daily Servings (Except as Noted)	Serving Sizes	Examples and Notes	Significance of Each Food Group to the DASH Eating Plan
		1 Tbsp lowfat mayonnaise 2 Tbsp light salad dressing 1 tsp vegetable oil	dressing, vegetable oil (such as olive, corn, canola, or safflower)	calories as fat, including fat in or added to foods
Sweets	5 per week	1 Tbsp sugar 1 Tbsp jelly or jam ½ oz jelly beans 8 oz lemonade	Maple syrup, sugar, jelly, jam, fruit-flavored gelatin, jelly beans, hard candy, fruit punch, sorbet, ices	Sweets should be low in fat

*Equals ½ to 1¼ cups, depending on cereal type. Check the product's Nutrition Facts Label.

†Fat content changes serving counts for fats and oils. For example, 1 Tbsp of regular salad dressing equals 1 serving; 2 Tbsp of a low-fat dressing equals ½ serving; 2 Tbsp of a fat-free dressing equals 0 servings.

From *Facts about the DASH Eating Plan.* Washington, DC: 2003. NIH, NHLBI.

sodium in the U.S. diet comes from processed foods. The DASH eating plan has been found to be more effective in reducing blood pressure if combined with a mild to moderate sodium restriction. A mild restriction would be a daily intake less than 100 mmol, or 2.4 g of sodium (6 g salt), and a moderate restriction would be 65 mmol, or 1.5 g of sodium (3.8 g salt). The American Heart Association also recommends that the general population consume no more than 2.4 g of sodium daily in order to reduce the risk of developing hypertension. Box 14-3 lists high-sodium foods that should be limited in sodium-restricted diets. Information to include in teaching about sodium restriction is as follows:

- The taste preference for salt usually decreases after about 2 to 3 months on a sodium-restricted diet.
- Herbs and spices (except high-sodium ones such as celery seeds and salt mixtures, e.g., garlic salt, onion salt, or celery salt) and fresh garlic and onions are good alternatives to salt in seasoning. Salt-free spice seasoning mixtures are available in supermarkets or can be homemade. Lemon juice and flavored vinegars are other good choices. Some foods and their suggested low-sodium accompaniments are provided in Table 14-7.
- Commercial salt substitutes contain potassium chloride rather than sodium chloride. The patient should consult with the physician about using them; generally their use is allowed if the individual has no renal impairment.
- Commercial mixes and convenience items (e.g., pasta or rice dishes, sauce mixes) are usually high in sodium and should be used rarely or never. Some low-salt versions are available, but check the nutrition label to be sure that the food can be used within the sodium allowance.
- Kosher meats contain two to three times as much sodium as nonkosher meats. Soaking meats in tap water for 1 hour, then discarding the water and cooking the food is effective in reducing the sodium content while still adhering to the Jewish food laws.
- Rinsing canned foods (e.g., tuna) can reduce sodium content.
- Some drugs, including antibiotics (especially the penicillins), sulfonamides, and barbiturates, are high in sodium. Their sodium content should be considered for the individual who is following a sodium-restricted diet. The pharmacist can provide information about the sodium content of these drugs. Individuals should be cautioned about using over-the-counter medications without

Table 14-7   Foods and Suggested Low-Sodium Accompaniments

Foods	Suggested Seasonings
Beef	Horseradish, dry mustard, cloves, pepper, bay, garlic
Poultry	Curry, sage, coriander, ginger, tarragon, rosemary
Stews	Bay, garlic, basil, oregano, thyme
Vegetables	Mace, nutmeg, dill, rosemary, savory

physician approval. Antacids (except those containing magaldrate), aspirins, cough medicines, and laxatives often contain sodium.

Congestive Heart Failure

Pathophysiology

Congestive heart failure (CHF), which results from decreased myocardial efficiency, is most commonly a result of hypertension and ischemic heart disease. Other causes include damage to the heart valves, thiamin deficiency, and congenital lesions of the heart. Renal blood flow may decrease, with impaired excretion of sodium and water. Peripheral edema, pulmonary edema, and ascites often result.

Treatment

Most of the medications used for treating hypertension are applicable to the treatment of CHF. ACE inhibitors and other vasodilatory agents and diuretics (used to reduce total body water) are used in the treatment of CHF. Inotropic agents such as digitalis are often given to improve cardiac contractility.

Nutritional Care

Prevention of CHF requires lifestyle changes to achieve good control of hypertension and LDL cholesterol. If CHF occurs, the goals of nutritional care are to reduce total body sodium and water to reduce the workload of the heart. Children with CHF frequently have impaired growth and poor weight gain. This condition may be caused by a combination of factors (see Table 14-2 for a listing). Improvement of growth is a major goal of their nutritional care.

Assessment

Assessment is summarized in Table 14-2.

Intervention and teaching

Decrease workload on the heart

Implement the following lifestyle changes to improve cardiac sufficiency:

- Achieve weight reduction if overweight. Obesity increases the likelihood of CHF among individuals at risk.
- Be physically active, as tolerated and with the physician's approval. Physical activity enhances weight reduction efforts and improves cardiac function.
- Divide daily food intake into five to six small meals. Small meals are often better tolerated by the dyspneic individual than three large meals a day.
- Reduce dietary sodium to decrease fluid retention. The usual sodium allowance is approximately 45 to 70 mg/kg/day in infants and 2 g/day in adults. Box 14-3 provides guidelines for achieving sodium restriction.
- Control fluid intake to help reduce circulatory volume, if necessary. The fluid allowance commonly ranges from 80 to 160 ml/kg/day in infants to 1.5 to 2 L/day in adults. This includes dietary sources, as well as fluids given with medications. Some foods that are solid at room temperature are liquid at body temperature. Gelatins can be considered to be 100% water, fruit ices 90%, pudding or custard 75%, sherbet 67%, and ice cream 50%. Nutrients must be provided in as small a volume as possible. If the person is fed by tube, then a formula providing at least 1.5 to 2 kcal/ml can be used.

Prevent or correct nutritional deficiencies

- Increase potassium intake to 4.5 to 7 g/day unless renal impairment is present. Diuretics increase potassium losses, and hypokalemia predisposes to digitalis toxicity. See Appendix A for potassium sources.

Box 14-3   Foods to Be Avoided on Sodium-Restricted Diets*

Mild Restriction (2-3 g/Day)

Do not use:

Salt at the table (use salt lightly in cooking; 1 tsp salt ≈2300 mg sodium)

Smoked, cured, or salt-preserved foods such as salted fish, ham, bacon, sausage, cold cuts, corned beef, kosher meats, sauerkraut, olives

Salted snack foods such as chips, pretzels, popcorn, nuts, crackers

Seasonings such as onion, garlic, and celery salt and monosodium glutamate, bouillon, and meat tenderizers; pickles; condiments such as catsup, prepared mustard, relishes, soy sauce, and Worcestershire sauce

Cheese, peanut butter

Moderate Restriction (1 g/Day)

Do not use:

Salt in cooking or at the table

Any food prohibited under Mild Restriction

Canned meat or fish, vegetables, and vegetable juice (except low-sodium)

Frozen fish filets or any frozen vegetables to which salt has been added

More than one serving of any of these in a day: artichoke, beet greens, beets, carrots, celery, dandelion greens, kale, mustard greens, spinach, Swiss chard, turnips

Buttermilk

Regular bread, rolls, crackers, doughnuts, pastries

Dry cereals (except puffed wheat, puffed rice, and shredded wheat); instant oatmeal and grits

Shellfish (except oysters)

Salted butter or margarine, commercial salad dressings and mayonnaise

Regular baking powder, baking soda, or any products containing them (e.g., biscuits, corn bread, muffins, cookies, cakes); self-rising flour

Prepared mixes such as breads, muffins, pancakes, entrees, cake, pudding, cocoa, frozen waffles, and French toast; instant flavored coffee

Box 14-3   Foods to Be Avoided on Sodium-Restricted
Diets*—cont'd

Water treated with a water softener

Bottled water (mineral, sparkling, spring, or other waters),
unless information obtained from the bottler indicates it is
low in sodium

Regular or diet soft drinks, unless information obtained
from the bottler indicates them to be low in sodium

Strict Restriction (0.5 g/Day)

Do not use:

Any food listed under Mild or Moderate Restrictions

More than 2 cups of milk per day

Commercial foods made with milk, such as yogurt, frozen
yogurt, ice cream, shakes

Artichokes, beet greens, beets, carrots, celery, dandelion
greens, kale, mustard greens, spinach, Swiss chard, turnips

Commercial candy, except hard candies, gumdrops, or
jelly beans (limit to 10 pieces daily)

*Low-sodium versions of many of the products are available. These may be
included in the diet.

■ If undernutrition is present, increase energy intake by mouth if possible (see Box 12-1). If oral feedings are not sufficient, malnourished individuals, especially children, have shown improved
growth without a worsening of CHF when given continuous tube
feedings. Modular ingredients (see Table 8-2) can be used to
increase the energy density of standard infant formulas to allow
provision of adequate energy within the fluid volume tolerated.

REFERENCES

Adult Treatment Panel (ATP) III. *Third Report of the National Cholesterol
    Education Program (NCEP) Expert Panel on Detection, Evaluation, and
    Treatment of High Blood Cholesterol in Adults (Adult Treatment Panel
    III)*, Washington, 2002, National Institutes of Health, National Heart,
    Lung and Blood Institute.

Erdman JW Jr: Soy protein and cardiovascular disease: A statement for
    healthcare professionals from the Nutrition Committee of the AHA,
    Circulation 102:2555, 2000.

Jenkins DJ et al: Effects of a dietary portfolio of cholesterol-lowering foods vs lovastatin on serum lipids and C-reactive protein, *JAMA* 290:502, 2003.

Kris-Etherton P et al: Lyon Diet Heart Study: Benefits of a Mediterranean-style, National Cholesterol Education Program/American Heart Association Step I Dietary Pattern on Cardiovascular Disease, *Circulation* 103:1823, 2001.

Kris-Etherton PM et al: Fish consumption, fish oil, omega-3 fatty acids, and cardiovascular disease, *Circulation* 106:2747, 2002.

Lichtenstein AH, Deckelbaum RJ (for the American Heart Association Nutrition Committee): Stanol/sterol ester-containing foods and blood cholesterol levels, *Circulation* 103:1177, 2001.

National High Blood Pressure Education Program: *The Seventh Report of the Joint National Committee on Prevention, Detection, Evaluation, and Treatment of High Blood Pressure (JNC 7),* Washington DC, 2003, National Institutes of Health, National Heart, Lung, and Blood Institute.

SELECTED BIBLIOGRAPHY

Colonna P et al: Nonpharmacologic care of heart failure: counseling, dietary restriction, rehabilitation, treatment of sleep apnea, and ultrafiltration, *Am J Cardiol* 91:41F, 2003.

Diet and cholesterol: why bother, *Harvard Men's Health Watch* 8(6):7, 2004.

He J et al: Dietary sodium intake and incidence of congestive heart failure in overweight US men and women: first National Health and Nutrition Examination Survey Epidemiologic Follow-up Study, *Arch Intern Med* 162:1619, 2002.

Hung T et al: Fat versus carbohydrate in insulin resistance, obesity, diabetes and cardiovascular disease, *Curr Opin Clin Nutr Metab Care* 6:165, 2003.

Pulmonary
Disease

15

Nutrition and acute or chronic respiratory failure interact in a variety of ways. The increased work of breathing in respiratory failure increases energy needs while dyspnea interferes with nutrient intake. These factors contribute to weight loss and inadequate nutritional status. Malnutrition adversely affects respiratory function by causing (1) wasting of the diaphragm and intercostal muscles, (2) decreased ventilatory response in response to hypoxia, (3) decreased surfactant production, (4) decreased replication of respiratory epithelium with predisposition to infection, (5) decreased cell-mediated immunity with increased susceptibility to pneumonia and other infections, and (6) decreased colloid osmotic pressure with increased likelihood of pulmonary edema. Moreover, phosphate is needed for adequate ATP to allow normal function of muscles, including those of the respiratory system, and for transport of oxygen by the red blood cells. Therefore, hypophosphatemia, which is common during protein-calorie malnutrition and/or the refeeding of malnourished individuals, further impairs respiratory function.

The total energy intake and the proportions of energy nutrients consumed also have an impact on respiratory function. Respiratory insufficiency is characterized by abnormal gas exchange, in particular the retention of carbon dioxide (CO_2). An excessive energy intake increases the metabolic rate and consequently elevates CO_2 production. The ratio of CO_2 produced to oxygen consumed is termed the **respiratory quotient (RQ).** Metabolism of carbohydrate yields the most CO_2, one mole for every mole of oxygen consumed, an RQ of 1. If excessive energy and carbohydrate are consumed, so that the body makes fat from the carbohydrate, then the RQ is greater than 1. The increase in CO_2 production resulting from overfeeding places a serious burden on an individual with a compromised respiratory system.

Chronic Obstructive Pulmonary Disease

Chronic obstructive pulmonary disease (COPD) is a group of diseases that includes asthma, bronchitis, emphysema, and bronchiectasis.

Pathophysiology

The common feature in COPD is chronic obstruction of airflow. Airflow obstruction can result from bronchospasm (asthma); overproduction of mucus in the respiratory system (bronchitis); destruction of elastin, the elastic lung tissue, with air trapping and poor gas exchange (emphysema); or bronchial obstruction caused by a tumor, foreign body, or infection (bronchiectasis).

Pulmonary vascular resistance tends to increase in patients with COPD as a result of vasoconstriction due to alveolar hypoxia. The pulmonary vasculature undergoes remodeling, with hypertrophy of muscles of the pulmonary artery walls and infiltration of smooth muscle into the normally nonmuscular smaller vessels of the pulmonary circulation. Chronic acidemia resulting from inadequate CO_2 removal also stimulates pulmonary vasoconstriction. This increases pressure within the pulmonary vasculature and the right cardiac ventricle, which can lead to enlargement of the ventricle (cor pulmonale).

Treatment

Bronchodilators, including the beta-agonists, anticholinergic agents, and theophylline, are mainstays in treatment of COPD. Antiinflammatory drugs are also widely used. Currently the glucocorticoids are the most commonly used, but other potential agents in trials or under development include immunomodulators (inhaled tacrolimus, rapamycin, and oxelclosporin), phosphodiesterase 4 inhibitors, cytokine inhibitors, antiinflammatory cytokines, and adhesion molecule blockers. Antibiotics are prescribed when secondary infections (e.g., pneumonia) occur. Chest percussion and postural drainage may be used in individuals producing large amounts of sputum. Long-term oxygen is recommended for those individuals with a resting arterial PO_2 level of 55 mm Hg or less while breathing room air. For those whose resting arterial PO_2 level is between 56 and 59 mm Hg, long-term oxygen therapy is indicated if they have excess red blood cell production (a hematocrit 55% or more) as a consequence of hypoxia or if they develop cor pulmonale. Oxygen therapy may be necessary during physical exertion for individuals with exercise-induced hypoxia.

Nutritional Care

Malnutrition is common among individuals with COPD, especially those with emphysema. As many as 70% of people with COPD have lost weight, are underweight, and/or show signs of muscle or fat wasting. Resting energy expenditure is increased in people with moderate to severe COPD because of the increased work of breathing.

Micronutrient levels are also of concern in people with COPD, especially the levels of the antioxidant vitamins and minerals. Low blood levels of vitamin A have been reported to be common among people with moderate to severe COPD. Moreover, some individuals with normal blood levels of vitamin A respond to vitamin A supplementation with improvements in respiratory function, indicating that there may be local deficiency of the vitamin in the lung in COPD. Deficiency of vitamin A reduces the replication of epithelial cells and causes degeneration of mucus-secreting cells in the respiratory tract, thus making the person more susceptible to infection. Poor vitamin C status has also been reported to be prevalent among individuals with COPD, which further predisposes them to infection. Epidemiologic data indicate that people with the highest fruit and vegetable intakes are least likely to suffer from COPD.

Assessment

Assessment is summarized in Table 15-1.

Intervention and teaching

Preventing or correcting underweight, if applicable

Teaching of the patient and family can include the following:

- Increase energy intake through use of energy-dense foods or supplements; Box 12-1 provides a list of suggestions. Individuals with moderate to severe dyspnea may prefer liquid supplements (shakes, instant breakfast, or other commercial nutrient drinks;

Table 15-1   Assessment in Pulmonary Disease

Area of Concern	Significant Findings
Protein-Energy Malnutrition (PEM)	*History* COPD: Poor intake of protein and energy resulting from pressure of a full stomach on the diaphragm, unpleasant taste in the mouth from chronic sputum production, gastric irritation from bronchodilator therapy, smoking, inadequate food preparation skills; increased needs because of increased work of breathing, frequent infections Acute respiratory failure: inadequate intake of protein and energy caused by upper airway intubation, altered state of consciousness, dyspnea; increase in protein and energy requirements because of increased work of breathing or acute pulmonary infections *Physical Examination* Evidence of weight loss (muscle wasting lack of fat); weight for height <90% of desirable or BMI <18.5; triceps skinfold <5th percentile *Laboratory Analysis* ↓ Serum albumin, transferrin, or prealbumin; ↓ creatinine-height index (all uncommon in COPD)
Overweight	*History* COPD: decreased energy needs resulting from decreased basal metabolic rate with aging, decreased activity to compensate for impaired respiratory function *Physical Examination* Weight for height >120% of desirable or BMI>25; triceps skinfold >95th percentile

Table 15-1   Assessment in Pulmonary Disease—cont'd

Area of Concern	Significant Findings
Vitamin Deficiencies	
A	*History* Failure to consume at least 1 serving of a food rich in vitamin A or its precursor, carotene, at least every other day
	Physical Examination Follicular hyperkeratosis; poor light-dark visual adaptation; dryness of the skin or cornea
	Laboratory Analysis ↓ Serum retinol
C	*History* Failure to consume at least one serving of vitamin C–rich foods per day
	Physical Examination Petechiae, ecchymoses; gingivitis
	Laboratory Analysis ↓ Serum or leukocyte ascorbic acid
Phosphate (P) Deficiency	*History* Previous undernutrition; refeeding with high-carbohydrate diet, tube feeding, or TPN; use of antacids that bind phosphate
	Physical Examination Muscle weakness; acute respiratory failure
	Laboratory Analysis ↓ Serum P
Magnesium (Mg) Deficiency	*History* Poor food intake, undernutrition
	Physical Examination Diminished ventilation, difficulty weaning from the ventilator

Continued

Table 15-1 Assessment in Pulmonary Disease—cont'd

Area of Concern	Significant Findings
	(decreased respiratory muscle strength)
	Laboratory Analysis
	↓ Serum Mg
Elevated Respiratory Quotient (RQ)	*History*
	Overfeeding
	Physical Examination
	Tachypnea (>20 breaths/min in a non–mechanically ventilated adult); shortness of breath
	Laboratory Analysis
	RQ ≥1; ↑ partial pressure of CO_2 (Pco_2)
Fluid Excess	*History*
	Administration of more than 35-50 ml fluid/kg/day in an adult, including fluids in IVs, medications, tube feedings, TPN, and oral intake; ventilator dependency, which causes ↑ release of antidiuretic hormone (ADH)
	Physical Examination
	Bounding pulse; sacral or peripheral edema; shortness of breath; pulmonary rales
	Laboratory Analysis
	↓ Serum Na
Excess IV Lipid	*History*
	Rapid administration (over 10 to 12 hours or less) of IV lipid emulsions, especially if >2 g lipid/kg/day is administered
	Laboratory Analysis
	↑ Serum triglycerides; ↓ PO_2, ↑ Pco_2

see Tables 8-1 and 8-2). Approaches to specific problems are outlined as follows:

- *Early satiety:* Eat high-energy foods first, then foods of low-energy density (beverages, raw vegetables) at the end of the meal or between meals. Experiment to see if foods served cold cause fewer problems.
- *Bloating:* Eat small, frequent meals and avoid hurrying through meals, to reduce air swallowing.
- *Anorexia:* Eat high-energy foods first and save lower-energy ones to eat at the end of the meal; have favorite foods available for snacks; use moderate amounts of fat-containing foods, which have higher energy density.
- *Dyspnea:* eat slowly; use pursed lip breathing between bites; avoid overeating; eat small, frequent snacks and meals; avoid excessive fat intake, which may delay gastric emptying (the diaphragm is more flattened in COPD than in the normal state, and a delay in gastric emptying prevents the diaphragm from fully extending).
- *Fatigue:* Rest before meals; eat larger meals in the morning or other times when less tired; have easy-to-prepare foods readily available for times when fatigued. Treatments and physical activity should be scheduled so that the individual has a chance to rest before meals.
- Ensure that patients have sufficient resources to secure an adequate diet. Many individuals with COPD are elderly or retired; they may have a limited income, or they may have a poor diet because of loneliness, apathy about food, or few food preparation skills (especially elderly men). They may need encouragement to eat at a group feeding site for the elderly (usually at senior citizen centers or in apartment houses for the elderly), or, if they are homebound, they may need referral to a program for home-delivered meals.
- Provide mouth care often or encourage the patient to perform mouth care, especially before meals, to clear the palate of the taste of sputum and improve the appetite.

Weight reduction (overweight or obese individuals)

Increasing activity within physical limitations is an important part of weight control. Walking, chair exercises, or water aerobics (if not oxygen dependent) may be tolerated. Start with short periods of low-intensity exercise if the person has been sedentary, and gradually increase the duration and intensity. Decrease energy intake by following the guidelines in Chapter 7.

Antioxidants

Some evidence suggests that levels of antioxidants (e.g., vitamins A, C, and E and beta-carotene) may be low in the respiratory tissues of individuals with COPD. Oxygen therapy increases the need for these nutrients. If dietary intake appears low, counseling should focus on increasing intake of the known antioxidants, and supplements may be needed.

Acute Respiratory Failure

Respiratory failure is one of the leading reasons for admission to intensive care units (ICUs). ICU patients are at increased risk of malnutrition, with more than 40% having signs of malnutrition at the time of admission.

Pathophysiology

Respiratory failure is not a disease but instead is a ventilatory disorder caused by a variety of different conditions. It can result from increased pulmonary capillary pressure or permeability (e.g., pulmonary edema, pneumonia, near drowning), inadequate excretion of carbon dioxide (e.g., chronic bronchitis, emphysema), and depression of the respiratory center or failure of neuromuscular transmission (e.g., drug overdose, spinal cord injury, multiple sclerosis).

Treatment

Treatment of respiratory failure includes administration of oxygen or use of mechanical ventilation to maintain near-normal partial pressures of oxygen and CO_2 in the blood; use of antibiotics if infection is present; and, frequently, use of corticosteroids to decrease pulmonary edema and stabilize pulmonary membranes.

Nutritional Care

Medical nutrition therapy is aimed at the prevention or correction of nutritional deficiencies or excesses that may worsen respiratory function and predispose the individual to secondary infections. Because individuals with acute respiratory failure tend to have multiple medical problems requiring simultaneous attention, it is easy to neglect nutrition. Persons with acute respiratory failure should be started on nutrition support within the first 3 or 4 days of hospitalization to prevent progression of nutritional deficits. Individuals given nutrition support are more readily weaned from ventilators than those given only intravenous (IV) glucose solutions.

Assessment

Assessment is summarized in Table 15-1.

Intervention

Preventing or correcting protein-calorie malnutrition

Patients able to eat are given a diet of nutrient-dense foods (see Box 12-1). Those unable to eat but who have functioning gastrointestinal (GI) tracts are often given nasogastric (NG) or nasoduodenal/nasojejunal (ND/NJ) feedings. Avoiding pulmonary aspiration of the formula is of key importance in delivering tube feedings in these patients. Measures to avoid pulmonary aspiration include ensuring that the tube is not in the respiratory tract before administering feedings; stopping feedings when the patient must be in Trendelenburg's position (e.g., during postural drainage); and possibly delivering feedings beyond the pyloric sphincter, directly into the duodenum or jejunum.

Those who are unable to be fully fed by the GI tract may be given total parenteral nutrition (TPN). Excessive amino acid administration should be avoided because it stimulates the ventilatory drive and may increase minute ventilation, fatigue respiratory muscles, and contribute to respiratory arrest.

Providing appropriate amounts of feedings

Patients should not be either underfed or overfed. Energy needs should be carefully evaluated so that the patient can be fed appropriately. Indirect calorimetry, which measures respiratory CO_2 release, is a common technique for assessing energy needs. Newer equipment that measures the metabolic rate using reflectance techniques, rather than CO_2 production, provides rapid, relatively inexpensive data. Calculations have been developed to estimate energy needs in critically ill patients where it is not possible to measure them (see Box 2-5), but individualized measurements are always preferable.

Overfeeding is particularly likely during nutrition support with enteral tube feedings or TPN because the feedings do not depend on the patient's voluntary food intake. Where indirect calorimetry is unavailable, physical examination and measurement of arterial blood gases can reveal some of the effects of overfeeding and high RQ. Elevated Pco_2 (partial pressure of CO_2 in the blood), unexpected difficulty in weaning from the ventilator, and tachypnea and shortness of breath (if non-ventilator-dependent patient) can be signs of overfeeding.

Avoiding fluid excess

The fluid required for delivery of tube feedings or TPN, along with medications, to patients with acute respiratory failure puts them at risk for overhydration. Fat is a concentrated source of energy, and therefore, using fat to supply most of the nonprotein energy in the diet also helps to control fluid intake. Tube feeding formulas with an increased nutrient density can be used for individuals receiving tube feedings. The formulas designed specifically for respiratory failure (Chapter 8) have an increased nutrient density, providing 1.5 kcal/ml. For individuals receiving TPN, 20% or 30% lipid emulsions can be used daily as an energy source. These emulsions supply 2 or 3 kcal/ml, whereas 10% emulsions provide only 1.1 kcal/ml.

Avoiding lipid excess

Rapid infusion of intravenous lipid emulsions may interfere with pulmonary diffusion capacity in individuals with respiratory impairment. Neonates are at increased risk. Assess the patient's serum triglyceride level after each increase in the infusion rate and at regular intervals thereafter to determine if the lipid infusion rate needs to be reduced. Schedule the delivery of the lipid over 12 to 24 hours each day, which allows the lowest possible infusion rate.

Providing adequate antioxidants

An increase in oxidative stress (e.g., oxygen therapy) increases the needs for antioxidants, including vitamins A, C, and E; beta-carotene; and selenium. Supplements of antioxidants should be provided if dietary intake appears to be low.

If tube feedings are necessary, formulas enriched with antioxidants (e.g., OXEPA) have been demonstrated to decrease ventilator days and days in intensive care in patients with acute respiratory failure.

SELECTED BIBLIOGRAPHY

Borum ML et al: The effect of nutritional supplementation on survival in seriously ill hospitalized adults: an evaluation of the SUPPORT data. Study to Understand Prognoses and Preferences for Outcomes and Risks of Treatments, *J Am Geriatr Soc* 48:S33, 2000.

Chailleux E, Laaban JP, Veale D: Prognostic value of nutritional depletion in patients with COPD treated by long-term oxygen therapy: data from the ANTADIR observatory, *Chest* 123:1460, 2003.

Denny SI, Thompson RL, Margetts BM: Dietary factors in the pathogenesis of asthma and chronic obstructive pulmonary disease, *Curr Allergy Asthma Rep* 3:130, 2003.

Eaton S, Martin G: Clinical developments for treating ARDS, *Expert Opin Investig Drugs* 11:37, 2002.

Suchner U et al: Effects of intravenous fat emulsions on lung function in patients with acute respiratory distress syndrome or sepsis, *Crit Care Med* 29:1569, 2001.

Thomas DR: Dietary prescription for chronic obstructive pulmonary disease, *Clin Geriatr Med* 18:835, 2002.

Renal Disease

16

A variety of diseases can affect the kidneys, including renal failure, **nephrotic syndrome**, and **nephrolithiasis**. The kidneys are responsible for maintaining the optimal chemical composition of body fluids. When renal failure occurs, there is difficulty in controlling the body content of sodium, potassium, and nitrogenous byproducts of metabolism. In nephrotic syndrome, large amounts of protein are lost in the urine. *Nephrolithiasis*, or renal calculi formation, refers to the precipitation of stones in the urinary tract.

Acute or Chronic Renal Failure

Pathophysiology

In acute renal failure (ARF), a sudden reduction in glomerular filtration rate occurs, with impairment in excretion of wastes. Causes for this sudden reduction include inadequate renal perfusion (e.g., hemorrhage); acute tubular necrosis following trauma, surgery, or sepsis; nephrotoxic drugs or chemicals; acute glomerulonephritis; and obstruction (e.g., stricture of a ureter). There are two phases: an oliguric phase with urinary output usually less than 400 ml/day (less than 0.5 to 1 ml/kg/hr in children), followed by a diuretic phase when urine output increases. ARF may resolve or it may instead progress to chronic renal failure (CRF). CRF is defined as having poor renal function (glomerular filtration rate, or GFR, ≤60 ml/min/1.73 m^2) for 3 months or more. GFR is expressed as a rate (ml/min) corrected for the body surface area.

The leading cause of CRF in North America is diabetes, and good metabolic control of diabetes is the most effective means of prevention. In renal insufficiency or failure, the glomerular filtration rate falls. The kidney is responsible for excretion of urea and creatinine derived from protein metabolism. With impaired renal function, circulating blood urea nitrogen (BUN) and creatinine levels rise, and retention of fluid, potassium, sodium, phosphorus, and other solutes normally excreted by the kidney occurs. CRF is divided into stages, based on the GFR. The stages are as follows: *stage 1*, or mild CRF, GFR ≥90 ml/min/1.73 m^2; *stage 2*, GFR 60 to 89; *stage 3*, GFR 30 to 59; *stage 4*, GFR 15 to 29; and *stage 5*, GFR <15 (or patient on dialysis).

Nutrition-related problems are prevalent in renal failure. Anorexia is common in the presence of high BUN and creatinine levels. In addition, the kidney normally activates erythropoietin, which is required for red blood cell formation, and vitamin D, which regulates calcium and phosphorus absorption and bone calcium stores. Anemia, hypocalcemia, bone loss (osteodystrophy), and hyperphosphatemia are common. Retention of sodium and water contributes to hypertension, and potassium retention may lead to cardiac dysrhythmia. Impaired ability to excrete the organic acids produced in metabolic reactions and/or inadequate ability to conserve bicarbonate by the kidney results in metabolic acidosis. Atherosclerosis is especially widespread among individuals with CRF. This may be related to the prevalence of diabetes among individuals with CRF and also to the existence of an inflammatory state, which appears to contribute to atherosclerotic heart disease, associated with CRF. Levels of interleukin-6 and C-reactive protein, two markers of inflammation, are frequently elevated in those with renal failure.

Treatment

Treatment involves removal or, if possible, correction of the cause of renal failure. The major complications during the oliguric phase include acidosis, hyperkalemia, infection, hyperphosphatemia, hypertension, and anemia. Alkalinizing agents (e.g., sodium bicarbonate or Shohl's solution), cation-exchange resins to bind potassium, antibiotics, phosphate-binding drugs, antihypertensive agents, and diuretics are the most commonly used treatment measures.

Dialysis or hemofiltration is needed if these measures, combined with dietary restrictions, are insufficient to prevent or control hyperkalemia, fluid overload, symptomatic uremia (drowsiness, nausea, vomiting, and tremors), or rapidly rising BUN and creatinine levels. Different dialysis modalities are available, depending on individual needs. These treatments include hemodialysis, chronic ambulatory peritoneal dialysis (CAPD), or automated peritoneal dialysis (APD). Transplantation is an option for some individuals with end-stage renal disease.

Nutritional Care

The goals of medical nutrition therapy are to reduce the production of wastes that must be excreted by the kidney; avoid excessive fluid and electrolyte intake that will contribute to hypertension; prevent or correct nutritional deficits; prevent or delay development of osteodystrophy; and control hyperlipidemia, which often occurs in these individuals.

Assessment

Assessment is summarized in Table 16-1. Because of the complexity of kidney disease and the impact that chronic illness can have on nutrition-related parameters, the National Kidney Foundation Disease Outcomes Quality Initiative (K/DOQI, 2000) recommends that a variety of measures, rather than only one or two, be used to evaluate protein-energy nutritional status in patients with chronic renal failure. The recommended schedule for maintenance dialysis patients is as follows: serum albumin (predialysis or "stabilized" [after hemodialysis or after drainage of peritoneal dialysate]), monthly; body weight (as a percentage of the usual postdialysis or postdrain body weight), monthly; body weight as a percentage of standard body weight (see Appendix C), every 4 months; subjective global assessment (described in the following text), every 6 months; dietary interview and/or diary, every 6 months; protein equivalent of total nitrogen appearance (protein catabolic rate) normalized to body weight, monthly for hemodialysis and every 2 months for continuous peritoneal dialysis. Other measures that may be obtained as needed are prealbumin (predialysis or stabilized); skinfold thicknesses; dual energy x-ray absorptiometry; serum creatinine, urea nitrogen, and cholesterol (predialysis or stabilized; these parameters fall in malnourished renal patients); and creatinine-height index (as an indicator of muscle mass). The protein equivalent of total nitrogen appearance in a stable patient provides an estimate of protein intake and of tissue **catabolism** and is calculated (in g/kg/day) as follows: $6.25 \times (UNA + 1.81 + 0.31)$, where UNA, or urea nitrogen appearance, is the total urea nitrogen output (measured in

Text continued on p. 427

Table 16-1   Assessment in Renal Disease

Area of Concern	Significant Findings
Protein-Energy Malnutrition (PEM)	*History* Poor intake of protein-containing and energy-containing foods as a result of dietary restrictions or anorexia from uremia, abdominal fullness from peritoneal dialysate, zinc deficiency, or depression; losses of amino acids or serum proteins caused by dialysis (hemodialysis losses ≈ 14 g/session, CAPD losses ≈ 5 to 15 g/day), steroid-induced tissue catabolism, and proteinuria; increased needs during infection *Physical Examination* Muscle wasting; thinning of hair; dry weight <90% of desirable, BMI <18.5, or decline in growth percentile for height or weight (children) (see Appendix D); triceps skinfold <5th percentile; NOTE: Loss of weight or decrease in subcutaneous fat may be masked by edema *Laboratory Analysis* ↓ Serum albumin, transferrin, or prealbumin;[*] nitrogen (N_2) losses in urine and dialysate greater than intake (negative N_2 balance)
Altered Lipid Metabolism	*History* Nephrotic syndrome, excessive consumption of carbohydrates (CHO) caused by dietary emphasis on CHO as an energy source or use of glucose as an osmotic agent in dialysis *Laboratory Analysis* ↑ Serum cholesterol, LDL and VLDL cholesterol, serum triglycerides

Continued

Table 16-1   Assessment in Renal Disease—cont'd

Area of Concern	Significant Findings
Fluid Excess	*History* Oliguria or anuria *Physical Examination* Edema; hypertension; acute weight gain (=1%-2% of body weight) *Laboratory Analysis* ↓ Hct
Potential for Mineral/ Electrolyte Imbalance	
Phosphorus (P) excess	*History* Oliguria or anuria *Physical Examination* Tetany *Laboratory Analysis* ↑ Serum P; Ca × P product (Ca in mg/dl × P in mg/dl) >55; renal calcification on radiographs
Calcium (Ca) deficit	*History* Metabolic acidosis; hyperphosphatemia *Physical Examination* Renal osteodystrophy with bone pain and deformities; tetany *Laboratory Analysis* ↓ Serum Ca (NOTE: ≈45% of Ca is bound to albumin; if the person is hypoalbuminemic, then the Ca level will be misleading; it can be "corrected" by adding 0.8 mg/dl to the total Ca level for each 1 g/dl decrease in albumin below 4 g/dl)
Zinc (Zc) deficit	*History* ↓ Intake caused by dietary restrictions; loss during dialysis

Table 16-1   Assessment in Renal Disease—cont'd

Area of Concern	Significant Findings
	Physical Examination Distorted taste, poor sense of taste; poor wound healing; alopecia; seborrheic dermatitis
	Laboratory Analysis ↓ Serum Zn
Iron (Fe) deficit	*History* Decreased intake as a result of dietary restrictions
	Physical Examination Fatigue; pallor
	Laboratory Analysis ↓ Hct, Hgb,† MCV, ↓ serum ferritin
Sodium (Na) excess	*History* Oliguria or anuria
	Physical Examination Edema; hypertension
Potassium (K^+) excess	*History* Oliguria or anuria
	Physical Examination Weakness, flaccid muscles
	Laboratory Analysis ↑ Serum K^+; electrocardiogram: elevated T wave, depressed ST segment
Aluminum (Al) excess	*History* Use of Al-containing phosphate binders, especially if Al dosages are >30 mg/kg/day; Al contamination in dialysis fluids or supplies
	Physical Examination Ataxia, seizures, dementia; renal osteodystrophy with bone pain and deformities
	Laboratory Analysis Plasma Al >100 µg/L

Continued

Table 16-1   Assessment in Renal Disease—cont'd

Area of Concern	Significant Findings
Potential for Vitamin Imbalance	
A excess	*History*
	Oliguria or anuria
	Physical Examination
	Anorexia, fatigue; alopecia, dry skin; hepatomegaly; irritability (progressing to hydrocephalus and vomiting in infants and children)
	Laboratory Analysis
	↑ Serum retinol
C deficit	*History*
	Losses in dialysis; ↓ intake caused by restriction of fruits and vegetables
	Physical Examination
	Gingivitis; petechiae, ecchymoses
	Laboratory Analysis
	↓ Serum or leukocyte ascorbic acid
B_6 deficit	*History*
	Failure of the diseased kidney to phosphorylate (activate) B_6; loss in dialysis
	Physical Examination
	Dermatitis; ataxia, irritability, seizures
	Laboratory Analysis
	↓ Plasma pyridoxal phosphate (PLP)
Folate	*History*
	Loss of folate during dialysis; ↓ intake caused by restriction of fruits, vegetables, and meats
	Physical Examination
	Glossitis (inflamed tongue); pallor
	Laboratory Analysis
	↓ Hct, ↑ MCV; ↓ serum and RBC folate

Table 16-1   Assessment in Renal Disease—cont'd

Area of Concern	Significant Findings
D deficit	*History* Failure of the diseased kidney to activate vitamin D, poor intake because of restrictions of dairy products *Physical Examination* Rickets (children), osteomalacia *Laboratory Analysis* ↓ 1,25-OH$_2$ vitamin D

*Serum proteins also fall in inflammation, which is common in renal failure.
†Decreased Hct, Hgb may occur because of decreased production of erythropoietic factor by diseased kidney.

the urine and the dialysate fluid). For pediatric patients, include measurement of height or length, and measure head circumference if 3 years old or less (K/DOQI, 2000).

The subjective global assessment (SGA), which requires no laboratory testing or specialized equipment, is useful in many disease states (e.g., cancer) and not just renal failure patients. However, the K/DOQI has formally recommended its regular use in patients with chronic renal failure and maintenance dialysis. The SGA consists of four parts: weight change over the past 6 months, dietary intake and gastrointestinal symptoms, visual assessment of subcutaneous tissue, and muscle mass. The SGA is carried out by a trained examiner (physician, dietitian, or nurse). Each part is scored subjectively on a scale of 1 to 7, where 1 or 2 is severe malnutrition, 3 to 5 is moderate to mild malnutrition, and 6 to 7 is mild malnutrition to normal nutritional status (Table 16-2). The scores for the four parts can then be totaled to yield an estimate of the overall degree of malnutrition. An overall score of 4 to 8 reflects severe malnutrition; a score of 12 to 20 reflects moderate malnutrition or a patient suspected of being malnourished, and a score of 24 to 28 indicates little or no evidence of malnutrition. Scores between these categories (i.e., 9 to 11 and 21 to 23) reflect intermediate degrees of malnutrition between the major categories.

Table 16-2   Subjective Global Assessment

Findings	Score
Weight loss over the last 6 months (percentage of usual body weight)[*]	
10% or more	1 to 2
5%-10%	3 to 5
Less than 5%	6 to 7
Dietary intake and gastrointestinal (GI) symptoms	
Appetite poor; intake poor compared with usual and recommended intakes; and/or nausea, vomiting or diarrhea (moderate to severe) lasting 2 weeks or more	1 to 2
Appetite and intake moderately decreased and/or mild to moderate GI symptoms lasting 2 weeks or more	3 to 5
Appetite and intake good or improving; no GI symptoms	6 to 7
Subcutaneous tissue[†]	
Severely depleted	1 to 2
Moderately to slightly depleted	3 to 5
Little or no depletion	6 to 7
Muscle mass and wasting[‡]	
Severe wasting	1 to 2
Moderate wasting	3 to 5
Little or no wasting	6 to 7

References: National Kidney Foundation Disease Outcomes Quality Initiative: Clinical practice guidelines for nutrition in chronic renal failure, *Am J Kidney Dis* 35 (6 suppl 2):S1, 2000; Canada-USA (CANUSA) Peritoneal Dialysis Study Group: Adequacy of dialysis and nutrition in continuous peritoneal dialysis: Association with clinical outcomes, *J Am Soc Nephrol* 7:198-207, 1996; Detsky AS et al: What is subjective global assessment of nutritional status? *J Parent Ent Nutr* 11:8, 1987.

[*]Give a higher score (less malnourished) if weight loss was intentional or if there has been recent weight regain that does not appear to be related to fluid retention.
[†]Examine fat pads directly below the eyes; they should have a slight bulge in a normally nourished person but a "hollow" appearance in malnutrition. Pinch the skin above the triceps and biceps gently (do not measure the skinfold); subjectively score the fat layer. In a depleted individual, there will be no cushioning between the layers of skin.
[‡]Assess the temporalis muscle (over the temples), the prominence of the clavicles, the contour of the shoulders (rounded indicates well-nourished; squared indicates malnutrition), visibility of the scapula and ribs, the quadriceps muscle, and the muscle mass between the thumb and forefinger.

Intervention and teaching

Modifications of fluid, electrolyte, mineral, and protein intakes are often needed because of the impairment of the kidney's ability to excrete fluid and wastes. Nutrition therapy is designed to reduce edema, hypertension, and uremia. Guidelines for daily nutrient allowances are given in Table 16-3, but individual needs vary, and continual monitoring and reassessment of the patient is the best guide. Malnutrition is associated with a poor prognosis in the patient with chronic renal failure, emphasizing the importance of aggressive nutrition intervention in these patients. Individuals with type 2 diabetes and renal failure are apt to be overweight or obese, which should not be allowed to obscure evidence of undernutrition.

The renal diet is complex, and the dietitian is the professional best prepared to plan the diet and perform initial teaching. Individualization of the diet as much as possible (to incorporate favorite foods and respond to the demands of the individual's lifestyle) improves quality of life and compliance with the diet. Intensive nutrition counseling is needed, with follow-up at least every 1 to 2 months and updating of the plan of care at least every 3 to 4 months.

Fluid needs

Fluid restriction is necessary when oliguria occurs. For the oliguric adult, the daily fluid allowance is approximately 500 ml (to account for insensible losses) plus the volume lost from urine, diarrhea, vomitus, and any other sources during the previous 24 hours. For children, the fluid allowance is equal to output plus a small amount to cover insensible losses. Hemodialysis allows fluid intake to be somewhat more liberal. Peritoneal dialysis is very effective at removing fluid, allowing an increased intake. Acute weight changes are the best guide to fluid deficits and excesses. Body weight should be measured daily, with the oral fluid intake adjusted so that gain is no more than 0.45 to 1 kg (1 to 2 lb) per day for adults on the days between dialyses.

Foods that are liquids at room temperature must be included in the fluid allowance. Water contents of some common foods are as follows: gelatins, 100% water; fruit ices, 90%; pudding or custard, 75%; sherbet, 67%; and ice cream, 50%.

Protein needs

Table 16-3 provides estimates of protein needs; intake should be adjusted as needed, depending on nutritional evaluation and

Table 16-3   Guidelines for Daily Nutrient Intakes in Renal Failure

Nutrient	Adults		Children
	Clinically stable	*Acutely ill*	
Energy	<60 years: 35 kcal/kg ≥60 years: 30-35 kcal/kg	<60 years: ≥35 kcal/kg ≥60 years: ≥30-35 kcal/kg	DRI for age*
Protein	*Clinically stable* UD: 0.6-0.75 g/kg[†] HD: 1.2 g/kg PD: 1.2-1.3 g/kg	*Acutely ill* HD: ≥1.2 g/kg PD: ≥1.3 g/kg	HD: DRI for age + 0.4 g/kg/day PD: DRI for age + amount equal to estimated losses in dialysis
Phosphorus	800-1000 mg (or 10-12 mg/kg) if serum phosphorus is elevated (>4.6 mEq/l in stages 3 and 4, or >5.5 mEq/l in stage 5) OR serum intact parathyroid hormone is elevated above target range[‡]		800 mg if serum phosphorus is >5.5 mEq/L *Note:* infants may require higher serum phosphorus for bone mineralization
Calcium	800-1200 mg (do not exceed 2000 mg in food, supplements, and phosphate binders)		DRI for age (do not exceed 2500 mg in food, supplements, and phosphate binders)

| Sodium | Individualize, 1-3 g | <20 kg: 2-3 g
>20 kg: 3-4 g |
| Potassium | Individualize to maintain serum potassium ≤5 mEq/L | Individualize to maintain serum potassium ≤5 mEq/L |

References: American Dietetic Association: *Chronic kidney disease (non-dialysis) medical nutrition therapy protocol*, Chicago, 2002, American Dietetic Association; National Kidney Foundation Disease Outcomes Quality Initiative (K/DOQI): Clinical practice guidelines for nutrition in chronic renal failure, *Am J Kidney Dis* 35(6 suppl 2):S1, 2000; Kleinman RE, ed: *Pediatric nutrition handbook*, ed 5, Elk Grove Village, IL, 2004, American Academy of Pediatrics.

Note: The numbers in this table represent an initial prescription and should be individualized as necessary based on the patient's response. Recommendations based on kg of body weight refer to dry weight.

UD, undialyzed; *HD,* hemodialysis; *PD,* peritoneal dialysis.

*Dietary Reference Intake (see Table 1-1).

†0.6 is preferred; 0.75 for individuals who will not accept the more severe limitation or cannot maintain adequate energy intake with protein intake at 0.6 g/kg/day.

‡Target ranges for intact parathyroid hormone: *stage 3,* 35-70 pg/ml; *stage 4,* 70-110 pg/ml; *stage 5,* 150-300 pg/ml. In addition, restrict phosphorus if serum calcium × phosphorus product (Ca in mg/dl × P in mg/dl) is greater than 55.

measures of renal function. At least half of dietary protein should be high in biologic value. **High-biologic-value (HBV) protein** is rich in essential amino acids (those not synthesized in sufficient amounts by the body) in proportions that are favorable for synthesis and maintenance of human tissues. Good sources of HBV protein are eggs, meat, poultry, fish, soy, and milk products. Approximately 7 g of HBV protein is contained in 1 oz of meat, fish, poultry; ¼ cup cooked soybeans or tofu (60 g); 1 egg; or 210 ml (7 fluid oz) of whole, low-fat, or skim milk. Cereals, breads, and vegetables, on the other hand, are sources of protein that is lower in HBV.

Low-protein pasta and bread products—available via mail order, some pharmacies, and some larger grocery chains—are a source of complex carbohydrate for the person on a very-limited-protein diet (usually the undialyzed patient). An alternative approach to the low-protein diet is to use a very-low-protein diet (~0.3 g/kg/day), primarily from vegetarian sources, supplemented with essential amino acids or a mixture of essential amino acids and ketoacid analogs (~0.3 g/kg/day). However, there is an increased risk of malnutrition among individuals consuming a highly restricted diet. It is especially important to consume adequate energy (see Table 16-3) to ensure that the amino acids in the diet are available for protein synthesis and not utilized for energy. Close monitoring of nutritional status is essential; the patient should not be allowed to become malnourished simply to delay the time when dialysis must be started.

Protein and amino acid losses during dialysis can result in protein malnutrition. One approach during peritoneal dialysis is to use a 1.1% amino acid mixture as the primary osmotic agent in one dialysis exchange per day. The amino acids are an effective osmotic agent, and net absorption of amino acids across the peritoneum exceeds the losses of protein and amino acids in the dialysate.

Energy needs

Enough energy must be consumed to prevent catabolism because this process not only reduces the amount of functional tissue but also releases nitrogen, which must be excreted by the kidney. In most cases, fat provides about 25% to 30% of the energy intake and carbohydrate provides approximately 50% to 60%. Hypertriglyceridemia affects a significant number of patients, and most carbohydrate should be complex (starches) to reduce the likelihood of hypertriglyceridemia .

In peritoneal dialysis, 1.5% to 4.25% glucose solutions (containing 1.5 or 4.25 g glucose/dl) are commonly used as an osmotic agent to remove body fluid. About 70% of the glucose is absorbed by the body and must be considered in the energy allowance. Glucose monohydrate used in the dialysate provides 3.4 kcal/g. Thus the individual receives the following:

$$42.5 \text{ g/L} \times 70\% \times 3.4 \text{ kcal/g} = 101 \text{ kcal/L of } 4.25\% \text{ dialysate}$$

or

$$15 \text{ g/L} \times 70\% \times 3.4 \text{ kcal/g} = 36 \text{ kcal/L of } 1.5\% \text{ dialysate}$$

Supplements may be necessary to achieve an adequate energy intake while adhering to the dietary restrictions. These supplements usually contain glucose oligosaccharides and/or vegetable oils. See Table 8-2 for modular ingredients that can be used to increase energy intake.

Electrolytes, minerals, and vitamins

Sodium and potassium. Sodium intake is restricted as necessary to reduce fluid retention, edema, and hypertension. Box 14-3 provides guidelines for different levels of sodium restriction, and Chapter 14 provides further information for the person needing a sodium-restricted diet. The need for potassium restriction can be gauged from the serum potassium levels, which may not rise substantially until the glomerular filtration rate falls to 10 ml/hr. In teaching about potassium restriction, include the following points:

- Salt substitutes are not usually used in renal failure because most are high in potassium. Low-sodium herbs and herb mixtures (see Table 14-7) and flavored vinegars are good choices for seasoning foods.
- The richest potassium sources are fruits and vegetables, meats, and dairy products. Choose canned, drained fruits or vegetables (processed without salt), rather than fresh or frozen. Decrease potassium in fresh vegetables and fruits by cutting them into small pieces and soaking or cooking them in a large amount of water, then discarding the water.

Phosphorus. Progression of renal insufficiency is delayed if phosphorus intake is limited; adults should consume no more than 800 to 1000 mg (or about 10 to 12 mg phosphorus per g of protein consumed) daily if serum phosphorus is elevated (see Table 16-3). Sources rich in phosphorus include legumes, tofu, milk and other dairy products, meats, poultry, fish, eggs, whole grains, nuts (tree and peanuts), seeds, and peanut butter. In the past, aluminum hydroxide antacids were used as phosphate binders to reduce the absorption of phosphate, but their long-term use has resulted in aluminum toxicity, with ataxia, dementia, and worsening of renal osteodystrophy. Consequently, they are no longer used except for short-term treatment when other therapy is ineffective in reducing phosphorus levels. Calcium carbonate or calcium acetate antacids are commonly used as phosphate binders, but there are risks in the use of large doses of calcium when phosphate levels are very high, especially the possibility that the combination of high levels of calcium and phosphorus will cause calcification of the soft tissues. Sevelamer hydrochloride is a phosphate binder that does not contain calcium, magnesium, or aluminum. It has the added advantage that it lowers levels of both total and LDL cholesterol.

Calcium. Calcium is needed to prevent or delay the progression of renal osteodystrophy, or loss of minerals from the bones, resulting from chronic acidosis (from inability to excrete acids produced in metabolism) and impaired vitamin D metabolism. Restriction of dairy products may be necessary to reduce phosphorus and protein intake, so a calcium supplement (e.g., calcium carbonate or citrate) may be needed to achieve the recommended level of intake (see Table 16-3). Calcium-containing phosphate binders are also a good source of calcium. The peritoneal dialysate contains calcium; normally it is at a concentration that does not cause calcium uptake or output, but the dialysate concentration can be increased to allow calcium to be absorbed by the individual if needed. Correction of metabolic acidosis also reduces bone loss.

Vitamin-mineral supplementation. Supplements providing the DRI for water-soluble vitamins, copper, and zinc should be given to ensure there are no deficiencies resulting from dietary restrictions or losses in dialysis (DOQI, 2000). An oral iron supplement may also be used if the individual is not receiving parenteral iron. Vitamin A levels should be assessed; if they are high, no supplements containing vitamin A should be used.

Iron, folic acid, and vitamin B_{12} intake must be adequate in the person receiving recombinant human erythropoietin to allow for adequate red blood cell formation (see discussion of anemia that follows). If dietary intake is inadequate, then supplements should be used. Calcitriol, a synthetic form of 1,25-dihydroxyvitamin D_3, is often prescribed to prevent renal osteodystrophy in individuals undergoing dialysis. Calcium intake must be at least 800 to 1200 mg/day for calcitriol to be effective.

Individualized diet plan

An example of an individualized diet plan is shown in Table 16-4. The diet order in this case is for 45 g of protein (34 g of which should be HBV), 1000 mg of sodium, 1650 mg of potassium, 2650 kcal or more, and 720 ml of fluid per day.

Anemia

Premenopausal women and prepubertal individuals with chronic renal failure should have a hemoglobin of 11 g/dl or greater (or hematocrit of 33% or greater). Men and postmenopausal women should maintain a hemoglobin of 12 g/dl or greater (or hematocrit of 37% or greater). If there is no obvious source of blood loss, patients with anemia should undergo a complete evaluation, including red blood cell indices (mean cell volume), reticulocyte count, serum iron, total iron binding capacity, percent transferrin saturation (serum iron divided by total iron binding capacity and multiplied by 100), serum ferritin, and test for occult blood in the stool (K/DOQI, 2001).

- Differentiating among anemias
  - *Microcytic, hypochromic:* Iron deficiency is common, and it causes a microcytic, hypochromic (small red blood cells [RBC], light in color) anemia, as does aluminum toxicity. Iron deficiency is associated with a low percent transferrin saturation and serum ferritin).
  - *Macrocytosis:* Folate or vitamin B_{12} deficiency is generally associated with macrocytosis (large, immature RBC). An increase in the reticulocyte count, as occurs with hemolytic conditions such as acute hemolytic-uremic syndrome, also causes macrocytosis.
  - *Normocytic, normochromic:* Anemia of erythropoietin deficiency is usually associated with RBC of normal size and color.

Table 16-4   Meal Plan of Man with Chronic Renal Failure (CRF)

Menu	Pro (g)	Na (mg)	K (mg)	kcal
Breakfast				
Shredded wheat, ½ cup	2	1	38	70
Frozen strawberries, ½ cup	0.5	1.5	115	80
Sugar, 1 tsp	—	—	—	16
Half and half, ½ cup	4	60	170	160
Cinnamon toast:				
Low-protein bread, 1 slice	0.1	9	9	100
Margarine, 2 tsp	—	100	2	90
Sugar, 2 tsp	—	—	—	32
Snack				
Jelly beans, 1 oz	0.1	9	9	100
Lunch				
Shrimp salad:				
Shrimp, 2 oz	13.8	60	190	150
Mayonnaise, 3 tsp	—	150	3	135
Lettuce, ¼ cup shredded	0.5	4.5	57	13
Matzo, 1 piece	2	1	38	70
Margarine, 2 tsp	—	100	2	95
Cranberry juice, 1 cup	0.1	9	9	100
With Polycose powder, 1 tbsp	—	6	—	31
Tangerine, 1 medium	0.5	1.5	115	40
Snack				
Hard candy, 1 oz	0.1	9	9	100
Dinner				
Grilled chicken, 2 oz	13.8	60	190	75
Rigatoni, low protein, ½ cup	0.1	9	9	100

Table 16-4   Meal Plan of Man with Chronic Renal Failure (CRF)—cont'd

Menu	Pro (g)	Na (mg)	K (mg)	kcal
With margarine, 2 tsp	—	100	2	90
Stir-fried vegetables:				
Mushrooms, ½ cup	1	9	113	25
Zucchini, ½ cup	1	9	113	25
Oil, 3 tsp	—	—	—	115
Hi-C, 1 cup	0.1	9	9	100
With Polycose powder, 1 Tbsp	—	6	—	31
Peaches, ½ cup, canned, drained	0.7	3.5	215	75
Sugar mints, 37	0.1	9	9	100
Snack				
Low-protein toast, 2 slices	0.2	18	18	200
Margarine, 3 tsp	—	150	3	135
Honey, 1 Tbsp	0.1	9	9	100
Milk, whole, ½ cup	4	60	184	80
With Polycose powder, 1 Tbsp	—	6	—	31
Totals	**44.8**	**979**	**1640**	**2664**

HBV protein = 35.6 g; fluid = 720 ml.

Pro, Protein; *Na*, sodium; *K*, potassium.

A normocytic, normochromic anemia in a patient with serum creatinine of 2 mg/dl or greater (or in one with a lower serum creatinine but marked muscle wasting), in whom no other cause of anemia is present, should be assumed to have deficiency of erythropoietin (EPO) resulting from renal failure. There is usually no need to measure erythropoietin.

- Treating anemias
  - *Iron deficiency:* The initial treatment should be oral iron supplementation (200 mg elemental iron/day in adults; 2-3 mg/kg daily in children). The cause of the deficiency must also be sought (usually occult blood loss). If the anemia is corrected with this, the patient's iron status should then be monitored

every 3 to 6 months to ensure that iron deficiency does not recur. If iron status improves but anemia persists, EPO deficiency is likely.

- *EPO deficiency:* EPO therapy should be initiated and titrated as necessary to maintain the hemoglobin in a target range of 11 to 12 g/dl.
  - *Iron supplementation:* Most patients will require iron supplementation to prevent anemia during EPO therapy. An oral supplement, as described above, can be used initially, but parenteral iron supplementation will be needed if the patient is unable to maintain adequate iron status (transferrin saturation ≥20% and serum ferritin level ≤100 ng/ml) with the oral supplement.
  - *Inadequate response to EPO and iron therapy:* If the patient is unable to maintain the hemoglobin in the target range with EPO treatment, or requires recombinant human erythropoietin (rHuEPO) dosages of more than 300 units/kg/week intravenously or more than 200 units/kg/week subcutaneously (or an equivalent dose of a related product), in spite of adequate iron stores (transferrin saturation >20%, ferritin >100 ng/ml), carnitine deficiency may be present.

Carnitine

Carnitine is an essential cofactor in fatty acid metabolism, and fatty acids are important metabolic fuels for the cardiac and skeletal muscles. Carnitine is normally synthesized in the body, but it is also found in foods of animal origin. Dietary restrictions in patients with CRF can result in low dietary carnitine intakes. Synthesis may be low in infants, as well as in individuals with chronic liver and kidney diseases. (Carnitine is synthesized primarily in the kidney, liver, and brain; other tissues must extract carnitine from the blood.) Moreover, carnitine is lost during dialysis, and these losses contribute to *dialysis-related carnitine disorder (DCD)*, characterized by low plasma free carnitine concentrations, an increase in the plasma ratio of acylcarnitine to free carnitine, anemia that is poorly responsive to treatment with recombinant human erythropoietin, severe hypotension during dialysis, cardiomyopathy, and skeletal muscle weakness (severe enough to interfere with quality of life).

The current recommendations of the National Kidney Foundation (Eknoyan et al., 2003) regarding DCD include the following:

- Measurement of carnitine and acylcarnitine concentrations is not necessary for diagnosis of the disorder or assessment of response to carnitine therapy. Carnitine supplementation is recommended for individuals that have the symptoms listed earlier (and for whom no other cause of the disorder can be identified).

- Treatment of DCD should consist of L-carnitine given intravenously at 20 mg/kg body weight following the dialysis procedure (to minimize losses). Insufficient data are available regarding the benefits and dosages to make any recommendation for oral therapy. D-carnitine can be toxic. Over-the-counter preparations of carnitine may contain both D- and L-carnitine, and these should be avoided.

- Response to L-carnitine therapy should be evaluated every 3 months, with the dosage titrated as low as possible to achieve the desired response, and it should be discontinued in 9 to 12 months if no clinical improvement is apparent.

Dyslipidemia

Arteriosclerotic heart disease is common among individuals with renal failure. Dietary fat is a valuable energy source, but saturated fats raise serum cholesterol levels and should be limited to no more than approximately 7% of total energy intake. Cholesterol intake should be restricted to 200 mg/dl. Individuals with hypercholesterolemia should use oils and soft margarines high in monounsaturated and polyunsaturated fats (those containing primarily liquid canola [rapeseed], olive, safflower, sunflower, corn, soybean, or cottonseed oils); lean meats, fish, or skinned poultry; and skim milk products. (See Chapter 14 for a more extensive discussion of dietary instruction in hypercholesterolemia.) Unfortunately, hypercholesterolemia often continues even after renal transplant. Nutritional problems in the posttransplant patient are discussed in Chapter 10.

Simple carbohydrates—such as sugar, jam, syrup, hard candy, gumdrops, jelly beans, and popsicles—are widely used as energy sources for the person who is not receiving dialysis, because they contribute little or no sodium, potassium, and protein. However, simple carbohydrates must be limited if hypertriglyceridemia occurs. To compensate, complex carbohydrates (breads, cereals, and vegetables) can be used, up to the amount allowed by the protein restriction. Fat intake, with emphasis on monounsaturated fatty acids (found in olive, canola, and peanut oils, for example;

see Chapter 14), can be increased to approximately 40% of energy intake and carbohydrate intake can be correspondingly decreased in order to reduce triglyceride levels. Alcohol intake should be restricted (preferably to none or only an occasional drink, but in no case more than 1 to 2 drinks a day) if hypertriglyceridemia occurs.

Constipation

The low fiber intake resulting from the need to limit complex carbohydrates to remain within the protein restriction may contribute to constipation. To reduce constipation, obtain regular physical activity. In addition, regular use of phosphate binding medications can contribute to constipation. Restrict dietary phosphorus so that use of phosphate binders can be decreased.

Nutrition support

Anorexia resulting from uremia, medications, or depression; the restrictions of the renal diet; abdominal fullness from the peritoneal dialysis; infections or inflammation; metabolic acidosis that stimulates protein degradation; and electrolyte imbalances or circulatory instability associated with renal failure or dialysis are all factors that can interact to impair nutritional status. Enteral tube feeding is preferred if specialized nutritional support is needed. Specialized formulas for renal failure, with low protein, phosphorus, and electrolyte content, are available if needed by the undialyzed patient (see Table 8-1). Usually, the dialyzed patient needs the higher protein and mineral content of a formula designed for general use. Some general-use formulas are available in concentrated forms (2 kcal/ml) for individuals needing fluid restriction.

Individuals who do not tolerate enteral feedings may require total parenteral nutrition (TPN). Specialized amino acid mixtures, containing reduced amounts of **nonessential amino acids,** are available for renal failure; however, the dialyzed patient usually tolerates a balanced amino acid solution containing both essential and nonessential amino acids. Intradialytic TPN (TPN administered during hemodialysis, usually three times weekly) is used to supply supplemental nutrition to some patients. The hemodialysis period provides a convenient time for nutrient infusion, and ultrafiltration during dialysis prevents development of fluid overload from the TPN.

Essential amino acid formulations are available for patients that require tube feeding or total parenteral nutrition. Essential amino acids have a theoretical advantage in renal failure because the lack of nonessential amino acids in the diet should encourage the use of nitrogenous products within the body for synthesis of nonessential amino acids. Nevertheless, balanced amino acid formulations containing both essential and nonessential amino acids are preferred for most individuals with renal failure who can tolerate them. Nonessential amino acids are required for protein formation, and the rate of nonessential amino acid synthesis may not be adequate to meet the body's needs, particularly in ill individuals.

Impaired growth is very common among children with renal failure. Intensive dietary counseling, oral supplements, and enteral tube feeding can be used as needed to maximize nutrient intake. In addition, growth hormone is approved for use in children with short stature associated with renal failure.

Nephrotic Syndrome

Pathophysiology

Nephrotic syndrome results from an increase in permeability of the glomerular capillary membrane. It is associated with proteinuria (2 g/day or more), hypoalbuminemia, edema, and hyperlipidemia. It may be idiopathic or may result from conditions such as glomerulonephritis, diabetes mellitus, collagen vascular diseases, or sickle cell anemia. The disorder can resolve spontaneously or follow a pattern of remissions and relapses.

Treatment

Drug therapy includes corticosteroids, which help lessen proteinuria, and diuretics. If hyperlipidemia is severe, medical therapy is used—for example, inhibitors of cholesterol synthesis (statins) for hypercholesterolemia and gemfibrozil or fenofibrate for hypertriglyceridemia.

Nutritional Care

Medical nutrition therapy in nephrotic syndrome is designed to maintain adequate nutritional status and to help control edema and hyperlipidemia.

Assessment

Assessment is summarized in Table 16-1.

Intervention and teaching

Sodium intake

A diet restricted in sodium is the most effective way to reduce the edema. The sodium allowance is usually 1 to 2 g (40 to 90 mEq) per day until the edema is reduced. See Box 14-3 for this level of restriction. If the edema resolves, then the sodium intake can be liberalized.

Protein intake

Increasing protein intake to replace urinary losses is ineffective and results in increased proteinuria. A diet providing approximately the DRI for protein usually supplies adequate protein.

Hyperlipidemia

A diet that is low in saturated fat and cholesterol is needed to reduce serum cholesterol. Good choices include oils and soft margarines high in monounsaturated and polyunsaturated fats (those containing primarily liquid canola [rapeseed], olive, safflower, sunflower, corn, soybean, or cottonseed oils); lean meats, fish, or skinned poultry; and skim milk products. A moderate intake of fat (30% of energy) is recommended because diets extremely low in fat (and consequently high in carbohydrates) could worsen hypertriglyceridemia. A diet rich in monounsaturated fats and in omega-3 fatty acids helps to reduce hypertriglyceridemia. If the person is overweight, modest weight reduction through lifestyle changes such as a reduction in energy intake and increase in physical activity usually helps reduce serum lipid levels. Alcohol should be avoided or consumed only occasionally in hypertriglyceridemia if possible, but if this is unacceptable to the patient, then intake should not exceed 1 to 2 drinks daily.

Hyperglycemia

Corticosteroid use can lead to impaired glucose tolerance and hyperglycemia. To control glycemia, reduce intake of simple carbohydrates such as dessert items, candy, soft drinks, and pastries. Complex carbohydrates such as whole-grain breads, cereals, legumes, and starchy vegetables provide energy while making less of a contribution to hyperglycemia. Maintaining a moderate fat intake (approximately 30% of energy intake) helps to control hyperglycemia.

Renal Calculi, or Nephrolithiasis

Pathophysiology

Calculi, or stones, can precipitate in any part of the urinary tract when the urine becomes supersaturated with the solute. The most important solutes, in terms of nephrolithiasis, are calcium, oxalate, and uric acid. Approximately 70% to 88% of all stones contain calcium, and 36% to 70% of stones are composed of calcium oxalate. Normal urine contains inhibitors of stone formation, and some people with stones have been found to have abnormalities of inhibitor production. In other individuals with stones, however, no abnormalities can be found. Risk factors for stone formation include recurrent urinary tract infections, hyperparathyroidism, prolonged immobilization, ileostomy, Crohn's disease, laxative abuse, gout (excessive uric acid production), paraplegia, and milk-alkali syndrome (excessive intake of milk or other dietary calcium sources, along with antacids).

Treatment

Many calculi pass through the urinary tract spontaneously, and therapy consists of analgesics to relieve the pain associated with calculi and treatment of any underlying causative factors such as urinary tract infection, obstruction, or gout. Some stones that do not pass spontaneously can be fragmented through lithotripsy to make it possible for the smaller fragments to be excreted. Calculi that are very large, too hard to be fragmented, or in an inappropriate location for lithotripsy can be removed either endoscopically or surgically.

Nutritional Care

Nutrition therapy can reduce the risk of recurrence of stones in some individuals. The most important aspect of nutritional care is maintaining an adequate fluid intake.

Assessment

Assess the quantity of fluids usually consumed, and determine whether there is a history of previous stone formation. The composition of any stones excreted should be determined, if possible, to provide a basis for recommending dietary changes.

Intervention and teaching
Fluid intake

Fluid intake should be sufficient to produce at least 2 liters of dilute urine (specific gravity <1.010) daily, which reduces the risk of precipitation of calculi. Water should be encouraged, but juices, herbal teas, and soft drinks can provide some of the liquid. It is especially important to consume fluids at bedtime because the urine tends to become concentrated during the night. People who are unconscious, unaware of thirst, or unable to drink fluids need to receive sufficient fluid via a feeding tube or intravenous infusions to produce dilute urine.

Dietary substrates contributing to calculi formation

Calcium-containing stones. In the past, it was common to use calcium-restricted diets in an effort to reduce the recurrence of calculi in people who formed calcium-containing stones. It is now recognized that hypercalciuria (excessive calcium excretion in the urine) is common among individuals with a history of stone formation, but only a subset of individuals benefit from calcium restriction. This subset includes people with absorptive hypercalciuria type II. For these individuals, dietary calcium may need to be restricted to approximately 400 to 500 mg/day. This can be accomplished by limiting milk products and deep green leafy vegetables to about one serving each per day. A high-fiber diet has also been suggested as a way to reduce calcium absorption.

Excessive intakes of protein and sodium increase urinary calcium losses and might contribute to stone formation. Limiting protein intake to no more than the Dietary Reference Intake and sodium intake to no more than 2 to 3 g/day may reduce the risk of recurrence of stone formation.

Oxalate-containing stones. Many foods contain oxalates, but only a few have been proven to increase urinary excretion of oxalate significantly. These foods include spinach, beets, rhubarb, chocolate, peanuts and peanut butter, strawberries, black or green tea, and wheat bran; these items are best avoided by people who form oxalate stones. At present, it is not clear whether it is safe to consume other foods rich in oxalates such as plums, berries other than strawberries, tomatoes, celery, beans (dried, baked, green, and wax), deep green leafy vegetables (spinach, kale, and collards), tofu and other soy products, almonds, and cashews. Vitamin C yields oxalate when it is metabolized. It has not been proven that vitamin C promotes stone formation, but the safest course is for people who form oxalate stones to avoid megadoses (1 g or more per day) of vitamin C.

If hypercalciuria is not present, then a high calcium intake may be beneficial. Calcium decreases oxalate absorption in the intestine. If the person has fat malabsorption, then a low-fat diet or reduction of long-chain triglycerides in the diet and supplementation with medium-chain triglycerides may be effective. Excessive calcium is lost in the feces during fat malabsorption because calcium becomes bound to fat that is not absorbed, and thus the calcium is also lost in feces. Fecal calcium loss permits enhanced oxalate absorption.

"Ash" from diets. Foods are metabolized in the body to yield acid or alkaline "ash," or end products. The original pH of the food has no relationship to the acidity or alkalinity of its end products. Medications are often used to change urine pH, but acid- or alkaline-ash diets are prescribed occasionally. Acid-ash diets help acidify the urine and prevent precipitation of calcium stones. Acid urine also reduces the growth of bacteria in the bladder, and prevention of urinary tract infections decreases the risk of stone formation. On the other hand, alkaline-ash diets are sometimes used to prevent recurrence of uric acid and cystine stones. Individuals on these diets make most of their food choices from the acid- or alkaline-ash food groups, as appropriate:

- *Acid-ash foods:* meat, whole grains, eggs, cheese, cranberries, prunes, and plums
- *Alkaline-ash foods:* milk; vegetables; fruits except cranberries, prunes, and plums

Physical activity

Whenever possible, individuals should have daily weight-bearing exercise. The stress of this type of exercise helps prevent release of calcium from the bone, with a resulting increase in urinary calcium loss. It is especially important that caregivers in long-term care and rehabilitation facilities be aware of this problem and make every attempt to assist patients to be physically active as tolerated.

REFERENCES

Eknoyan G, Latos DL, Lindberg J: Practice recommendations for the use of L-carnitine in dialysis-related carnitine disorder: National Kidney Foundation Carnitine Consensus Conference, *Am J Kidney Dis* 41: 868, 2003.

National Kidney Foundation Disease Outcomes Quality Initiative (K/DOQI): Clinical practice guidelines for nutrition in chronic renal failure, *Am J Kidney Dis* 35(6 suppl 2):S1, 2000.

National Kidney Foundation Disease Outcomes Quality Initiative (K/DOQI): National Kidney Foundation clinical practice guidelines for bone metabolism and disease in chronic kidney disease, 2003. Accessed January 27, 2004 at www.kidney.org/professionals/kdoqi/guidelines_bone/index.htm.

National Kidney Foundation Disease Outcomes Quality Initiative (K/DOQI): Clinical practice guidelines for anemia of chronic kidney disease: update 2000, *Am J Kidney Dis* 37(1 suppl 1):S182, 2001.

SELECTED BIBLIOGRAPHY

Bernardi A et al: Long-term protein intake control in kidney transplant recipients: effect in kidney graft function and in nutritional status, *Am J Kidney Dis* 41:S146, 2003.

Boudville N et al: Oral nutritional supplementation increases caloric and protein intake in peritoneal dialysis patients, *Am J Kidney Dis* 41:658, 2003.

Brem AS et al: Prevalence of protein malnutrition in children maintained on peritoneal dialysis, *Pediatr Nephrol* 17:527, 2002.

Caglar K et al: Approaches to the reversal of malnutrition, inflammation, and atherosclerosis in end-stage renal disease, *Nutr Rev* 60:378, 2002.

Delvechhio FC, Preminger GM: Medical management of stone disease, *Curr Opin Urol* 13:229, 2003.

Dwyer JT et al: Nutritional status affects quality of life in Hemodialysis (HEMO) Study patients at baseline, *J Ren Nutr* 12:213, 2002.

Fouque D et al: Advances in anabolic interventions for malnourished dialysis patients, *J Ren Nutr* 13:161, 2003.

Giordano M et al: Effects of dietary protein restriction on fibrinogen and albumin metabolism in nephrotic patients, *Kidney Int* 60:235, 2001.

Jones CH, Wolfenden RC, Wells LM: Is subjective global assessment a reliable measure of nutritional status in hemodialysis?, *J Renal Nutr* 14:26, 2004.

Pifer TB et al: Mortality risk in hemodialysis patients and changes in nutritional indicators: DOPPS, *Kidney Int* 62:2238, 2002.

Pupim LB, Ikizler TA: Uremic malnutrition: new insights into an old problem, *Seminars in Dialysis* 16:224, 2003.

Diabetes Mellitus

17

Diabetes mellitus is a disorder characterized by impaired carbohydrate, fat, and protein metabolism. Hyperglycemia and glucosuria commonly occur in untreated diabetes (Box 17-1).

Pathophysiology

Diabetes is classified according to its etiology:

- *Type 1 diabetes* (previously known as *insulin-dependent diabetes*) is characterized by insulin deficiency that results from destruction of the beta cells of the pancreas. Most individuals with type 1 diabetes are normal weight or underweight at the time of diagnosis. Classic symptoms of untreated type 1 diabetes include polyuria, polydipsia (increased fluid intake), polyphagia (increased food intake), and weight loss.
- *Type 2 diabetes* (previously known as *non-insulin-dependent diabetes*) is characterized by insulin resistance, or decreased tissue uptake of glucose in response to insulin, along with an insulin secretory defect that makes it impossible for the individual to release enough insulin to compensate for the insulin resistance. Type 2 diabetes is much more common than type 1 diabetes, accounting for about 90% of the diabetes in the United States and Canada, and most individuals with type 2 diabetes are overweight or obese.
- *Other specific types of diabetes* is a broad category that encompasses genetic defects in pancreatic beta cell function (including maturity onset diabetes of youth, or MODY); genetic defects in insulin action; diseases of the exocrine pancreas that damage the pancreas and thus impair beta cell function (e.g., pancreatitis, neoplasia, cystic fibrosis, hemochromatosis); endocrinopathies

---

Box 17-1   Criteria for Diagnosis of Diabetes Mellitus in Adults

---

Two of these findings, on different days (either two different tests, or two abnormal findings with the same test) are required for the diagnosis of diabetes:

■ Casual (any time of day without regard to time since the last meal) plasma glucose level of ≥200 mg/dl (11.1 mM) plus symptoms of diabetes such as excessive thirst and urination and unplanned weight loss.

OR

■ Fasting plasma glucose level of ≥126 mg/dl (7.0 mM). "Fasting" means no energy intake for at least 8 hours.

OR

■ Plasma glucose level of ≥200 mg/dl (11.1 mM) 2 hours after consuming a 75 g glucose load.*

From American Diabetes Association: Diagnosis and classification of diabetes mellitus, *Diabetes Care* 27(suppl 1):S9, 2004.

*Oral glucose tolerance test; this is not recommended for routine clinical use.

---

such as acromegaly; drug- or chemical-induced diabetes (e.g., glucocorticoids, injected pentamidine, thyroid hormone); and diabetes induced by infectious agents, uncommon immune-related illnesses, or genetic disorders.

■ *Gestational diabetes mellitus* is the term given to any glucose intolerance that first occurs or is recognized during pregnancy.

Impaired glucose tolerance (IGT) and impaired fasting glucose (IFG) are considered prediabetes, intermediate stages between the normal state and frank diabetes. They are components of the metabolic syndrome described in Chapter 5 and are risk factors for later development of diabetes and cardiovascular disease. IGT is defined as a glucose concentration ≥140 mg/dl (7.8 mmol/L) but <200 mg/dl (11.1 mmol/L) 2 hours after ingestion of a 75 g glucose load. IFG is present when fasting (no food intake for at least 8 hours) plasma glucose is ≥110 mg/dl (6.1 mmol/L) and <126 mg/dl (7.0 mmol/L).

Diabetes is associated with many complications. The major chronic ones are accelerated coronary heart disease, peripheral vascular disease, cerebrovascular disease, retinopathy, nephropathy, and neuropathy. Gastrointestinal (GI) motility disorders occur in 20% to 76% of people with diabetes, with **gastroparesis** or delayed gastric emptying being the most common of these disorders. Symptoms of gastroparesis include early satiety, abdominal discomfort and/or distension, bloating, nausea, vomiting, anorexia, and unexplained hypoglycemia. The cause of these motility disorders is not fully understood, although neuropathy probably plays a role, at least in some individuals.

Acute complications of type 1 diabetes include diabetic ketoacidosis (DKA) and hypoglycemia, and those of type 2 diabetes include hyperglycemic hyperosmolar nonketotic syndrome (HHNS) and infections such as pneumonia, cellulitis, bacteriuria, and vulvovaginitis. DKA results from insulin deficiency—too small a dosage; omission of a dose or doses; increased need for insulin; or elevation of the insulin-antagonizing counterregulatory hormones (glucagon, catecholamines, cortisol, and growth hormone), as occurs during infection or trauma. In response to the insulin deficiency, hyperglycemia and glucosuria occur. Glucosuria leads to an osmotic diuresis with resulting dehydration and loss of electrolytes. The insulin deficit also allows increased lipolysis, or release of fatty acids from storage sites. Accelerated synthesis of ketones from the fatty acids results in ketosis (increased blood ketone levels because of increased production of ketones from fatty acids), and acidosis (because ketones are acidic). HHNS, on the other hand, is almost always precipitated by some stressor that increases blood glucose levels (surgery, trauma, burns, chronic disease, infection, drugs such as corticosteroids or diuretics, dialysis). Insulin levels are high, although they are not high enough to normalize the blood glucose. HHNS results in marked hyperglycemia (often greater than 1000 mg/dl), elevation of serum osmolality, glucosuria, and dehydration. Ketosis is absent or only very mild.

Treatment

Treatment of diabetes hinges on an appropriate plan for meals and physical activity, as well as medications if necessary. The Diabetes Control and Complications Trial showed that intensive management of diabetes to maintain blood glucose levels as near normal as possible reduces retinopathy, nephropathy, and neuropathy in type 1 diabetes (American Diabetes Association [ADA], 2003).

Furthermore, data from the United Kingdom Prospective Diabetes Study (the largest and longest study ever performed on patients with type 2 diabetes) demonstrate that reduction of the occurrence of retinopathy, nephropathy, and possibly neuropathy in this form of diabetes is possible with intensive treatment to achieve near-normal blood glucose concentrations (Genuth et al., 2003).

Diabetes care is a team effort that usually involves several health professionals—one or more physicians, dietitians, nurses, and other professionals such as a podiatrist and optometrist or ophthalmologist—as well as the patient and family members. Certified diabetes educators (CDEs) are physicians, nurses, dietitians, or others who have received extensive education in diabetes care and have passed a certification examination to show that they have special qualifications for patient teaching related to diabetes.

Nutrition Therapy

Medical nutrition therapy is an essential component of the care of all people with diabetes. A registered dietitian (RD) who is knowledgeable in diabetes care is the best person to carry out nutrition planning and teaching. All health professionals on the team should be familiar with the principles of nutrition care in diabetes so that they can reinforce the instruction provided by the dietitian, however.

Medications

Insulin or oral hypoglycemic agents may be needed to help control hyperglycemia and excessive hepatic glucose production. Current practice is to recommend intensive therapy for all people with diabetes who are able to manage it. The goal of intensive therapy is to reduce long-term complications by maintaining glucose at normal or near-normal levels almost all the time. For intensive therapy of type 1 diabetes, several insulin injections are usually needed daily. Insulin is available in four forms: (1) ultra-short-acting, (2) short-acting, (3) intermediate-acting, and (4) long-acting (Table 17-1). Injections of ultra-short- or short-acting insulin are taken before each meal, often combined with one or two daily injections of long- or intermediate-acting insulin. Alternatively, motivated individuals may use continuous subcutaneous insulin infusion (CSII), or insulin pump therapy, which delivers short-acting insulin continuously to provide basal levels and allows the patient to administer boluses as needed with meals or snacks. Hypoglycemia is more

Table 17-1 Activity of Human Insulin Preparations*

Insulin	Approximate Number of Hours after Injection		
	Onset	Peak	Duration
Ultra-Short Acting			
Aspart	<0.25	1-3	4-6
Lispro	<0.25	0.5-1.5	4-6
Short-Acting			
Regular	0.5-1	2-4	6-8
Intermediate-Acting			
NPH	1.5-5	4-12	14-18
Lente	2.5-5	4-12	16-20
Long-Acting			
Glargine	1.5	—[†]	18-24
Ultralente	4-10	8-16[†]	20-24

*The times of onset, peak activity, and duration may vary widely from individual to individual and at different times in the same individual. These times are guidelines only.

[†]Glargine has no peak of activity. The effect reaches a plateau after 3 to 4 hours. Ultralente has a minimal peak effect. These long-acting insulins provide a basal level of insulin activity, and additional doses of short- or ultra-short-acting insulin are given to provide peaks of insulin at the time of nutrient absorption and assimilation.

prevalent with intensive therapy than with less intensive therapy. Also, the individual is more likely to become overweight with intensive therapy than with traditional therapy. With their diabetes under better control, patients lose less glucose in the urine, and insulin stimulates storage of glucose as fat.

Intensive management is not recommended for patients who are unwilling to participate actively in their care. The risk of hypoglycemia is heightened with intensive therapy. Thus intensive management is also not recommended for children under 2 years of age and only with caution for those 2 to 7 years old because hypoglycemia may impair normal brain development. Hypoglycemia may precipitate strokes or heart attacks if atherosclerosis is present, and thus older adults or others with significant atherosclerosis need to be especially careful if they choose to use intensive therapy.

Oral hypoglycemic agents—including metformin, repaglinide, the sulfonylureas (tolbutamide, chlorpropamide, tolazamide, glipizide, and glyburide), and the thiazolidinediones (pioglitazone and rosiglitazone)—are used in treatment of some individuals with type

2 diabetes. Metformin decreases hepatic glucose production, decreases intestinal absorption of glucose (and may cause diarrhea and some weight loss as a consequence), and improves insulin sensitivity by increasing peripheral glucose uptake and utilization. Repaglinide and the sulfonylureas stimulate insulin release from the pancreas; thus they require a functioning pancreas. Insulin release with the sulfonylureas, in particular, is not linked to increases in blood glucose, as it is in the healthy individual, and thus these drugs are prone to cause hypoglycemia. Acarbose is a medication that delays the digestion of starches and other complex carbohydrates, thus reducing the peak postprandial blood glucose concentrations. The thiazolidinediones decrease liver glucose production and increase insulin sensitivity of muscle cells. Some individuals with type 2 diabetes require daily insulin injections to maintain good control of blood glucose.

Monitoring Blood Glucose

The American Diabetes Association (2004) has suggested goals for glycemic control as follows: preprandial plasma glucose, 90 to 130 mg/dl (5 to 7.2 mmol/L); postprandial plasma glucose (1 to 2 hours after the start of a meal), less than 180 mg/dl (10 mmol/L); and **glycosylated hemoglobin** (HbA$_{1c}$ or simply A1C, which reflects the blood glucose levels over the 2- to 3-month period before the test was performed), less than 7%. However, goals must be individualized. The elderly, pregnant women, and children, in particular, require special consideration. The glycemic goals may need to be relaxed if hypoglycemia is frequent or severe. Motivated patients may strive for an A1C in the normal range (less than 6%), with the understanding that there is an increased risk of hypoglycemia, especially in patients receiving insulin. If A1C goals are not met even though preprandial glucose is in the target range, efforts may be made to reduce postprandial glucose concentrations.

Self-monitoring of blood glucose (SMBG) is an important tool for glycemic goals. The frequency of monitoring depends upon the individual's needs and goals, but SMBG is usually done at least three times daily in type 1 diabetes. SMBG is recommended for patients with type 2 diabetes who are treated with insulin and is desirable for those treated with sulfonylureas and those who are not achieving their blood glucose goals. Whenever therapy is being modified, SMBG is recommended for both type 1 and type 2 diabetes. Whether stable patients with type 2 diabetes who can control their glucose levels with dietary modifications alone should perform routine SMBG is controversial.

Decreasing the Risk of Comorbidities

The American Diabetes Association (2004) recommends that blood pressure be maintained at less than 130/80. Serum lipids should be controlled as follows: low-density lipoprotein (LDL) cholesterol less than 100 mg/dl (2.6 mmol/L), triglycerides less than 150 mg/dl (1.7 mmol/L), and high-density lipoprotein (HDL) cholesterol greater than 40 mg/dl (1.1 mmol/L).

Nutritional Care

Assessment

A diet history to determine the usual intake and activity level is an essential part of planning nutritional care for the individual with either type 1 diabetes or type 2 diabetes. Other aspects of assessment are summarized in Table 17-2.

Intervention and Teaching

The goals of nutrition intervention and teaching are as follows: (1) attain and maintain optimal metabolic outcomes, including blood pressure, glucose, and lipid levels, as close to normal as possible to prevent or reduce the risk for complications; (2) prevent and treat chronic complications of diabetes; (3) improve health through healthy food choices and physical activity; and (4) address individual needs (cultural, lifestyle, financial, willingness to change).

Nutrition guidelines in type 1 diabetes

Planning of care begins with a diet history to determine the person's usual pattern of food intake and physical activity, which is used to develop an individualized meal plan and schedule of insulin therapy. It is recommended that all individuals taking insulin perform SMBG so that hypoglycemia and hyperglycemia are detected early and insulin dosages can be adjusted as needed. Food intake and the pharmacodynamic pattern of the insulin used must be synchronized (see Table 17-1). For example, if a dose of NPH insulin is taken at 6:00 am, then breakfast should be eaten by 7:30 AM, when the onset of insulin activity could occur. Both lunch and an afternoon snack are needed because the peak insulin activity will occur between

Table 17-2   Assessment in Diabetes Mellitus

Area of Concern	Significant Findings
Overweight	*History* Type 2 diabetes; sedentary lifestyle; excessive insulin or energy intake *Physical Examination* Weight >120% of desirable or BMI >25; triceps skinfold >95th percentile; blood pressure >130/80; waist circumference >40 inches (102 cm) in males or >35 inches (88 cm) in females
Underweight	*History* Type 1 diabetes; polydipsia, polyuria, excessive hunger *Physical Examination* Weight < 90% of desirable or BMI <18.5; triceps skinfold <5th percentile; failure of children to follow established growth patterns (see Appendix D)
Glucose Tolerance Hyperglycemia	*History* Type 1 and 2 diabetes with inadequate treatment (too low a drug dosage or too great an energy intake), noncompliance to the treatment regimen, or stress such as infection or surgery *Physical Examination* Flushed skin, thirst, polyuria, poor skin turgor; drowsiness, dizziness, weakness; pain in abdomen; nausea, vomiting *Laboratory Analysis* ↑ Blood glucose; urine positive for ketones (in ketoacidosis); ↑ serum osmolality (in nonketotic hyperosmolar coma); Hb A_{1c} >7%

Continued

Table 17-2   Assessment in Diabetes Mellitus—cont'd

Area of Concern	Significant Findings
Hypoglycemia	*History* Excessive intake of insulin; unusual exertion without increased food intake; omission of scheduled meal or snack; gastroenteritis or other illness with vomiting; excessive alcohol use; use of drugs that reduce blood glucose (e.g., salicylates, chloramphenicol) *Physical Examination* Hunger, headache, trembling, excessive perspiration, faintness, double vision *Laboratory Analysis* ↓ Blood glucose
Adequacy of Mineral Nutriture	
Zinc (Zn)	*History* ↑ Excretion *Physical Examination* Anorexia; diminished sense of taste; altered taste sensation; poor wound healing; diarrhea; dermatitis *Laboratory Analysis* ↓ Serum Zn
Magnesium (Mg)	*History* ↑ Excretion, especially in ketoacidosis *Physical Examination* Weakness, muscle pain, disorientation *Laboratory Analysis* ↓ Serum Mg

noon and late afternoon, and a bedtime snack is needed because insulin activity can last 24 hours. For people who are willing to participate in intensive therapy, with multiple daily insulin injections or CSII, there is more flexibility in the timing and composition of meals and snacks. Insulin dosages and administration times can be adjusted to compensate for changes in the meal plan. Ultra-short-acting insulin, taken at the time of a meal or snack, allows for quick changes in plans. Insulin glargine is a newer insulin analog that is slowly absorbed from the subcutaneous tissue and provides a long-lasting basal amount of insulin. When insulin glargine is used, shorter-acting insulins are used at the time of food intake to provide peaks of insulin activity during absorption.

Nutrition guidelines in type 2 diabetes

Nutritional care in type 2 diabetes is aimed at controlling blood glucose, lipids, and blood pressure. Most individuals with type 2 diabetes are overweight or obese, and weight loss improves metabolic control, but efforts to achieve and maintain an ideal body weight are often unsuccessful. A nutritionally adequate meal plan low in saturated fat and cholesterol and providing 250 to 500 kcal less than the calculated energy needs, along with an increase in physical activity, will stimulate weight loss. A weight loss of only 5 to 9 kg (10 to 20 lb), regardless of the starting weight, usually reduces blood glucose levels, dyslipidemia, and blood pressure. The focus should be on making lifestyle changes, rather than being on a diet. Stress reduction techniques, regular physical activity, making healthy food choices, and smoking cessation (if applicable) are key measures in reducing health risks in diabetes.

Preconception care in diabetes

The infant of a diabetic woman in poor control at the time of conception is at risk for fetal malformations or death, prematurity, respiratory distress syndrome, and macrosomia (excessive body size). Very good control of blood glucose during pregnancy reduces the risk of complications in the infant. To prevent congenital anomalies, it is best if intensive therapy begins before conception because most organ formation occurs very early in pregnancy. The woman must be counseled about the need for effective contraception until glycemia is well controlled; made aware of the risks to both fetus and mother if glycemia is poorly controlled; and taught to perform SMBG, if she is not doing this already. Human insulin is the most common agent used if medications are needed to control glycemia. Women should maintain their premeal capillary plasma glucose (i.e., SMBG readings) between 80 and 110 mg/dl (4.4 to 6.1 mmol/L). Conception should not occur until a woman exhibits stable glycemic control, as evidenced by HbA_{1c} level. All women with potential for childbearing should consume at least 400 µg folic acid per day from supplements or fortified foods, in addition to consuming good food sources of folate.

Diabetes care during pregnancy and lactation

Both diabetes existing before pregnancy and gestational diabetes mellitus (GDM) increase the risk of fetal macrosomia, maternal hypertensive disorders, and need for cesarean delivery, as well as complications in the neonatal period, including hypoglycemia, hypocalcemia, and polycythemia. Good metabolic control reduces these risks, and the remainder of this section represents a summary of the ADA Clinical Practice Recommendations (2003a) to achieve good control during pregnancy. Daily SMBG is an important part of diabetic care in pregnancy. The goal is to maintain plasma glucose concentrations as follows: fasting, 105 mg/dl (5.8 mmol/L) or less; 1-hour postprandial, 155 mg/dl (8.6 mmol/L) or less; and 2-hour postprandial, 130 mg/dl (7.2 mmol/l) or less. Fetal demise is more common in pregnancies where fasting plasma glucose is >105 mg/dl. Ideally, women with GDM will be counseled by a registered dietitian to adhere to a meal plan that provides adequate energy and nutrients to promote normal growth of the fetus and achieve blood glucose levels consistent with the goals that have been established. Guidelines for weight gain during pregnancy are provided in Chapter 3. Medical nutrition therapy should be individualized based on patient height and weight and blood glucose goals. For normal-weight women, no increase in energy intake is recommended during the first trimester of pregnancy; during the second and third trimesters, an increase of about 300 kcal (1255 kJ) daily over their prepregnant intake is usually adequate to support fetal growth. Obese women (BMI >30) have had improved glucose and triglyceride levels without an increase in ketone levels when following a moderately energy-restricted diet (approximately 25 kcal/kg actual body weight per day, or approximately 30% less than estimated energy needs). Limiting carbohydrate intake to 35% to 40% of energy intake improves maternal glucose concentrations and maternal and fetal outcomes. Adequate protein is usually provided by an intake of 0.75 g/kg/day plus an additional 10 g/day.

Regular meals and snacks are necessary to reduce the risk of hypoglycemia because of the fetus's continual requirement for nutrients. A bedtime snack helps to decrease the likelihood of hypoglycemia during sleep. Carbohydrate is distributed into three small to moderate meals and two to four snacks daily; distributing it as evenly as possible throughout the day reduces the incidence of severe hyperglycemia. Physical activity can be encouraged as a means of improving control of blood glucose in women without medical or obstetric complications that would contraindicate it, although there is inadequate evidence to make a firm recommendation about the type of exercise. Some evidence suggests that excessive ketone levels may have adverse effects on the fetus, and therefore, urine monitoring of ketones may be of benefit in determining the adequacy of energy intake and/or insulin dosages.

Breastfeeding should be encouraged, both because it can be associated with improved maternal postpartum weight loss and blood glucose control and because it has been shown to have emotional benefits for mother and infant and health benefits for the infant. Breastfeeding lowers blood glucose, and consequently women taking insulin may need a snack before or after breastfeeding. An energy intake of approximately 200 kcal/day over pregnancy needs (but usually no more than about 1800 kcal/day) meets the needs of most women during the first 6 months of lactation.

Components of the diet in diabetes

Protein

Adults with diabetes and normal renal function are believed to have protein needs similar to those of the general population, and a protein intake providing 10% to 20% of caloric intake is usually considered appropriate. If nephropathy develops but the glomerular filtration rate (GFR) is still normal, then the diabetes care team may consider limiting protein intake to no more than 0.8 g/kg/day (the adult Dietary Reference Intake [DRI], and approximately 10% of energy intake). Once the GFR begins to fall, restricting protein intake to no more than 0.6 g/kg/day may slow the progression of the nephropathy in some patients.

Fat

Diabetes is a risk factor for dyslipidemias and coronary heart disease, and overweight and obesity are very common among people with diabetes. To help control these problems, saturated fats should provide less than 10% of the total energy intake, and monounsaturated fats such as olive and canola should be emphasized. Cholesterol intake should be limited to 300 mg/day (see Chapter 14). If serum triglyceride levels are elevated, steps to reduce them include an increase in monounsaturated fat and a decrease in carbohydrate intake, avoiding alcohol, weight reduction (if overweight or obese), and an increase in physical activity. Omega-3 fat from fish or supplements (fish oil) may be beneficial in diabetic individuals with very high triglycerides.

Carbohydrate

Carbohydrate usually accounts for 50% or more of the energy consumed. Even when insulin is not used, carbohydrate (and other energy nutrients) should be spread as evenly as possible among the meals, and meals should be far enough apart (4 to 5 hours) to allow blood glucose to return to basal concentrations before each meal. Although most of the carbohydrate should come from nutritious foods within the meal plan, sugars can be substituted for other carbohydrate foods without impairing metabolic control. Soluble fiber from oats, legumes, fruits, and vegetables may help to reduce serum lipid levels. Diabetic individuals should consume at least 25 to 30 g of fiber daily, as should the general population. Even higher fiber intakes (up to 38 g daily) are recommended for males 14 to 50 years of age, who have higher energy needs than other groups.

Some foods have been identified as having a low **glycemic index**—that is, they cause less change in the blood glucose than some reference carbohydrate (usually white bread or glucose). Rice is a food of relatively high glycemic index, and legumes are low, for example; however, the speed of digestion is a major determinant of how much blood glucose changes, and many factors affect the speed of digestion, including preparation method, the presence of fat in the meal or snack, and the ripeness of fruits or vegetables. It is not clear whether there is long-term benefit from a diet of low glycemic index. Some individuals may wish to plan their diets with a focus on foods of low glycemic index, but many others find it more practical to control total carbohydrate intake than to try to control the glycemic index. A compilation of glycemic index data for various foods is available (Foster-Powell & Miller, 1995). The American Diabetes Association states that the total amount of carbohydrate consumed is more important than the source and type (ADA Clinical Practice Recommendations, 2004).

Nonnutritive sweeteners (those containing negligible or no calories) include aspartame, acesulfame K, sucralose, and saccharin. These sweeteners can be consumed within the limits recommended by the Food and Drug Administration. Individuals with phenylke-tonuria should not use aspartame (Nutrasweet). Nutritive sugar sub-stitutes such as sugar alcohols (e.g., sorbitol) are sometimes used in products marketed to people with diabetes. They provide about half the energy per gram as sugars do, but their energy contribution must be considered as part of the meal plan. Excessive amounts may cause diarrhea.

Alcohol

Limited amounts of alcohol can be included in the meal plans of most diabetic individuals if they so desire. Alcohol is not metabo-lized to glucose, and it inhibits gluconeogenesis (formation of glu-cose from noncarbohydrates, i.e., amino acids and glycerol). Alcohol should be consumed with food, because drinking on an empty stomach raises the risk of hypoglycemia. The daily limit on consumption should be no more than two drinks for men and one for women (1 drink ≥12 oz [360 ml] of beer, 5 oz [150 ml] of wine, or 1.5 oz [45 ml] of distilled spirits). Pregnant women, children, and people with a history of alcohol abuse should not consume alcohol, and individuals with pancreatitis or hypertriglyceridemia should avoid it as well. Hypertensive individuals should limit their alcohol intake to one drink a day or less.

Vitamins and minerals

No sound evidence suggests that individuals with diabetes have an increased need for vitamins, compared with nondiabetic adults. Deficiencies of two minerals, chromium and magnesium, are asso-ciated with resistance to the effects of insulin and glucose intoler-ance. Supplements may improve glucose tolerance if the individual is deficient in these nutrients, but there is no benefit from supple-mentation if stores are adequate. Deficiencies of these minerals do not appear widespread, because they can readily be obtained from a varied diet including whole grains, legumes, fruits, vegetables, and nuts. Older adults, especially those with low energy intakes, may benefit from a multivitamin-multimineral supplement, and they should consume at least 1200 mg calcium in food or supple-ments daily.

Sodium

Recommendations for sodium intake for nonhypertensive people with diabetes are the same as for the general population—no more than 2400 to 3000 mg/day. If mild to moderate hypertension is present, limiting daily sodium intake to 2400 mg or less may be beneficial. For the person with hypertension and nephropathy, an intake of 2000 mg/day or less is reasonable. Box 14-3 provides guidelines for these levels of sodium restriction.

Tools for meal planning

Making healthy food choices should be emphasized in the diet of the diabetic individual, just as it is for all others. Teaching in regard to meal planning can be relatively simple or extremely detailed and complex, depending on factors such as the skills and abilities of the individual and his/her significant others, motivation, and goals of therapy. At its most basic, nutrition teaching includes wise food choices; portion control; and principles of a healthy lifestyle such as smoking cessation, physical activity, and moderation in alcohol intake. Eating Healthy with Diabetes (American Diabetes Association & American Dietetic Association, 2003c), which is suited for individuals with limited reading skills, is appropriate for teaching in meal planning at this basic level. This approach has proven as effective as more structured meal planning in some instances, particularly among older individuals with type 2 diabetes.

Some individuals prefer to follow more structured meal plans and may need these plans to achieve optimal glucose control. One approach is described in the Exchange Lists for Meal Planning (American Diabetes Association & American Dietetic Association, 2003d), in which foods are grouped according to similarities in their carbohydrate, protein, and fat content. An alternative resource, the Exchange Lists for Weight Management (American Diabetes Association & American Dietetic Association, 2003e), includes all the information from the Exchange Lists for Meal Planning, along with guidelines for controlling energy intake and increasing physical activity. This is useful for overweight individuals, whether or not they have diabetes. In working with the person with diabetes to develop a meal plan, the dietitian considers the person's optimal energy intake (~20 to 25 kcal/kg desirable body weight for an adult, plus 30% more energy for a sedentary individual, 50% more for a moderately active person, and 100% more for a strenuously active person). For children and pregnant and lactating women, use the DRI (see Chapter 1) for a guideline. The desirable proportions of carbohydrate, protein, and fat in the diet are determined as described previously. Once these parameters are established, the number of exchanges (servings) from each group can be identified, and the exchanges can be assigned to specific meals and snacks so that the carbohydrate is spread evenly throughout the day. Starch, milk, and fruit exchanges contain approximately the same amount of carbohydrate (12 to 15 g/exchange) and can be substituted for one another.

Carbohydrate counting is a technique that focuses on the carbohydrate content of foods consumed. Carbohydrate is the main component of the diet that affects postprandial blood glucose levels and insulin requirements. Depending on the skills and interest of the diabetic individual, carbohydrate counting can be a very simple or very complex technique. At its simplest, the dietitian teaches the person with diabetes to identify sources of carbohydrate in the diet, and they work together to make carbohydrate intake at a meal consistent from day to day. Keeping food records is encouraged to help the person recognize the relationship between carbohydrate intake and blood glucose levels. At an intermediate level, the person further develops record-keeping skills, comparing blood glucose records with food intake records. The person learns to recognize patterns in blood glucose readings and to understand how they relate to food intake, physical activity, and diabetes medications. At its most complex level, carbohydrate counting is appropriate for people with type 1 diabetes who are receiving intensive insulin therapy. At this level, the person with diabetes matches insulin dosages precisely with carbohydrate intake, decreasing or increasing the insulin dosage to allow consumption of less or more carbohydrate than usual. Publications to help the beginning and more advanced carbohydrate counter develop their skills are available (American Diabetes Association & American Dietetic Association, 2003a, 2003b).

Exercise

Regular exercise (continuous activity lasting at least 20 to 30 minutes and performed at least 3 to 4 days a week) can promote weight control, reduce the risk of cardiovascular disease, help relieve psychologic stress, and increase the sensitivity of the tissues to insulin. The guidelines in Chapter 6 for becoming and remaining physically fit are appropriate for individuals with diabetes, as long as they first have the approval of their physicians. Impact exercises such as jogging, treadmill running, and step exercises are generally less desirable when neuropathy or retinopathy is present, but swimming, cycling, rowing, or other low-impact activities are good alternatives.

Individuals with type 1 diabetes should monitor their blood glucose before and after exercise to determine whether insulin or food intake needs to be adjusted. The person should not exercise if the blood glucose is >250 mg/dl (13.9 mmol/L) and ketosis is present and use caution if the blood glucose is >300 mg/dl (16.6 mmol/L) whether or not ketosis is present (American Diabetes Association, 2004). If the preexercise blood glucose concentration is less than 100 mg/dl (5.6 mmol/L), then the individual needs to consume a carbohydrate-containing snack before exercise. Snacks may be needed every 30 to 60 minutes to prevent hypoglycemia during exercise lasting more than 30 minutes. Appropriate snacks provide approximately 10 to 15 g of rapidly absorbed carbohydrate. Examples include 1 small apple or banana, 1/2 cup of regular soft drink, 1/2 bagel, or 4 to 6 oz of fruit juice. Some individuals become hypoglycemic several hours after exercise ends, and they need a snack or meal after exercise. Strenuous activity lasting 45 minutes or longer may result in a need to decrease the insulin dosage.

Coping with acute illness

Individuals with diabetes must have anticipatory teaching about how to cope with sick days (e.g., acute viral illnesses):

- Check blood glucose and urine ketones frequently, every 2 to 4 hours or as indicated.
- Consume approximately 45 to 50 g of carbohydrate (adults), or approximately three carbohydrate choices (Box 17-2) every 3 to 4 hours. When vomiting, diarrhea, or fever is present, small amounts of liquids every 15 to 30 minutes help to prevent dehydration, replace electrolyte losses, and provide energy.
- Notify the health care provider if it is impossible to take and retain carbohydrate-containing foods and fluids for 4 hours or more, if blood glucose is difficult to control or ketonuria is present, if persistent diarrhea occurs, if severe abdominal pain is present, or if the illness lasts more than 24 hours.

Minimizing acute complications

Hypoglycemia

Hypoglycemia is most common in people treated with insulin but can also occur with oral hypoglycemic therapy. Instruction

Box 17-2   Foods and Fluids for Sick Days*

½ cup (120 ml) regular gelatin dessert
½ cup (120 ml) fat-free, light, or regular ice cream
½ cup (120 ml) sherbet or sorbet
1 frozen fruit juice bar
6 saltine crackers
4 slices melba toast
1 cup (240 ml) tomato, vegetable, chicken noodle, or cream soup
½ cup (120 ml) sugar-free (or ¼ cup regular) pudding
¾ cup (180 ml) regular ginger ale
½ cup (120 ml) regular cola or lemon-lime soda
½ cup (120 ml) orange juice

*Each serving provides approximately 15 g of carbohydrate.

should be planned to help the person (and significant others, as appropriate):

- Be aware of and avoid precipitating factors: failing to eat scheduled meals and snacks, eating meals or snacks late, vomiting or poor food intake during acute illness, prolonged or intense physical activity without a compensatory increase in carbohydrate intake or decrease in insulin dosage, alcohol intake, and impaired mentation and self-care skills resulting from alcohol intoxication or illicit drug use.

- Recognize signs and symptoms of hypoglycemia: hunger, irritability, headache, shakiness, sweating, and altered neurologic status ranging from drowsiness to unconsciousness and convulsions. Repeated episodes of hypoglycemia can cause symptom unawareness; for example, if hypoglycemia occurs one day, then the person with diabetes may be unaware of symptoms if an episode of hypoglycemia occurs the following day.

- Test blood glucose regularly and any time signs of hypoglycemia appear.

- Correct hypoglycemia (blood glucose <70 mg/dl [3.8 mmol/L]) if it occurs. During insulin-induced hypoglycemia, 10 g of carbohydrate can raise the blood glucose ~40 mg/dl (2.2 mmol/L), and 20 g can raise the blood glucose ~60 mg/dl (American Diabetes

Association, 2004). Blood glucose levels will fall ~60 minutes after glucose ingestion. Glucose is available as a gel or in tablets, but any carbohydrate that will supply glucose is acceptable. Ten grams of carbohydrate is found in 1.5 tbsp of raisins, 3 oz (90 ml) of apple juice, 3.3 oz (100 ml) of regular cola beverage, or 3 jelly beans or gum drops. Fat can slow gastric emptying, and therefore consuming fat with the carbohydrate (e.g., a chocolate bar) may delay recovery from hypoglycemia.

- Wear a Medic-Alert bracelet so that treatment can be given if the individual becomes confused or unconscious.

Diabetic ketoacidosis

This complication occurs primarily in individuals with type 1 diabetes. Instruction should include the following:

- Be aware of precipitating factors, such as acute infectious illnesses or failure to take the prescribed dosage of insulin or oral hypoglycemic agents.
- Recognize the signs and symptoms such as elevated blood glucose, thirst, warm dry skin, nausea and vomiting, "fruity"-smelling breath, pain in abdomen, drowsiness, and polyuria.
- Check blood glucose if the symptoms occur, and obtain medical treatment if blood glucose is excessively elevated.

Hyperglycemic hyperosmolar nonketotic syndrome

This complication is more common in the individual with type 2 diabetes. Instruction should include the following:

- Be aware of precipitating factors, such as infections or other stress.
- Recognize the symptoms such as excessive thirst, polyuria, dehydration, shallow respirations, and altered sensorium.
- Check blood glucose if symptoms occur, and obtain medical attention if the blood glucose level is excessive.

Coping with diabetic gastroparesis

Prokinetic agents, including metoclopramide and the investigational drug domperidone, can be effective in stimulating GI motility in some instances. Correcting hyperglycemia can help relieve symptoms because hyperglycemia has an inhibitory effect on gastric emptying. People with gastroparesis should be encouraged to keep detailed food intake, blood glucose, and symptom records so that insulin administration can be fitted to peak absorption times. Use of short-acting and ultra-short-acting insulin increases flexibility in coping with the problem (e.g., a dose of insulin lispro can be injected postprandially if SMBG reveals that blood glucose is excessively high).

Medical nutrition therapy in gastroparesis includes counseling to reduce fat intake because fat tends to delay gastric emptying. People with gastroparesis are at risk for formation of gastric bezoars (hardened gastrointestinal contents, often containing food fibers), and individuals with severe gastroparesis may find it necessary to decrease the intake of insoluble fiber (e.g., wheat bran, whole wheat, brown rice, vegetable and fruit skins, prunes, and raisins). Small, frequent meals may be better tolerated than large meals if early satiety is a problem. Food should be chewed thoroughly. Maintaining an upright posture for at least 30 to 60 minutes after a meal allows gravity to facilitate gastric emptying (Valentine et al., 1998).

REFERENCES

American Diabetes Association: Clinical practice recommendations 2004, *Diabetes Care* 27(suppl 1):S1, 2004.

American Diabetes Association: Implications of the diabetes control and complications trial, *Diabetes Care* 26(suppl 1):S25, 2003.

American Diabetes Association, American Dietetic Association: *Advanced carbohydrate counting*, Alexandria, VA, and Chicago, 2003a, The Associations.

American Diabetes Association, American Dietetic Association: *Basic carbohydrate counting,* Alexandria, VA, and Chicago, 2003b, The Associations.

American Diabetes Association, American Dietetic Association: *Eating healthy with diabetes,* Alexandria, VA, and Chicago, 2003c, The Associations.

American Diabetes Association, American Dietetic Association: *Exchange lists for meal planning,* Alexandria, VA, and Chicago, 2003d, The Associations.

American Diabetes Association, American Dietetic Association: *Exchange lists for weight management,* Alexandria, VA, and Chicago, 2003e, The Associations.

Foster-Powell K, Miller JB: International tables of glycemic index, *Am J Clin Nutr* 62:871S, 1995.

Genuth S et al: Implications of the United Kingdom prospective diabetes study, *Diabetes Care* 26(suppl 1):S28, 2003.

Valentine V, Barone JA, Hill JVC: Gastropathy in patients with diabetes: current concepts and treatment recommendations, *Diabetes Spectrum* 11:248, 1998.

Selected Bibliography

Benjamin SM et al: Estimated number of adults with prediabetes in the U.S. in 2000: opportunities for prevention, *Diabetes Care* 26:645, 2003.

Costacou T, Mayer-Davis EJ: Nutrition and prevention of type 2 diabetes, *Annu Rev Nutr* 23:147, 2003.

Franz MJ et al: Evolution of diabetes medical nutrition therapy, *Postgrad Med J* 79:30, 2003.

Gadsby R: Promoting self-management in diabetes, *Practitioner* 247:318, 2003.

Howard BV: Dietary fat and diabetes: a consensus view, *Am J Med* 113(suppl 9B):38S, 2002.

Alcohol-Related, Mental, and Neurologic Disorders

18

Alcohol Abuse and Alcoholism
Pathophysiology

Alcohol abuse can be defined as heavy drinking with an increasing tolerance for ethanol but no withdrawal symptoms when drinking stops. **Alcoholism** refers to a strong craving for ethanol, associated with increasing tolerance to alcohol's intoxicating effects and symptoms of withdrawal when drinking is discontinued. Approximately two thirds of adults in the United States drink alcohol, but heavy drinkers (about 10% of those who drink or 7% of the total adult population) account for most of the social and physical problems associated with alcoholism and alcohol abuse. Both genetic and environmental factors appear to contribute to development of alcoholism and alcohol abuse.

Heavy alcohol use has adverse effects on nutrition both because it displaces other, more nutritious, foods in the diet and because chronic use impairs absorption and metabolism of many nutrients. The most common nutritional problems in heavy drinkers include deficiencies of protein, thiamin, folic acid, vitamin B_6 (pyridoxine), niacin, riboflavin, magnesium, zinc, and calcium. The protein deficiency, along with generalized nutritional deficits, contributes to the development of fatty liver. Fatty liver occurs when inadequate protein is available to form lipoproteins for the transport of lipids out of the liver, causing the lipids synthesized in the liver to be stored there.

The effect of heavy alcohol use on body weight has been a controversial issue. Ethanol is energy-rich, containing 7.1 kcal/g (Table 18-1). Approximately 75% of this energy in alcohol is usable when alcohol is metabolized via the alcohol dehydrogenase pathway, which is responsible for most ethanol metabolism when drinking is light to moderate. A second alcohol metabolizing pathway, the microsomal ethanol oxidizing system (MEOS), is inducible, meaning that its activity increases with heavy drinking. Less than 50% of the energy contained in alcohol is available to the body when it is metabolized via the MEOS (Suter, 2000). Resting energy expenditure has been reported to be higher in alcohol abusers than in nonabusers in one report (Levine et al., 2000), indicating that the energy-wasting effects of the MEOS

Table 18-1   Approximate Alcohol and Kilocalorie Content of Some Common Alcohol Beverages

Beverage and Serving Size	Alcohol (g/Serving)	kcal/ Serving
Beer, Ale, and Malt Liquor		
Beer, 12 fl oz	3	150
Beer, light, 12 fl oz	11	100
Beer, low-alcohol, 12 fl oz	6.5	75
Malt liquor or ale, 12 fl oz	15	150
Cocktails*		
Bloody Mary, 5 fl oz	14	120
Gin and tonic, 7.5 fl oz	16	170
Martini, 2.5 fl oz	22	160
Piña colada, 4.5 fl oz	20	260
Distilled Spirits (Gin, Rum, Vodka, Whiskey), 1.5 fl oz Jigger		
80 proof	14	97
90 proof	16	110
100 proof	18	124
Wines		
Dessert, 2 fl oz	9	75
Table, 3.5 fl oz	9.6	75

fl oz, Fluid ounce (approximately 30 ml).
Components: Bloody Mary = tomato juice, vodka, and lemon juice; gin and tonic = tonic water, gin, and lime juice; martini = gin and vermouth; piña colada = pineapple juice, rum, sugar, and coconut cream.

and of an elevated metabolic rate might minimize the net energy gain from heavy alcohol use. In some investigations, heavy drinkers have been found to have lower weights than people who drank less (reviewed in Lieber, 2000). However, studies taking into account confounding variables, particularly smoking behavior, suggest that individuals with the heaviest alcohol intakes are more likely to exhibit weight gain and be overweight than lighter drinkers (Kaplan et al., 2003; Wannamethee & Shaper, 2003). Alcohol abuse appears to be especially likely to promote fat accumulation in the trunk. In women, the pattern of drinking may be especially important; women were more likely to have an increase in abdominal obesity if they consumed large amounts of alcohol sporadically (e.g., 4 drinks/day on weekends, none on weekdays) than if they consumed small amounts (1 drink or less) daily (Dorn et al., 2003).

In addition to the nutritional deficiencies associated with alcohol abuse, the metabolism of alcohol can result in metabolic complications such as hypoglycemia, lactic acidosis, hyperuricemia (contributing to gout), hypertriglyceridemia, and ketoacidosis.

A variety of other medical problems are associated with heavy alcohol use, including cirrhosis of the liver, hepatic encephalopathy, pancreatitis, gastritis, cerebral atrophy, hypertension, osteopenia (thinning of the bones), and neuropathy associated with demyelination of the nerves. **Wernicke-Korsakoff syndrome** is a serious disorder of the central nervous system that can occur in alcoholism. Symptoms are confusion, memory loss, confabulation (filling in memory gaps with inaccurate, fabricated, and often implausible information), ataxia, abnormal ocular motility (ophthalmoplegia and nystagmus), and peripheral neuropathy. The cause of Wernicke-Korsakoff syndrome appears to be multifactorial, but both genetic susceptibility and thiamin deficiency play roles in its development.

Treatment

Alcoholics tend to deny that they have a problem. Effective therapy for alcoholism comes only after the individual has acknowledged the illness. Comprehensive therapy includes individual or group counseling, usually involving family members and/or close friends, and a nutritious diet. Prolonged follow-up (e.g., through participation in a group such as Alcoholics

Anonymous) is necessary for most recovering alcoholics. Pharmacologic agents are often used early in treatment of alcoholism. Antianxiety agents such as diazepam may be used to reduce anxiety during alcohol withdrawal. Disulfiram (Antabuse), which interferes with the metabolism of alcohol, is sometimes administered for several weeks or months to help the individual resist the compulsion to drink. When alcohol is ingested by the person taking disulfiram, acetaldehyde levels in the blood rise, causing many unpleasant symptoms (see previous Pathophysiology discussion).

Nutritional Care

Most forms of alcohol are low in micronutrients (vitamins and minerals). Chronic alcohol abuse can cause low hepatic stores of folate, niacin, and vitamins B_6 (pyridoxine) and B_{12}, as well as impaired utilization of folate and vitamins B_1 (thiamin) and B_6. In addition, zinc and magnesium levels may be low as a result of increased urinary excretion of these minerals during heavy drinking. Bone loss may occur because of increased calcium loss in the urine. Organ damage associated with alcohol abuse—including hepatitis, hepatic cirrhosis, and pancreatitis—interferes with absorption of fat, fat-soluble vitamins, and minerals. Gastritis related to alcohol abuse may result in iron-deficiency anemia from blood loss. Goals of medical nutrition therapy are to support the individual in avoiding alcohol and to correct nutritional deficits.

Assessment

Assessment is summarized in Table 18-2.

Intervention and teaching

Promoting hepatic regeneration and correcting nutritional deficits

The most important dietary change is abstinence from alcohol to allow the liver to heal. People who abuse alcohol are likely to have a variety of nutritional deficits, as described previously. A nutritious diet adequate in energy, protein, and micronutrients can promote hepatic regeneration. If esophageal varices are present, foods that are soft in texture reduce the risk of bleeding varices. Medical nutrition therapy of hepatitis, hepatic encephalopathy,

Table 18-2   Assessment in Alcoholism and Disruptions of Mental Health

Area of Concern	Significant Findings
Protein-Energy Malnutrition (PEM)	*History* Chronic alcohol or other drug abuse (inadequate intake of nutritious foods or impaired absorption of nutrients); paranoia, delusions (e.g., fear that food is poisoned); confusion, disorientation, inability to care for self (e.g., schizophrenia, Alzheimer's disease); anorexia, nausea, vomiting, or diarrhea related to medication usage (e.g., cholinesterase inhibitors in Alzheimer's) *Physical Examination* Hepatomegaly (can be from both malnutrition and toxic effects of alcohol); ascites, edema; muscle wasting; triceps skinfold <5th percentile; weight <90% of desirable or BMI <18.5 (↓ body weight may be masked by presence of ascites and edema) *Laboratory Analysis* ↓ Serum albumin, transferrin, or prealbumin (↓ levels may indicate liver failure instead of or in addition to malnutrition); ↓ creatinine-height index
Overweight/ Obesity	*History* Excessive intake of energy (sometimes occurs in depression or alcoholism) *Physical Examination* Weight >120% of desirable or BMI >25; triceps skinfold >95th percentile

Continued

Table 18-2   Assessment in Alcoholism and Disruptions of Mental Health—cont'd

Area of Concern	Significant Findings
Vitamin Deficiencies	
B complex, especially B_1, B_6, folate	*History* Alcohol abuse; excessive ethanol or carbohydrate intake without adequate vitamins; severely restricted diet (e.g., canned soups, soft drinks, candy, snack foods) *Physical Examination* Peripheral neuropathy; dermatitis; glossitis, cheilosis; edema, congestive heart failure; confusion, memory loss *Laboratory Analysis* ↓ Hct, ↑ MCV, ↓ serum or RBC folate (NOTE: Laboratory assessment of vitamins B_1 and B_6 is rarely done; these vitamins have low toxicity; large doses are given and response is evaluated clinically.)
Mineral Deficiencies	
Zinc (Zn)	*History* Alcohol abuse, with poor intake and ↑ excretion of Zn *Physical Examination* Poor sense of taste, distorted taste; alopecia; poor wound healing; diarrhea; dermatitis *Laboratory Analysis* ↓ Serum Zn
Magnesium (Mg)	*History* Alcohol abuse with poor intake and ↑ excretion of Mg

Table 18-2   Assessment in Alcoholism and Disruptions of Mental Health—cont'd

Area of Concern	Significant Findings
	Physical Examination Tremor, ataxia; mental disorientation
	Laboratory Analysis ↓ Serum Mg
Calcium (Ca)	*History* Alcohol abuse, with poor intake and ↑ excretion of Ca
	Laboratory Analysis Osteopenia on radiograph

and steatorrhea related to alcohol abuse are described in Chapter 11. If ascites are present, then a sodium restriction (usually 1 g/day) is commonly used (see Box 14-3).

In the severely malnourished alcoholic, especially if Wernicke-Korsakoff syndrome is suspected, thiamin (50 to 100 mg/day) is given parenterally for 3 to 7 days because absorption is likely to be impaired. After the initial treatment, oral thiamin (10 to 50 mg/day) is recommended for a period of weeks to months, until cardiovascular and neurologic symptoms have resolved or it is clear there will be no further improvement (Russell, 2001). The other B vitamins (particularly folic acid and vitamin B_6), zinc, and magnesium are administered orally at dosages two to three times the Dietary Reference Intake (DRI) for several weeks, to replenish the tissue stores of these nutrients. A daily oral multivitamin-multimineral supplement providing the DRI is usually prescribed for several months thereafter.

Recovered alcoholics need continued help, particularly advice for coping with social events and holidays when alcohol is usually served. Role-playing before these occasions can be helpful. The likelihood of success is increased by involvement of family and friends. Organizations such as Al-Anon can be of great benefit in providing support to family and friends and in helping them to learn how to help the recovering alcoholic.

Disorders of Mental Health
Pathophysiology

Mental illnesses have a variety of diverse origins too extensive to describe here. It is important to note that most mental illnesses have no nutritional cause. "Orthomolecular psychiatry," a treatment approach using vitamin supplements containing 10 to 500 times the recommended intakes, is not supported by scientific evidence or recognized as acceptable therapy by the American Psychiatric Association. There is also no reason to believe, as some individuals do, that many cases of mental illness arise from allergies or hypersensitivity to common foods. In most cases, nutritional care is primarily a supportive measure during the treatment of mental health disorders.

Treatment

A variety of treatment modalities may be used in mental disorders, including psychoanalysis, behavioral therapy, and family therapy. Some of the medications used are major and minor tranquilizers and lithium. Appendix H lists effects of these drugs on appetite and nutrient needs.

Nutritional Care

The goal of care is for the person to be able to cope with nutrition-related symptoms often seen in disruptions of mental health.

Assessment

Table 18-2 describes assessment in mental disorders.

Intervention

A variety of nutrition-related symptoms are found among individuals with disruptions of mental health. Most of these conditions are corrected when the individual receives adequate treatment for the underlying disorder; however, Table 18-3 summarizes approaches that can be used until the person has responded to treatment.

Neurologic Disorders
Convulsive (Seizure) Disorders
Pathophysiology

Numerous types of convulsive disorders (generally referred to as epilepsy) occur. Partial seizures affect only one cerebral hemisphere

Table 18-3   Intervention in Mental Disorders

Symptoms	Example of Mental Disorders	Suggested Interventions
Anorexia/apathy about food	Depression	Provide small, frequent feedings of foods high in energy; determine likes and dislikes, and try to accommodate these; serve foods in an attractive manner; use nutritional supplements (see Tables 8-1 and 8-2) as needed.
Constipation	Depression	Encourage high-fiber foods and liberal fluid intake.
Overeating	Depression	Make low-energy foods available, but avoid emphasizing weight control until mental condition stabilizes.
Confusion/disorientation	Schizophrenia, organic brain syndrome, Alzheimer's disease (senile dementia)	Remind individual to eat, if necessary; may need to direct him to take each bite; feed in an unhurried manner if self-feeding is not possible.
Excessive activity with "no time to eat"	Manic behavior	Provide high-energy foods that can be carried with the person who is too active to sit for a meal: sandwiches; muffins; cheese; fruit,

Continued

Table 18-3   Intervention in Mental Disorders—cont'd

Symptoms	Example of Mental Disorders	Suggested Interventions
Delusions (e.g., fear that food is poisoned or, conversely, belief that certain foods have magical powers)	Schizophrenia	custard, or pudding served in unbreakable containers; liquid nutritional supplements (see Table 8-1) in plastic containers. Allow individual to choose foods and beverages until delusions have responded to treatment; try to avoid tube feeding of persons with paranoia because this may increase the feeling of persecution.

so that consciousness is maintained but some cognitive functions such as speech are transiently lost. Generalized seizures affect the brain as a whole, and consciousness is lost, but the loss of consciousness may be so brief that it is barely noticeable. Signs of convulsive disorders range from subtle (a blank stare or a brief twitching of the mouth or eyelids) to severe (tonic-clonic seizures, with alternate sustained contraction and relaxation of the muscles). Convulsive disorders may occur as a result of hypoxia or central nervous system trauma, malformations, neoplasms, or infections. A variety of metabolic disorders (hypoglycemia, hypocalcemia, hypomagnesemia, water intoxication, lead poisoning, medication side effects) can cause seizures; in these cases, correcting the underlying disorder is the primary treatment. A significant percentage of convulsive disorders are idiopathic (have no known cause).

Treatment

Anticonvulsant medications are the primary means of treatment. Anticonvulsants used include carbamazepine, hydantoins (phenytoin and ethotoin), ethosuximide, valproic acid, and phenobarbital.

Nutritional care

Long-term use of anticonvulsant medications increases the risk of drug-nutrient interactions and may impair nutritional status. In some instances, medications are unsuccessful in controlling seizures. Ketosis, achieved with a "ketogenic" high-fat diet, has been found to improve control in some individuals with seizures that respond poorly to medication.

Assessment

Nutritional assessment is summarized in Table 18-4.

Intervention and teaching

Anticonvulsant medications. Many commonly used anticonvulsants—including phenytoin, phenobarbital, and primidone—accelerate the turnover of vitamin D and can contribute to poor bone mineralization (osteomalacia). Intake of the anticonvulsants and calcium at the same time impairs the absorption of both the drug and the nutrient. Vitamin D and calcium supplements may be needed by people who take these medications, but they should not be taken at the same time as the medications.

Table 18-4   Assessment in Neurologic Disorders

Area of Concern	Significant Findings
Protein-Energy Malnutrition (PEM)	*History* Restricted protein intake; unpalatable diet (e.g., ketogenic diet); feeding/swallowing difficulties such as dribbling of food and beverages from the mouth, dysphagia, weakness of muscles required for chewing, incoordination or spasticity interfering with chewing and swallowing; dementia or memory loss (refusing or forgetting to eat); use of corticosteroids
	Physical Examination Muscle wasting; triceps skinfold <5th percentile; weight <90% of desirable or BMI <18.5; or BMI, weight for height, or weight for age <5th percentile (children); edema, ascites
	Laboratory Analysis ↓ Serum albumin, transferrin, or prealbumin; ↓ creatinine-height index
Overweight/ Obesity	*History* ↓ Energy needs resulting from inactivity; reliance on soft or pureed foods, which are often more dense in energy than higher-fiber foods
	Physical Examination Triceps skinfold >95th percentile; weight >120% of desirable or BMI >25 (adults); or BMI, weight for height, or weight for age >85th percentile (children)

Table 18-4   Assessment in Neurologic Disorders—cont'd

Area of Concern	Significant Findings
Vitamin and Mineral Deficiencies	
Folate	*History* Phenytoin use *Physical Examination* Pallor; glossitis *Laboratory Analysis* ↓ Hct, ↑ MCV; ↓ serum and RBC folate
D	*History* Use of phenobarbital, primidone, or phenytoin, especially when combined with ketogenic diet; lack of sun exposure (e.g., institutionalization) *Physical Examination* Rickets; osteomalacia *Laboratory Analysis* ↓ Serum 1,25-dihydroxyvitamin D; ↑ alkaline phosphatase
Iron (Fe)	*History* Inadequate intake (ketogenic diet used in seizure disorders, difficulty chewing meats) *Physical Examination* Pallor, blue sclerae; spoon-shaped nails *Laboratory Analysis* ↓ Hct, Hgb, MCV; ↓ serum ferritin
Zinc (Zn)	*History* Inadequate intake (ketogenic diet, difficulty chewing meats) *Physical Examination* Diarrhea; dermatitis; poor sense of taste, distorted taste; alopecia; delayed wound healing

Continued

Table 18-4   Assessment in Neurologic Disorders—cont'd

Area of Concern	Significant Findings
	Laboratory Analysis ↓ Serum Zn
Calcium (Ca)	*History* Phenytoin use (↓ Ca absorption) or corticosteroid use with increased losses; inadequate intake (lactose intolerance)
	Physical Examination Rickets; osteomalacia
	Laboratory Analysis ↓ Serum Ca (uncommon); ↑ serum alkaline phosphate
Fluid Deficit	*History* Poor intake caused by difficulty swallowing fluids (as in CP or ALS) or inability to express thirst
	Physical Examination Poor skin turgor; ↓urinary output; dry, sticky mucous membranes
	Laboratory Analysis ↑ Serum Na, serum osmolality, BUN, Hct, urine specific gravity

Ketogenic diet. High levels of blood ketones produced from the metabolism of fat appear to decrease seizure activity. A diet that stimulates ketone production (a **ketogenic diet**) is used by selected children who exhibit a poor response to anticonvulsant medications. The effect of the diet has not been well studied in adults. Nearly 30% of children on the diet were found to be free of seizures or have at least a 90% reduction in seizures, and many were able to discontinue or reduce use of medications (Hemingway, 2001). The diet is effective only if adherence is rigid because a small excess of carbohydrate will inhibit ketosis. Adherence becomes much more difficult as children age, unless they are severely retarded. The high fat intake is unpalatable to many individuals, and the strict diet can be a burden. Potential side effects include kidney stones and hypocalcemia. These side effects probably occur because the diet is so high in fat that absorption is incomplete, and calcium is trapped in the fat in the feces. Calcium in the intestine reduces the absorption of oxalate, whereas loss of calcium in the stools allows increased absorption of oxalate. Oxalate is a component of many kidney stones. The diet may also result in acidic urine that promotes formation of uric acid stones. Drugs that make the urine alkaline inhibit uric acid stone formation. Additionally, the diet can result in poor growth, especially in young children, who must be especially carefully monitored for growth delays.

To accelerate development of ketosis, the diet is usually initiated after a 36- to 48-hour period of fasting, or a period of partial fasting (50 kcal/kg/day for young children). The diet is introduced over a period of 3 to 4 days to reduce the likelihood of nausea and vomiting. In the classic diet, the ratio of dietary fat to the combined carbohydrate and protein intake is between 3:1 and 4:1 (3 to 4 g of fat for every gram of carbohydrate plus protein). The diet commonly includes a protein allowance of 1.2 g/kg desirable body weight for children under 2 years of age and 1 g for children between 2 and 19 years. To promote ketosis, energy intake is limited to approximately 75 kcal/kg/day for children ages 1 to 3, 68 kcal/kg/day for children ages 4 to 6, and 60 kcal/kg/day for children ages 7 to 10. (For more information, consult Freeman MJ et al: *The Ketogenic Diet: A Treatment for Epilepsy*, ed 3, New York, 1999, Demos Medical Publishing.) A downloadable ketogenic diet meal planner is available at *www.stanford.edu/group/ketodiet/,* and an alternative planner is available by contacting the Ketogenic Diet Program, c/o Epilepsy Association of Maryland, 300 East Joppa Road, Suite 1103, Towson, MD 21286-3018 ([410] 828-7700). The ketogenic diet is usually low in vitamins C, A, and B complex and in iron, zinc, and calcium. A daily supplement providing the DRI for the person's age is advisable. Many medications, including vitamin and mineral supplements, contain carbohydrates, which must be considered in calculating the diet; see Lebel et al. (2001) for a compilation.

Heavy cream and margarine or butter are key components of most ketogenic diets. Hypercholesterolemia is common, and there is a concern about promotion of arteriosclerotic heart disease. Soft (tub or squeeze bottle) margarine and polyunsaturated and monounsaturated oils such as corn, soybean, safflower, sunflower, canola, and olive oil can be substituted for butter and cream if serum cholesterol becomes excessive. The risk of promotion of atherosclerotic heart disease by the diet must be balanced against the benefit; the ketogenic diet is normally prescribed only for individuals who have poor control of seizures even with optimal drug therapy.

Fluids are restricted to approximately 600 to 1200 ml/day, with no more than 120 ml taken in a 2-hour period, to prevent expansion of plasma volume with dilution of the ketones. The urine should not be dilute; the specific gravity must be maintained at approximately 1.025.

Some clinicians prefer the use of MCTs to long-chain triglycerides (LCTs). MCTs appear to be more ketogenic than the LCTs found in most common foods, which allows the combined carbohydrate and protein content of the diet to be increased to 20% to 40% of the total energy intake and the energy and fluid allowances to be more liberal. Results are still better if moderate energy and fluid restrictions are practiced, however. There are disadvantages to the MCT diet. MCTs are more expensive than LCTs, and excessive intakes of MCTs can result in abdominal cramping and diarrhea. Incorporating MCTs into the diet can be accomplished by blending them into skim milk, using them in place of other cooking oils, making salad dressing from them, or mixing them into unsweetened applesauce, scrambled eggs, meat or pasta salads, or casseroles. Gastrointestinal side effects are lessened and seizure control is improved if small amounts are served throughout the day, rather than larger amounts once or twice daily. A modification of the MCT diet supplies approximately 30% of the kcal as MCT and 41% as LCT, with the remainder of the kcal from protein and carbohydrate. Constipation, a common problem with the ketogenic diet, is less prevalent when MCTs are used.

Cerebral Palsy

Pathophysiology

Cerebral palsy (CP) is usually the result of hypoxia during the perinatal period. Motor centers of the brain are affected, with resulting incoordination, physical disabilities, and sometimes impairments of speech, sight, and hearing. There are several types of CP: *spastic paralysis*, with hyperactivity of the extensor muscles; *choreoathetosis*, with involuntary muscle movements; *ataxia*, or incoordination; and *flaccidity*, or decreased muscle tone.

Treatment

Physical therapy and judicious use of devices, such as computers that make communication by nonverbal individuals possible, can help people with CP achieve their maximum potential. Orthopedic surgery is sometimes used to correct deformities.

Nutritional care

Goals of care are to maintain adequate intake of nutrients and to prevent obesity, which further impairs mobility in individuals with CP.

Assessment

Assessment is summarized in Table 18-4.

Intervention and teaching

Chewing and swallowing problems. Provision of adequate nutrients may be difficult because of neuromuscular impairments and persistence of primitive reflexes. To minimize these problems, follow these guidelines:

- Individuals with CP should be placed in good anatomic position for feeding. Those with spastic CP are especially likely to hyperextend their necks, which makes swallowing difficult. Positioning them with back straight and hips and knees flexed reduces hyperextension. Separating the legs promotes stability.
- Underweight is a common problem, largely because of difficulty ingesting food. Parents and caregivers may spend 3 or more hours daily feeding an individual with CP. Because of the prolonged mealtimes, provision of snacks is often not effective in increasing intake. Thus, increasing the energy content of foods eaten at mealtimes is the best alternative. Skim milk powder, margarine, oils, or modular ingredients (see Table 8-2) can be added to foods to increase energy density. Gastrostomy feedings are beneficial for many children who cannot eat enough to maintain their nutritional status and obtain adequate nutrients to support growth.
- Additional suggestions can be found in Box 18-1.

Promoting self-feeding. To make it easier for people with CP to feed themselves, follow these guidelines:

Box 18-1   Common Nutritional Problems in Patients with Neurologic Disorders

Constipation

- Increase intake of fiber-containing foods.
  - Bran, whole-grain cereals and breads, legumes, vegetables, and fresh and dried fruits are good sources (see Appendix B).
  - Set a goal of 30 g fiber or more daily.
  - Use fiber-containing formulas if enteral tube feedings are necessary.
- Maintain a liberal fluid intake (30 to 50 ml per kg [14 to 23 ml/lb] for adults, unless contraindicated) to encourage formation of soft, bulky stools.
- Consume dried plums (prunes) or prune juice regularly for their natural laxative properties.
- Obtain regular physical activity (preferably at least 30 minutes daily) as tolerated to stimulate gastrointestinal motility.

Dysphagia or Difficulty Swallowing

- Try thickened liquids.
  - Thin liquids such as water or tea are often among the most difficult items to swallow.
  - Shakes, commercial supplements, or beverages thickened with infant cereals, cornstarch, or instant potatoes may be easier to swallow.
  - Sherbet, sorbet, fruit ices, and frozen yogurt or ice cream can be used to supply some of the individual's fluid needs if they do not result in excessive energy intake.
  - Commercial thickened water, coffee, and juices are available, as well as thickeners to be added to regular foods and beverages; different levels of thickening can be achieved, depending on the patient's needs.*
- Avoid dry, hard foods.
  - Use soft, moist foods such as casseroles, meats and vegetables with gravies and sauces, mashed potatoes, applesauce, and cooked cereals.
- Avoid slick foods such as gelatin or pasta salad if these appear to cause difficulty.
- Maintain an upright position during and for at least 30 minutes after meals.

> ### Box 18-1   Common Nutritional Problems in Patients with Neurologic Disorders—cont'd
>
> - Keep the chin positioned slightly downward.
> - Consult speech or physical therapists for suggestions on techniques to improve swallowing effectiveness.
> - Do not rush while eating.
> - Avoid eating alone, if possible, and have suction equipment available.
> - Consider percutaneous endoscopic gastrostomy (PEG) or other enteral tube feeding techniques if necessary to deliver nutrients safely.

*For example, Resource ThickenUp (Novartis Nutrition) and Thick & Easy (Hormel HealthLabs).

- Utilize plates with rims to allow food to be scooped up by pushing it against the rim.
- Use specially made silverware with thick handles or insert the spoon or fork handle into a rolled washcloth to make it easier to grip.
- Prevent scooting of plates or bowls by putting suction cups, such as those used for soap holders, under them.

Preventing or correcting obesity. Individuals who are very inactive, such as those with severe motor impairments who are confined to a wheelchair, may become overweight or obese. The following guidelines help to prevent or alleviate this problem:

- Try reducing fat in the diet. Choose lean meat and skinless poultry; use skim or low-fat milk and dairy products made with skim or low-fat milk; limit intake of fried or fatty foods; serve pastries, doughnuts, and high-fat cookies and cakes rarely; use butter or margarine sparingly; use low-fat or fat-free salad dressings.
- Serve unsweetened beverages or those sweetened with sugar substitutes often. Beverages consumed before or with meals help the person feel full faster.
- Increase intake of fibers and starches. Whole grains and fresh fruits and vegetables are bulky and help the individual to feel full more quickly.

- Increase activity to the extent possible.
- See Chapter 7 for further suggestions.

Preventing or correcting constipation. See Box 18-1 for measures to relieve constipation.

Amyotrophic Lateral Sclerosis

Pathophysiology

Amyotrophic lateral sclerosis (ALS) is a progressive degenerative neurologic disease that results in atrophy of the muscles. Eventually, it affects most of the body, including the muscles involved in chewing and swallowing.

Treatment

Although there is no cure for ALS, riluzole, a neuroprotective drug, extends survival or delays the time until tracheotomy is needed. This drug has numerous gastrointestinal side effects including nausea, vomiting, dyspepsia, anorexia, and diarrhea. Physical therapy can help maintain as much muscle mass as possible as the disease progresses.

Nutritional care

Goals of care are to prevent nutritional deficits and maintain feeding safety (i.e., prevent choking or aspiration of foods and beverages into the lungs).

Assessment

Assessment is summarized in Table 18-4. Weight loss is inevitable because of muscle wasting. Nutritional deficits, however, accelerate loss. When weight loss in 6 months is greater than 10% of the usual body weight, energy deficits should be suspected. Chair or bed scales are often necessary to obtain weights. BMI may not be very useful in people with ALS because of the effects of muscle wasting on their body composition. Bioelectrical impedance has been used to assess lean body mass, and the effects of nutrition support maintenance of lean body mass, in individuals with ALS.

Intervention and teaching

Preventing nutritional deficits

- Encourage small, frequent feedings to maintain optimal intake. Box 12-1 offers suggestions for increasing energy intake.

Supplements in the form of puddings or thick liquids may be the easiest to consume.

- Try utensils with loops to fit over the hands to help prevent dropping of utensils and improve grip.
- Protein foods may be difficult to chew, especially if dry. Good protein sources are tender, chopped meats and poultry; moist casseroles made with meat, fish, or poultry; cheese and cottage cheese; yogurt; and poached, soft-cooked, or scrambled eggs. Gravies and sauces served with meats make chewing and swallowing easier.
- Commercial supplements (high-protein puddings and beverages or protein powders to be added to other foods; see Tables 8-1 and 8-2) are available, but home-prepared products are often tastier.
- Vitamins and minerals may be lacking because of impaired intake. A daily multivitamin-multimineral supplement can be recommended if assessment indicates a need.

Reducing dysphagia and potential for pulmonary aspiration. Box 18-1 includes suggestions for dealing with dysphagia. Many individuals with ALS require gastrostomy of other tube feedings when their swallowing ability deteriorates to the point that pulmonary aspiration is very likely.

Preventing constipation. Inactivity and muscle weakness contribute to decreased bowel motility and constipation. See Box 18-1 for measures to alleviate this problem.

Multiple Sclerosis

Pathophysiology

Multiple sclerosis (MS), a disease of the central nervous system, affects the myelinated nerve fibers and the muscles they innervate. Patches of the myelin surrounding the nerves degenerate, and the myelin is replaced by scars. MS tends to follow a pattern of exacerbations and remissions. It appears that the disease is autoimmune, with cell-mediated and humoral responses being generated against myelin proteins. The cause of MS is unknown, but evidence suggests that some individuals have a genetic susceptibility that makes them vulnerable to MS when exposed to certain environmental influences. Viruses or toxic substances have been proposed as possible environmental triggers for the disease. Some epidemiologic evidence indicates that a diet rich in plant foods (grains, fruits, and vegetables) is associated with a reduced risk for development of MS.

Treatment

Although there is no cure for MS, immunomodulators such as interferon beta-1a and -1b and immunosuppressives such as glatiramer acetate are used to reduce the likelihood of acute exacerbations of the disease. Steroids are frequently used for their antiinflammatory properties in acute exacerbation of the disease. Mitoxantrone, an antineoplastic agent, improves neurologic function and reduces relapses in selected patients with secondary (chronic) progressive, progressive relapsing, or worsening relapsing-remitting forms of the disease. These drugs may have nutritional impacts such as nausea, vomiting, diarrhea, and stomatitis. Numerous mediations are used for palliation of symptoms. Muscle spasms are a common problem that may be alleviated by baclofen. Diazepam may be used as an adjunct to potentiate the effects of baclofen. Dantrolene is an alternative antispastic drug. Clonazepam can be used if intention tremor is a problem. Urinary retention, which contributes to urinary tract infections, is another frequently encountered symptom, which can be treated with anticholinergic agents such as oxybutynin or propantheline. Nonsteroidal antiinflammatory drugs (NSAIDs, e.g., ibuprofen) relieve muscle and joint pain, and antidepressants such as amitriptyline may be effective in controlling emotional lability. Even small increases in environmental temperature may worsen symptoms, and thus cool showers or air conditioning may be effective in promoting comfort. It is suggested that avoidance of physical and psychologic stress helps prevent relapses.

Nutritional care

Assessment

Assessment is summarized in Table 18-4.

Intervention and teaching. There is no proof that a special diet is effective in alleviating the effects of MS; however, long-term use of a low-fat diet, especially one low in saturated fat, is postulated to reduce the number of acute exacerbations and slow the progress of the disease. Although firm evidence for the efficacy of this diet is lacking, it should not be harmful if individuals are carefully instructed so that the diet is nutritionally adequate.

Low-fat diet. The low-fat diet generally includes at least 60 to 70 g of protein and approximately 50 to 60 g of fat per day, with sufficient carbohydrates to provide the balance of needed energy. Saturated fat is restricted to 10 g/day. Meat, fish, and poultry intake is usually reduced to about 2 oz/day, and dairy products must be prepared from skim milk. Fish oil, 1 tsp/day (equivalent to 4.5 g of fat), is recommended. Other unsaturated fats included in the diet are safflower, sunflower, corn, soybean, olive, and cottonseed oils. Intake of calcium, iron, and zinc should be evaluated. Supplements are often needed because of the restriction of animal products.

Constipation. Constipation is reported by more than 40% of people with multiple sclerosis. Generalized muscle weakness, immobility, and constipating medications probably are etiologic factors. To help prevent or correct constipation, consult Box 18-1.

Parkinsonism (Parkinson's Disease)
Pathophysiology

Parkinsonism is a progressive neuromuscular disorder characterized by a low content of dopamine in the basal ganglia of the central nervous system. This results in tremor, rigidity, a characteristic "pill rolling" movement of the fingers, and hypoactivity. The cause is not known, but it has been speculated that oxidative damage from free radicals in the central nervous system may be involved. Two genes have been linked to parkinsonism, and it has been suggested that there is a genetic-environmental cause for this disorder—that is, a genetic susceptibility to develop the disease upon exposure to environmental factors, which might include toxins, smoking, or head trauma.

Treatment

Treatment is aimed at increasing dopamine levels or action in the nervous system. Levodopa, a precursor of dopamine, or a combination of levodopa and carbidopa are frequently used to treat parkinsonism. Dopamine receptor agonists such as pramipexole, ropinirole, and pergolide may be used alone in conjunction with levodopa and carbidopa. Selegiline and other inhibitors of monoamine oxidase, the enzyme that degrades dopamine, may be used with dopamine to prolong dopamine's actions; entacapone is used with carbidopa-containing preparations for the same purpose. Common nutrition-related side effects of levodopa and the drugs used as adjuncts to it are nausea, vomiting, anorexia, and dry mouth. Anticholinergic agents such as procyclidine, benztropine mesylate, and trihexyphenidyl may relieve excessive salivation and reduce the rigidity associated with the disease. The anticholinergics can cause the mouth to be excessively dry, increasing feeding problems; taking these drugs after meals may reduce difficulties in chewing and swallowing.

Nutritional care

People with Parkinson's disease may experience weight loss because the tremors and involuntary movements increase energy expenditure and may make it difficult for them to feed themselves adequately. Parkinson's disease may also impair the ability to swallow, interfering with intake of foods and beverages. In addition, levodopa has significant drug-nutrient interactions that must be understood in order to maximize the benefits of the medication.

Assessment

Assessment is summarized in Table 18-4.

Intervention and teaching

Preventing or correcting weight loss

- Monitor weight regularly.
- Encourage the individual to consume energy sufficient to reach the upper limit of the recommendation for age and sex (usually approximately 25 to 30 kcal/kg).
- Choose foods that are easy to get to the mouth (sandwiches and other foods eaten with the hands, or foods that can be impaled with a fork such as chunks of fruit or vegetables). Soups or other foods that must be balanced on a utensil are difficult and embarrassing for the person with a tremor to consume.
- Keep foods warm and palatable for slow eaters by using insulated dishes or a warming tray.
- Avoid interruptions (e.g., medication administration) during meals and snacks. Any distraction can cause the elderly person with parkinsonism to lose focus on eating and have difficulty starting again.
- Plate guards (a high rim around the plate) may be needed to help affected people scoop up food and bring it to their mouths.
- Avoid especially tough, hard, and chewy foods.

Optimizing drug therapy

- Take levodopa 1 hour before or 2 hours after meals. Protein consumed at the same time as levodopa impairs its action.
- Avoid excessive amounts of vitamin B_6 (pyridoxine), which antagonize levodopa action. Use vitamin supplements that provide no more than the DRI of vitamin B_6. Consume only moderate amounts of high-pyridoxine foods: avocados, bacon, bran, beef kidney, beef liver, kidney beans, lentils, lima beans, malted milk, molasses, navy beans, oatmeal, pork, sweet potatoes, fresh salmon, soy beans, split peas, tuna, walnuts, yeast.
- Avoid taking iron supplements at the same time as levodopa, because iron can impair levodopa absorption.
- After several years of levodopa therapy, individuals may become less responsive to the drug. If this occurs, the first step should be to assess protein intake. The North American diet often includes twice the DRI for protein, which may reduce effectiveness of levodopa. It may be necessary to change the diet pattern to improve the drug action:
  - Limit protein intake from morning through afternoon to ≤7 g (approximately three servings of grain products or starchy vegetables). Fruits, green leafy vegetables, juices, candies, and small amounts of bread, cereal, or starchy vegetables can be consumed.
  - Consume legumes, meats, and dairy products at dinner because control of parkinsonism symptoms is less important during the night.
  - Monitor weight and evaluate intake of protein, calcium, iron, riboflavin, and niacin if this pattern is followed. Calcium or other supplements may be needed.

Preventing constipation. The disease itself or medications used may result in constipation. Consult Box 18-1 for measures to relieve constipation.

Cerebrovascular Accident (Stroke)
Pathophysiology

Cerebrovascular accident (CVA), or stroke, refers to neurologic symptoms resulting from the interruption of blood flow to the brain. Stroke can result from ischemia (diminished blood flow usually related to blood vessel occlusion) or hemorrhage (sub-arachnoid or intracerebral). Symptoms vary, depending on the extent and location of the CVA. Some individuals experience hemiplegia, or paralysis of one side of the body; visual field defects (e.g., hemianopia, or failure to see half of the visual field); apraxia (inability to perform a known task in response to verbal instructions); and dysphagia. Cerebral edema, increasing the intracranial pressure and damage to the brain, occurs in about 10% to 20% of individuals with ischemic stroke. Vasospasm, or narrowing of the cerebral arteries, is common following hemorrhagic stroke.

Treatment

Pharmacologic therapy is aimed at decreasing or preventing extension of the damage. Use of recombinant tissue plasminogen activator (rt-PA), a thrombolytic agent, within 3 hours of the stroke has been effective in minimizing the effect of ischemic stroke. Ticlopidine hydrochloride and aspirin with dipyridamole inhibit platelet aggregation and may be used in strokes due to thrombosis. Nausea, diarrhea, and abdominal discomfort are common side effects of these drugs. Steroids or osmotic agents such as mannitol may be used to reduce cerebral edema. The calcium channel blocker nimodipine is used to decrease cerebral vasospasm in individuals with subarachnoid hemorrhage. Blood pressure–lowering drugs are used in therapy of intracerebral hemorrhage.

Nutritional care

The extent and location of the CVA will determine the severity and exact type of problems experienced. Thorough assessment to provide the basis for an individualized plan of care is thus essential.

Assessment

Assessment is summarized in Table 18-4.

Intervention and teaching

Prevention of stroke. High blood levels of the amino acid homocysteine have been found to be predictors of cardiovascular diseases, including stroke, and adequate dietary folate is an important factor in maintaining low levels of homocysteine. Moreover, epidemiologic evidence indicates that the risk of stroke, particularly in people with hypertension, is lessened by a diet rich in potassium, magnesium, calcium, and fiber. It is not clear that potassium, magnesium, calcium, and fiber by themselves (i.e., taken in the form of a supplement) would be effective in prevention of strokes. It may be that they are simply markers of a nutritious diet and a healthful lifestyle. It appears, however, that a diet rich in fruits and vegetables (five or more servings a day) and grain products—which would provide good sources of fiber, minerals, and folate—might reduce the likelihood of stroke.

Coping with feeding difficulties after stroke

Hemiplegia

- Anticipate more difficulty in self-feeding if the dominant hand is affected.
- Provide unobtrusive help in opening packages of utensils or condiments, cutting or buttering foods, or feeding the person, if necessary.
- Check for "pocketing" of food in the cheek on the affected side during meals, which occurs because the individual cannot sense that the food is there.
- Provide good mouth care after meals. Teach the patient or home caregivers to do this before discharge.

Visual field defects.   The individual may fail to eat half the food on the tray because he or she does not see it. Teach the individual to compensate by scanning, or routinely turning the head and moving the eyes toward the affected side.

Dysphagia.   Muscle weakness or incoordination, impaired gag or swallowing reflexes, and impaired cough contribute to dysphagia. Dysphagia, in turn, reduces the adequacy of nutrient intake and increases the likelihood of pulmonary aspiration. (see Box 18-1).

Diet and medication side effects.

- The platelet inhibitors are especially likely to cause gastrointestinal side effects. To reduce these, do as follows:
  - Administer ticlopidine with food.

- Give aspirin with dipyridamole on an empty stomach with a full glass of water.
- Avoid grapefruit juice if taking nimodipine, because it can enhance the drug's action and cause toxicity. Use orange or other juices instead.

Correcting constipation. See Box 18-1 for measures to correct constipation.

Alzheimer's Disease and Dementia

Pathophysiology

Alzheimer's disease (AD) is the most common cause of dementia, or progressive loss of mental function because of an organic cause. The cause is not definitely known, but the most common findings in the brains of individuals with AD are cerebral atrophy, senile plaques, and neurofibrillary tangles, as well as low levels of the neurotransmitter acetylcholine. Genetic factors are believed to be involved in many cases of AD. Oxidative damage to the neurons has also been suggested as a likely cause. Affected people experience memory loss, shortened attention span, expressive and receptive language disorders, apraxia (inability to perform a task in response to verbal commands), loss of reasoning skills, and intolerance of frustration.

Treatment

A cure for AD is unavailable at this time, but some medications can improve symptoms. Cholinesterase inhibitors such as tacrine and donepezil are commonly prescribed for use in AD. Hormone replacement therapy in postmenopausal women was hypothesized to provide some benefit in delaying or preventing AD, but recent data indicate that estrogen and progestin therapy may actually increase the risk of dementia and has no benefit for cognitive impairment. NSAIDs and antioxidants (e.g., vitamins E and C, beta-carotene) remain under study for treatment of AD. Gingko biloba, an extract derived from the gingko tree, has antioxidant and anticholinesterase properties, but current findings do not indicate that gingko is beneficial for individuals with AD. Antipsychotropic medications may be needed to control the agitation experienced by some individuals with more advanced AD.

Nutritional care

Progressive loss of self-care skills affects food intake and nutritional status. Weight loss and underweight are common in individuals with Alzheimer's disease, and some investigators have suggested that the metabolic rate and energy needs may be increased in this condition.

Assessment

Assessment is summarized in Table 18-4.

Intervention and teaching

Nutrition interventions are designed to encourage an adequate intake in order to maintain weight and strength, lessen morbidity (e.g., decubitus ulcers, pneumonia), and optimize comfort.

Encouraging adequate intake. The following list summarizes nutritional management of some of the more common problems experienced by the individual with AD.

- *Memory loss:* The individual may forget to eat or to finish a meal. Provide verbal and nonverbal cues that it is mealtime (e.g., announce the meal to the person; put utensils in his or her hand). Eating in a group setting may improve intake because the individual observes models of eating behavior.
- *Poor swallowing:* Swallowing difficulties increase the risk of pulmonary aspiration. See Box 18-1 for suggestions for improving swallowing.
- *Poor intake:* Inadequate consumption is common even in the individual with no swallowing problems. Provide adequate time for the individual to eat, and avoid distractions during mealtimes. Many affected people experience "sundowning," or restlessness and agitation in the evening, and food intake is poor at this time. For these individuals, maximize intake at the noon and morning meals when cognitive abilities are better. The affected person may need to be fed. When feeding a person with AD, try alternating bites of sweetened with unsweetened foods to see if this improves intake. Sweet items may be preferred to other foods. Use diversions (singing, cheerful conversation, touching, holding hands) to redirect behavior if the person is combative or resistive when being fed.

REFERENCES

Dorn JM et al: Alcohol drinking patterns differentially affect central adiposity as measured by abdominal height in women and men, *J Nutr* 133:2655, 2003.

Hemingway C et al: The ketogenic diet: a 3- to 6-year follow-up of 150 children enrolled prospectively, *Pediatrics* 108:898, 2001.

Kaplan MS et al: Prevalence and correlates of overweight and obesity among older adults: findings from the Canadian National Population Health Survey, *J Gerontol A Biol Sci Med Sci* 58:M1018, 2003.

Lebel D et al: The carbohydrate and caloric content of concomitant medications for children with epilepsy on the ketogenic diet, *Can J Neurol Sci* 28:322, 2001.

Lieber CS: Alcohol: its metabolism and interaction with nutrients, *Ann Rev Nutr* 20:395, 2000.

Levine JA, Harris MM, Morgan MY: Energy expenditure in chronic alcohol abuse, *Eur J Clin Invest* 30:779, 2000.

Russell RM: *Vitamin and trace mineral deficiency and excess.* In Braunwald E et al, eds: *Harrison's principles of internal medicine online,* ed 15, New York: McGraw-Hill, 2001.

Suter PM: The paradox of the alcohol-paradox—another step towards the resolution of the "alcohol energy wastage" controversy, *Eur J Clin Invest* 30:749, 2000.

Wannamethee SG, Shaper AG: Alcohol, body weight, and weight gain in middle-aged men, *Am J Clin Nutr* 77:1312, 2003.

SELECTED BIBLIOGRAPHY

Cameron A, Rosenfeld J: Nutritional issues and supplements in amyotrophic lateral sclerosis and other neurodegenerative disorders, *Curr Opin Clin Nutr Metab Care* 5:631, 2002.

Engelhart MJ et al: Dietary intake of antioxidants and risk of Alzheimer's disease, *JAMA* 287:3223, 2002.

Fung EB et al: Feeding dysfunction is associated with poor growth and health status in children with cerebral palsy, *J Am Diet Assoc* 102:361, 2002.

Hardiman O: Symptomatic treatment of respiratory and nutritional failure in amyotrophic lateral sclerosis, *J Neurol* 247:245, 2000.

Kidd PM: Multiple sclerosis, an autoimmune inflammatory disease: prospects for its integrative management, *Altern Med Rev* 6:540, 2001.

Kraus JJ, Metzler MD, Coplin WM: Critical care issues in stroke and subarachnoid hemorrhage, *Neurol Res* 24(suppl 1):S47, 2002.

Kwiterovitch PO et al: Effect of a high-fat ketogenic diet on plasma levels of lipids, lipoproteins, and apolipoproteins in children, *JAMA* 290:912, 2003.

Leboeuf R: Homocysteine and Alzheimer's disease, *J Am Diet Assoc* 103:304, 2003.

Levy R, Cooper P: Ketogenic diet for epilepsy, *Cochrane Database Syst Rev* (3):CD001903, 2003.

Markowitz JS, McRae AL, Sonne SC: Oral nutritional supplementation for the alcoholic patient: a brief overview, *Ann Clin Psychiatry* 12:153, 2000.

Payne A: Nutrition and diet in the clinical management of multiple sclerosis, *J Hum Nutr Diet* 14:349, 2001.

Perry L, McLaren LS: Nutritional support in acute stroke: the impact of evidence-based guidelines, *Clin Nutr* 22:283-293, 2003.

Samson-Fang L et al: Relationship of nutritional status to health and societal participation in children with cerebral palsy, *J Pediatr* 141:637, 2002.

Thomas FJ, Wiles CM: Dysphagia and nutritional status in multiple sclerosis, *J Neurol* 246:677, 1999.

Wilkinson TJ et al: Tolerance of early diet textures as indicators of recovery from dysphagia after stroke, *Dysphagia* 17:227, 2002.

Zhang SM et al: Intakes of carotenoids, vitamin C, and vitamin E and MS risk among two large cohorts of women, *Neurology* 57:75, 2001.

Eating Disorders

19

Anorexia nervosa and bulimia nervosa are eating disorders most commonly diagnosed in adolescent and young adult females. The prevalence of these eating disorders among females is about 8 to 10 times higher than among males. Even though the disorders are commonly diagnosed in the young, they may persist throughout life.

Pathophysiology
Characteristics of Eating Disorders

Anorexia nervosa and bulimia nervosa have distinguishing characteristics, as described as follows and in Table 19-1; however, it is relatively common for a combination of these two disorders to exist in the same individual. Moreover, the person who has one of these disorders may later develop the other. A person with anorexia nervosa, for example, may recover sufficiently to maintain a stable body weight but may continue to practice the bingeing and purging behaviors associated with bulimia.

The characteristics of anorexia nervosa include excessive thinness (refusal to maintain weight at or above 85% of the expected weight for height and age); body image disturbances (e.g., misperceptions of body size or shape or denial of the degree of underweight present); serious fear of gaining weight or becoming fat, even though underweight; and amenorrhea for at least three menstrual cycles in a girl or woman who has previously menstruated. Fat accounts for approximately 17% to 27% of the body weight in most healthy women, and amenorrhea is likely when the body fat falls below 17%. Anorectic behaviors can be divided into restrictive (practices that limit energy intake) and purging (practices meant to remove food from the body, such as self-induced vomiting and laxative abuse). An affected individual may exhibit one type of behavior or a combination of the two.

Table 19-1   Distinguishing Between Anorexia Nervosa and Bulimia

Characteristics	Anorexia Nervosa	Bulimia
Age of onset (years)	12 to mid-30s; two peaks; 13-14 and 17-18	17-25
Attitude toward therapy	Denial that a problem exists	Often extremely secretive about bulimic behavior, but willing to accept help once the problem is admitted
Body weight	15% or more below usual or desirable body weight; BMI <5th percentile for age	May be at or only slightly below desirable body weight
Metabolic	Amenorrhea; inability to maintain body temperature in heat or cold stress	Irregular menses; amenorrhea in fewer that 20%
Gastrointestinal	Decreased gastric emptying; constipation; elevated hepatic enzymes	Parotid enlargement; dental enamel erosion; esophagitis; Mallory-Weiss tears
Cardiovascular	Bradycardia; hypotension; dysrhythmias	Ipecac poisoning (tachycardia, cardiac dysrhythmias)
Skeletal	Decreased bone density (correlated with degree of underweight)	

Bulimia is characterized by recurrent (at least twice a week for 3 months) binge eating, defined as eating much more during some period of time than a normal person would and feeling a loss of control over behavior at the same time. In the purging form of this disorder, bulimic individuals regularly induce vomiting or use laxatives or enemas to prevent weight gain. They may also exercise heavily or fast frequently. In the nonpurging form of bulimia, fasting and heavy exercise are quite common.

The American Psychiatric Association (2000) has established criteria for two other eating disorders related to anorexia nervosa and bulimia nervosa. These are "binge eating disorder" and "eating disorder not otherwise specified." The binge eating disorder (BED) involves binge eating episodes without compensatory behaviors such as purging or exercise. People with BED eat so much within a 2-hour period that they are uncomfortable, and they often eat alone when they binge because of their embarrassment over their behavior. Binge eating in BED occurs at least twice a week, and bingeing is followed by feelings of guilt, depression, or disgust. Eating disorders not otherwise specified (ED-NOS), as the name implies, are those that cannot easily be assigned to the other eating disorder diagnoses. Purging behaviors in ED-NOS are similar to those in bulimia nervosa, but binges occur less than twice a week. Some individuals with ED-NOS exhibit restrained eating, similar to the restrictive pattern in anorexia nervosa, but people with ED-NOS manage to maintain their body weight in or close to the normal range (even though they may have lost a substantial amount of weight) and have regular menses. Frequently, people with ED-NOS chew and spit out food. Depending on the symptoms that predominate in a particular case, BED and ED-NOS are treated similarly to anorexia nervosa or bulimia nervosa.

Etiology of Eating Disorders

The causes of eating disorders are not fully understood. Cultural factors (e.g., the abundance of food in developed countries coupled with society's emphasis on thinness as desirable and beautiful) probably play a role. A period of restricted eating for the purpose of trying to lose weight often triggers both anorexia nervosa and bulimia. It has been reported that people who diet very stringently may be as much as 18-fold more likely to develop eating disorders than people who have never dieted, and even those who have made only moderate attempts at dieting may be at fivefold greater risk of eating disorders. Binge eating behaviors are more than twice as common in adolescents who diet frequently as in those who diet infrequently or not at all.

Family dysfunction may contribute to development of the disorders. Families of individuals with eating disorders have been described as overprotective, rigid, lacking in conflict resolution skills, and displaying a lack of confidence in the affected individual. As a result, the children may grow up to be dependent, unassertive, excessively reliant on the approval of others, and low in self-esteem. Abnormal eating behaviors are often initiated as a response to feelings of insecurity and a distorted perception of the importance of body shape and size in determining self-worth. Behavioral theorists also note that anorexia nervosa is reinforced by the attention it receives. The individual becomes the center of attention and manipulates the environment through his or her behavior.

Treatment

Treatment of eating disorders can include individual psychotherapy, group therapy, family psychotherapy, and behavioral therapy. Bulimics, in particular, appear to have a high incidence of depression. Antidepressant medications, especially the selective serotonin reuptake inhibitors (SSRIs), such as fluoxetine, are frequently used in therapy. SSRIs have also been used in an effort to prevent binge eating and in maintenance therapy of anorexia nervosa. These drugs increase brain serotonin, a neurotransmitter involved in regulating eating behaviors. Two agents that are undergoing study for bulimia and binge eating disorder are the serotonin receptor antagonist ondansetron and the anticonvulsant topiramate. Sibutramine, a serotonin/norepinephrine/dopamine inhibitor, has also shown some promise in treatment of bulimia and binge eating disorder. Substance abuse is common among bulimics, and thus careful screening for alcohol and drug abuse is needed before they begin any pharmacotherapy.

Treatment may occur on an inpatient or outpatient basis. Some indications for hospitalization are as follows: (1) loss of 25% or more of body weight; this state is often life-threatening, and hospitalization for nutritional support and intensive psychiatric therapy is usually necessary; (2) presence or likelihood of serious electrolyte imbalance as a result of an inability to cope with daily living without use of laxatives, diuretics, diet pills, or self-induced vomiting;

(3) family tensions necessitating separation of the affected individual and family; (4) severe depression with strong potential for suicide; and (5) inability or unwillingness to cooperate during outpatient therapy.

Nutritional Care

Goals of care are for the individual to change weight gradually, change eating behaviors in an incremental manner until food intake patterns are normal, separate eating behaviors from feelings and psychologic issues, learn to maintain a weight that is healthful without using abnormal food- and weight-related behaviors, and develop more effective coping skills to deal with stress and conflict.

Assessment

Individuals with eating disorders may be deficient in any or all nutrients, depending on the extent of their illness. The nutritional problems addressed in Table 19-2 are the most common ones. With the exception of electrolyte disorders, nutritional deficits are more common in anorexia nervosa than in bulimia.

Intervention and Teaching

A team approach to intervention is usually the most successful technique. The team usually includes, at a minimum, a physician experienced in treating eating disorders, a therapist experienced in working with adolescents and their families, a dietitian, and a nurse. The team works together with the patient and family to develop and assess the plan of treatment. Care of the patient includes nutrition assessment and correction of nutritional deficits and electrolyte abnormalities; individual and family counseling; nutrition teaching; modeling of healthful eating and activity patterns, coping strategies, and assertiveness skills; pharmacologic intervention in some cases; and monitoring the patient's status and responses to therapy.

Nutrition therapy

Restoring body weight should be a major goal in the early treatment of underweight individuals. Weight gain, on its own, may improve symptoms of depression, irritability, social withdrawal, and menstrual and other endocrine abnormalities. The long-term goal is for weight to be at least 85% to 90% of that expected for height. Intermediate goals can be set, such as achieving the 10th, 15th,

Table 19-2   Assessment in Eating Disorders

Area of Concern	Significant Findings
Fluid and Electrolyte Imbalance	*History* Self-induced vomiting; laxative or diuretic abuse
	Physical Examination Poor skin turgor; weakness; signs of self-induced vomiting; parotid salivary gland enlargement, dental enamel erosion, esophagitis, upper GI bleeding (Mallory-Weiss tears), hoarseness or sore throat; tachycardia, cardiac dysrhythmias (ipecac poisoning, potassium [K^+] deficits); anal irritation (laxative abuse)
	Laboratory Analysis Signs of prolonged or frequent vomiting: $\downarrow$ serum K^+, $\downarrow$ serum Cl^-; metabolic alkalosis (blood pH >7.45, HCO_3^- >26 mEq/L); stools turn red upon addition of NaOH (caused by presence of phenolphthalein, an ingredient in some laxatives); $\downarrow$ BUN (dehydration)
Protein-Energy Malnutrition (PEM)	*History* Severely restricted food intake (especially over a period of several months or even years); self-induced vomiting; frequent and prolonged periods of physical exercise
	Physical Examination Weight <90% of standard for height; BMI <18.5 or <5th percentile; amenorrhea; edema; thinning of hair, changes in hair texture

Continued

Table 19-2   Assessment in Eating Disorders—cont'd

Area of Concern	Significant Findings
Mineral Deficiencies	
Zinc (Zn)	*History* Severely restricted food intake; self-induced vomiting; laxative or diuretic abuse
	Physical Examination Impaired sense of taste; alopecia
	Laboratory Analysis ↓ Serum Zn
Calcium (Ca)	*History* Severely restricted food intake; amenorrhea
	Physical Examination Skinfold measurements <5th percentile
	Laboratory Analysis Radiograph evidence of osteopenia; ↓ bone mineral density

25th, and finally the 50th percentile of weight for height (see Appendix D). Dietary rehabilitation usually begins with 1200 to 1500 kcal/day, although this depends on the patient's recent intake level. Energy intake is then increased by 200 kcal/day every 2 to 3 days until consistent weight gain occurs. The intensity of nutritional care in eating disorders is determined by the severity of the existing nutritional disorders.

In mild undernutrition, or early in development of an eating disorder, the body weight may be 85% or more of the desirable weight. The disorder is usually managed on an outpatient basis, with the weight gain goal being set at a gain of 0.45 to 0.9 kg (1 to 2 lb)/week. A contract between the patient and the team is usually established, setting out the expected rate of weight gain, the target weight, and the consequences of failing to achieve the weight gain goals. An example of a consequence is restriction of physical activity until consistent weight gain is achieved. Family members or significant others are involved in outpatient care. It may be necessary for them to prepare and place all food on the plate, then monitor eating behavior, to ensure that adequate servings are consumed.

In moderate undernutrition (weight 75% to 85% of desirable), vital signs are frequently unstable. Physical activity is restricted until vital signs stabilize and there is no bradycardia. Weight gain goals and patient–health care team contracts are established as for mild undernutrition. One intermediate goal that can be set is to achieve adequate weight gain and sufficiently stable condition so that physical activity can be carried out. Outpatients are seen by the team at least weekly, and the possibility of hospitalization if continued weight loss occurs is made clear to the patient.

In severe malnutrition (<75% of desirable body weight), hospitalization is almost always required, particularly if vital signs are unstable (e.g., orthostatic hypotension), bradycardia is present, and electrolyte and other laboratory values are seriously abnormal. The goal is to achieve a weight gain of 0.14 to 0.18 kg (0.3 to 0.4 lb)/day. Meals and snacks should be supervised to ensure that they are consumed and that food is not discarded or vomited. Bathroom visits should also be supervised to prevent purging or surreptitious exercising. Enteral tube feeding or total parenteral nutrition (TPN; see Chapters 8 and 9) is normally reserved for severe, life-threatening malnutrition and is never used as a punishment for failing to eat. Patients should not be aggressively refed and those with severe malnutrition must be carefully monitored for refeeding syndrome, especially hypophosphatemia, as anabolism begins. Edema (pulmonary or other sites), tachypnea, and cardiac arrhythmias can indicate overfeeding in the severely malnourished individual. Hospitalization goals are to stop weight loss and begin to achieve weight gain, to stabilize vital signs and correct serum chemistry values, and to begin the process of helping the patient to recognize and consume a healthful diet.

For all degrees of undernutrition the following guidelines apply:

■ Patient food preferences should be accommodated as much as possible, especially early in treatment. People with eating disorders usually have foods that are considered "bad" or are feared. Including these foods in the diet early in treatment may cause excessive stress. These foods can be introduced later in treatment, when the patient has developed trust that the health care team will not let her lose control of her eating and gain excessive weight.

- Adequate vitamins and minerals should be provided in the diet, or supplements should be used, with special attention given to zinc, calcium, iron, thiamin, and folic acid. Severely malnourished individuals, who are at risk of refeeding syndrome, generally need vitamin-mineral supplementation, with special care given to ensuring that adequate thiamin and folic acid is consumed.
- Patients usually deny hunger. They need adequate supervision to prevent the overuse of chewing gum, diet soft drinks, and foods modified to be low in energy, which may help them to avoid feelings of hunger.

Special concerns in bulimia nervosa

Bulimic individuals may be at or above their ideal body weights at the time they begin treatment, but they are likely to have electrolyte and other laboratory abnormalities that need to be corrected. Establishing a pattern of regular eating, with dieting being discouraged, is the first step in therapy. Weight maintenance is the initial goal. Only after bulimic behaviors are under control will it be safe for the individual to undertake a weight reduction diet, if weight needs to be lost. The following measures help the patient achieve weight maintenance and avoid bingeing:

- The patient needs to avoid becoming excessively hungry. Bulimic individuals have a great fear of losing control of eating, and excessive hunger can lead to a loss of control. A diet plan with meals or snacks approximately every 3 hours (i.e., three meals and two to three snacks a day) reduces the risk of hunger. A diet with adequate fiber and fat also helps to promote satiety.
- Education and supervision to help avoid unhealthy weight control strategies and excessive focus on body weight are needed. Weights should be measured only at scheduled intervals, usually no more than once a week. Excessive exercise and strategies such as calorie or fat gram counting need to be identified and corrected.
- The patient should be helped to include forbidden or "bad" foods in the diet, using behavioral strategies (discussed below). Health care providers can help the individual to plan ways to control stimuli and to plan ahead for situations that have resulted in bingeing in the past.
- Dietary record keeping is useful, because the patient and the health care team review the records for evidence of progress and of potential problems.

Behavioral strategies for avoiding binge eating

The patient can be taught to maintain control of eating behaviors by practicing the following habits:

- Identify activities that can serve as distractions when temptations or negative emotions prompt a desire to binge.
- Identify cues or stimuli that lead to overeating and alter these stimuli. For instance, if overeating is most likely to occur in the kitchen, avoid eating in the kitchen and instead eat only in the dining room.
- Learn what an appropriate serving size is (using scales, measuring cups, or food models), and eat that amount. Many individuals with eating disorders have spent most of their lives either eating almost nothing or gorging. They may have little knowledge of normal serving sizes.
- Eat slowly; bingeing is associated with rapid food intake.
- Eat at regular meal times. Skipping meals and becoming excessively hungry may trigger bingeing.
- Avoid repeated helpings of food. At meals, serve the food and then put leftovers away before beginning to eat. At parties, sit as far from the food as possible.
- Plan ahead for events when excessive energy intake can be expected. For instance, if the individual plans to go out for pizza with friends, she or he can reduce food intake throughout the day to compensate.
- Limit alcohol intake because it increases energy intake and may reduce control over behavior.

Increasing self-esteem and coping skills

The individual can be helped to develop a better self-image, greater assertiveness, and better problem-solving techniques through group or individual therapy. Professionals provide positive reinforcement for progress made toward weight goals and improving self-esteem and interactive skills. The patient and the health care team should recognize that setbacks are normal and should be accepted calmly. Social situations are often very stressful to people with an eating disorder. They need to learn healthy ways to cope with interpersonal interaction, rather than focusing on food.

Lifestyle changes to correct eating disorders

Most individuals with anorexia nervosa and bulimia have misconceptions about food and nutrition, as well as about physical activity level. It may have been several years since they consumed a balanced diet. They need help in recognizing and selecting a nutritious diet. Initially the diet may have to be planned and served to them, with the clear expectation that all of the food will be eaten. Gradually the patient can assume more responsibility for selecting an adequate diet. The goal is to establish the habit of eating a healthful diet while maintaining a balance with energy expenditure so that it will not be necessary to resort to unhealthy practices such as self-induced vomiting or excessive exercise to control weight. Changes should be made gradually to avoid increasing stress. Foods that are most feared (usually those likely to be associated with bingeing) should be introduced only after recovery is well under way. The person with an eating disorder needs to learn a new approach to food intake, focusing on the nutritional contributions and other desirable characteristics of foods, rather than on the energy content. In regard to physical activity, the goal is for the individual to view it as a means to optimize health and receive enjoyment, rather than focusing solely on exercise as a tool for weight control.

Monitoring progress and behavior

A system of contingencies for failing to follow the treatment plan and rewards for successfully adhering to the plan are established by contract. Contingencies are often the withholding of desired privileges, and rewards may be the receipt of the same privileges. Progress toward the goals should be carefully monitored.

- During intensive inpatient therapy, the individual should be observed closely to protect her and maximize therapy. Examples of behaviors that undermine treatment include absenting herself from group activities after meals to vomit, diluting tube feeding formulas to reduce energy intake, surreptitiously wearing weights during weight measurement, failing to void before daily weight measurement, or hiding uneaten food.
- All weights should be obtained at the same time of day and after the individual has voided. Weighing should be done in the same light clothes (i.e., gown) each time. The return of spontaneous menses is a key milestone in the nutritional rehabilitation of the anorectic individual.
- Outpatients have increased responsibility for self-monitoring. Individuals should weigh themselves only at scheduled intervals, usually once weekly, to interrupt unhealthy weighing behaviors

accompanying their intense fear of weight gain. Individuals record their dietary intakes, as well as any episodes of vomiting and diuretic or laxative use. Health professionals and the affected individual evaluate these records for signs of progress and to plan strategies for dealing with problems.

REFERENCE

American Psychiatric Association: Practice guideline for eating disorders (revision), *Am J Psychiatry* 157(suppl):1-39, 2000.

SELECTED BIBLIOGRAPHY

American Psychiatric Association: *Diagnostic and Statistical Manual of Mental Disorders (DSM-IV-TR)*, ed 4 (text revision), Washington, DC, 2000, American Psychiatric Association.

Field AE, Austin SB, Taylor CB, et al: Relation between dieting and weight change among preadolescents and adolescents, *Pediatrics* 112:900, 2003.

Greeno CG, Wing RR, Marcus MD: How many donuts is a "binge"? Women with BED eat more but do not have more restrictive standards than weight-matched non-BED women, *Addict Behav* 24:299, 1999.

Rome ES, Ammerman S, Rosen DS, et al: Children and adolescents with eating disorders: The state of the art, *Pediatrics* 111:e98, 2003.

Wolfe BE, Gimby LB: Caring for the hospitalized patient with an eating disorder, *Nurs Clin N Am* 38:75, 2003.

Pediatric Disorders 20

Many of the nutritional needs of infants and children with disease-related nutritional impairments have been discussed previously, in the relevant chapters (e.g., renal or gastrointestinal disease). This chapter will describe nutritional problems in selected disorders that either occur only in pediatrics or are likely to cause significant nutritional problems early in life.

Low-Birth-Weight Infants

Low-birth-weight (LBW) infants are those with birth weights less than 2500 g. They are premature and/or **small for gestational age (SGA)**. Preterm or premature infants are those born before 37 weeks of gestation. **Very-low-birth-weight (VLBW)** infants have birth weights less than 1500 g, and **extremely-low-birth-weight (ELBW)** infants weigh less than 1000 g at birth.

Pathophysiology

The smaller and the more premature the infant, the greater the nutritional risk. The following list provides some of the factors contributing to nutritional problems:

- *Decreased nutrient stores:* Most fat, glycogen, and minerals—such as iron, calcium, phosphorus, and zinc—are deposited during the last 8 weeks of pregnancy. Thus, preterm infants have increased potential for hypoglycemia, rickets, and anemia.
- *Increased energy and nutrient needs for growth:* The LBW infant requires approximately 120 kcal/kg/day, compared with the term neonate's 108 kcal/kg/day. Needs for protein and other nutrients are also increased (Table 20-1).
- *Immature mechanical function of the gastrointestinal (GI) tract:* A coordinated suck-and-swallow function, which is necessary for

Table 20-1   Daily Nutritional Recommendations for
Premature Infants Weighing Fewer Than 1000 g

Ingredient (Unit/Day)	Enteral	Parenteral
Water (ml/kg)	150-200	120-150
Energy (kcal/kg)[a]	110-130	90-100
Protein (g/kg)[b]	3-3.8	2.5-3.5
Carbohydrates (g/kg)	8-12	10-15
Fat (g/kg)	3-4	2-3.5
Sodium (mEq/kg)	2-4	2-3.5
Chloride (mEq/kg)	2-4	2-3.5
Potassium (mEq/kg)	2-3	2-3
Calcium (mg/kg)[c]	120-230	60-90
Phosphorus (mg/kg)[c]	60-140	40-70
Magnesium (mg/kg)	8-15	5-7
Iron (mg/kg)[d]	2-4	0.1-0.2
Vitamin A (μg)[e]	0.21-0.44	0.21-0.44
Vitamin D (μg)	10	3
Vitamin E (mg)[f]	6-12	2-4
Vitamin K (μg)	7-9	60
Vitamin C (mg)	20-60	25-50
Vitamin B_1 (mg)	0.2-0.7	0.4-0.8
Vitamin B_2 (mg)	0.3-0.8	0.4-0.9
Vitamin B_6 (mg)	0.3-0.7	0.3-0.7
Vitamin B_{12} (μg)	0.3-0.7	0.3-0.7
Niacin (mg)	5-12	5-12
Folic acid (μg)	50	40-90
Biotin (μg)	6-20	6-13
Zinc (μg/kg)	800-1000	400
Copper (μg/kg)	100-150	20
Selenium (μg/kg)	1.3-3	1.5-2
Chromium (μg/kg)	0.7-7.5	0.2
Manganese (μg/kg)	10-20	1
Molybdenum (μg/kg)	0.3	0.25
Iodine (μg/kg)	30-60	1

From Pereira GR: Nutritional care of the extremely premature infant, *Clin Perinatol*
22:62, 1995; Shils ME et al: *Modern nutrition in health and disease*, ed 9,
Philadelphia, 1999, Lippincott, Williams & Wilkins; *Federal Register* 65(no. 17):
4255, 2000.

[a]Adjust according to weight gain and stress factors.
[b]Requirements increase with increasing degree of prematurity.
[c]Inadequate amount in total parenteral nutrition solutions because of risk of precipitation.
[d]Initiate at 2 weeks of age. Higher values recommended for erythropoietin therapy.
[e]Supplementation might reduce incidence of bronchopulmonary dysplasia.
[f]Supplementation might reduce severity of retinopathy of prematurity.

nipple-feeding an infant, does not develop until 32 to 34 weeks of gestation. Delayed gastric emptying and poor intestinal motility are common in preterm infants.

- *Reduced digestive capability:* Preterm infants have a smaller pool of bile salts, which are required for fat digestion and absorption, than do term infants. Production of pancreatic amylase and lipase, enzymes involved in carbohydrate and fat digestion, is also reduced. Lactase (the enzyme required for milk sugar digestion) levels are low until about 34 weeks of gestation.

- *Immature lungs with increased work of breathing and increased energy needs:* Respiratory problems also interfere with enteral feedings. A tachypneic infant, with a respiratory rate greater than 60 breaths/min, cannot be safely nipple-fed, nor can an infant requiring mechanical ventilation.

- *Immature renal function:* The immature kidney is not able to produce a highly concentrated urine. Therefore, the renal solute load of the feedings must not be excessive. Renal solute load is largely a function of the protein and electrolytes in the feedings.

- *Potential for heat loss:* Preterm infants have a large body surface area in relation to body weight, as well as little subcutaneous fat to provide insulation. Loss of heat increases energy needs.

- *Susceptibility to **necrotizing enterocolitis (NEC)**:* NEC is a serious disease of the GI tract that can result in intestinal perforation and even death. The risk of developing NEC is increased by prematurity, birth asphyxia (as indicated by low Apgar scores), catheterization of the umbilical arteries (used for arterial blood gases), formula feedings, and hyperosmolar enteral intake (e.g., vitamin supplements, medications given as oral elixirs, and oral calcium or potassium supplements).

Treatment

Immaturity of the lungs (particularly inadequate surfactant production, resulting in respiratory distress syndrome or RDS) is the primary problem for many preterm infants. Surfactant replacement, oxygen therapy, and mechanical ventilation are mainstays of treatment. Oxygen therapy is an essential part of the care of many LBW infants; yet oxygen is toxic to the tissues, particularly the retina and lung. Retinopathy of prematurity and **bronchopulmonary dysplasia (BPD)** are two of the long-term consequences of oxygen administration. The use of mechanical ventilation in combination with supplemental oxygen increases the risk of BPD, a lung injury characterized by a persistent oxygen requirement beyond 36 weeks' gestational age. Right-sided heart failure is common in BPD, as are hypoxia, hypercarbia, and oxygen dependency. Severe BPD is associated with pulmonary fibrosis, bronchoconstriction, emphysematous changes, and a mismatch between ventilation and perfusion. Treatment includes diuretics, bronchodilators, steroids, and gradual weaning from oxygen.

Nutritional Care

Ideally, the infant would receive adequate nutrients to enable growth to occur as rapidly as it would have in the uterus, or approximately 15 to 20 g/day. Unfortunately, this goal is elusive in many sick, stressed, or extremely premature infants.

Assessment

Assessment is summarized in Table 20-2.

Intervention

Nutrition support

Total parenteral nutrition (TPN). TPN is used in a variety of conditions, including severe RDS, congenital bowel anomalies (e.g., intestinal atresia, where some portion of the lumen of the bowel fails to form), NEC, or intolerance of enteral feedings. It may be delivered through an umbilical artery catheter, a central venous catheter inserted into the subclavian vein, a peripherally inserted central catheter (PICC), or a peripheral vein (see Chapter 9).

Lipid emulsions (2 to 3 g/kg/day, or 10 to 15 ml/kg/day of 20% lipid emulsion) are often given to provide part of the needed energy. High levels of indirect bilirubin are toxic to the central nervous system (CNS). Most indirect bilirubin (a product of degradation of red blood cells) is transported by albumin in the blood, and as long as it remains bound to albumin, the bilirubin does not enter the CNS to any great extent. Elevated levels of free fatty acids in the blood (which can result from lipid infusion) can displace bilirubin from its albumin binding sites, increasing the likelihood of CNS damage. If lipid is delivered continuously over 24 hours daily, however, there seems to be little risk of increasing the free bilirubin levels in the jaundiced infant (Kleinman, 2004).

Complications of long-term TPN include osteopenia (inadequate calcification of the bones) and cholestasis (poor flow of bile, which can cause liver damage). Several factors may contribute to

Table 20-2   Assessment in Vulnerable Infants and Children

Area of Concern	Significant Findings
Undernutrition/ Inadequate Growth	*History* LBW infants: ↑ energy needs for growth and physiologic stress— cold, infection, respiratory disease; poor energy reserves; poor enteral feeding tolerance caused by immature GI function; impaired digestive ability; hypoxia with impaired absorption; limited fluid tolerance. Cleft palate: poor suck. SCD: impaired absorption due to hypoxia; ↑ resting energy expenditure; ↑ needs due to frequent infections; poor intake related to chronic pain (especially abdominal). *Physical Examination* Poor weight gain (in stable LBW infants, gain should average 20-30 g daily); length or height <5th percentile for age (see Appendix D for term infants and children; charts for preterm infants are available in Fanaroff and Martin, 2002)
Vitamin Deficiencies A	*History* LBW infants: poor stores; oxygen therapy, with ↑ need for antioxidants *Physical Examination* Poor growth *Laboraory Analysis* Serum retinol <20 µg/dl

Table 20-2   Assessment in Vulnerable Infants and
Children—cont'd

Area of Concern	Significant Findings
E	*History* LBW infants: Poor stores; use of oxygen, with ↑ need for antioxidants *Physical Examination* Pallor, tachycardia, mild generalized edema *Laboratory Analysis* ↓ Serum tocopherol, Hct, Hgb (hemolytic anemia)
Folate	*History* SCD: ↑ needs for RBC synthesis *Physical Examination* Pallor, fatigue *Laboratory Analysis* ↓ Hct, ↑ MCV, ↓ serum and RBC folate
Electrolyte/Mineral Deficiencies	
Sodium (Na)	*History* LBW infants: poor renal conservation caused by immaturity; increased Na needs for growth; use of diuretics *Laboratory Analysis* ↓ Serum Na
Iron (Fe)	*History* LBW infants: poor stores; losses from frequent testing; SCD: ↑ needs for RBC synthesis *Physical Examination* Pallor; tachycardia *Laboratory Analysis* ↓ Hct, Hgb, MCV, serum ferritin; ↑ TIBC

Continued

Table 20-2   Assessment in Vulnerable Infants and
Children—cont'd

Area of Concern	Significant Findings
Calcium (Ca)	*History* LBW infants: very high needs for bone mineralization; limited Ca/phosphorus solubility in TPN solutions *Laboratory Analysis* ↓ Serum Ca;* ↑ alkaline phosphatase; radiographic evidence of poor mineralization or fractures
Phosphorus (P)	*History* LBW infants: very high needs for bone mineralization; limited Ca/phosphorus solubility in TPN solutions *Laboratory Analysis* ↓ Serum P; ↑ alkaline phosphatase; radiographic evidence of poor mineralization or fractures; ↓ Hct (hemolysis)
Zinc (Zn)	*History* LBW infants: poor stores; ↑ needs for anabolism. Cleft palate and SCD: poor intake *Physical Examination* Delayed growth; diarrhea; seborrheic dermatitis; poor sense of taste, distorted taste; alopecia

LBW, Low birth weight; *SCD*, sickle cell disease; *TIBC*, total iron binding capacity.
*If serum albumin is low, Ca concentrations must be "corrected." Corrected Ca = Ca concentration + (0.8 mg/dl × [4 – albumin concentration in g/dl]).

osteopenia in LBW infants, including difficulty in providing adequate calcium and phosphorus in TPN because of problems related to insolubility, metabolic acidosis often present in very immature infants, and potential for impaired vitamin D metabolism due to immature kidney function.

Small amounts of enteral feedings seem to "prime" the GI tract by stimulating the GI mucosal development, GI motility, and gut hormone release. Therefore "minimal" or "trophic" enteral feedings of formula or human milk delivered at 0.5 to 24 ml/kg/day are often begun when TPN is still needed (Fanaroff & Martin, 2002).

Monitoring the response to TPN. LBW infants are especially vulnerable to mechanical and infectious complications of nutrient delivery. To prevent these complications, nutrition support must be carefully administered and monitored (see Chapters 8 and 9).

- Measure weight daily, and measure head circumference and length weekly.
- Monitor state of hydration continually. Fluid overload increases the workload on the heart and can interfere with normal postnatal closure of the ductus arteriosus. On the other hand, phototherapy and the use of radiant warmers increase fluid requirements because they increase insensible fluid losses.
- Check blood glucose every 4 to 8 hours or as indicated until stable. LBW infants often have poor glucose tolerance and a low renal glucose threshold. Thus, they can experience hyperglycemia and glucosuria, with loss of energy and osmotic diuresis, on relatively low doses of glucose.
- Check serum triglyceride levels in infants receiving lipid infusions daily until stable and then 2 to 3 times weekly and after any increase in lipid infusion rate, especially in infants with respiratory compromise and those with sepsis. Excessive lipid doses may decrease the partial pressure of oxygen in the blood (PO_2), and septic infants may have impaired ability to metabolize lipids.

Enteral tube feedings. Enteral tube feedings can be used when there are GI motility (active bowel sounds or passage of stools); no excessive abdominal distention; soft, nontender abdomen (indicating no signs of peritonitis); no bilious nasogastric drainage, which would indicate abnormal bowel motility; no evidence of GI bleeding; and no signs of intestinal obstruction.

Nonnutritive feeding, or sucking a pacifier, during tube feedings may calm the infant and improve oxygenation, and some researchers have reported that it speeds the transition to nipple feedings, improves growth, and shortens hospitalization.

Routes and types of tube feedings include the following:

- Intermittent oral-gastric or nasogastric (OG or NG) feedings

  Uses: Intermittent (gavage) feedings every 1 to 3 hours are frequently used for routine feeding of stable infants.

  Advantages: This is the most physiologic schedule for enteral tube feeding because intermittent feedings stimulate GI and pancreatic hormone secretion in a cyclic manner.

  Shortcomings: There is a potential for pulmonary aspiration. Bolus feedings are not tolerated well by infants with delayed gastric emptying and in some infants recovering from severe RDS, who have decreased arterial oxygen tension and lung volumes with bolus feedings. Nasogastric feeding tubes increase upper airway resistance and may compromise gas exchange in small infants. For this reason, orogastric tubes are preferred in infants weighing less than 2 kg, with transition to nasogastric tubes when the weight exceeds 2 kg (Fanaroff & Martin, 2002).

- Continuous OG or NG feedings

  Uses: Often used for infants recovering from severe RDS, those with diminished absorptive capacity (such as short-bowel syndrome), or gastroesophageal reflux.

  Advantages: Some data indicate there is a trend toward earlier discharge of infants <1000 g at birth and faster weight gain in infants <1250 g given continuous vs. intermittent feedings (Premji and Chessell, 2003).

  Shortcomings: There is a potential for pulmonary aspiration. Nasogastric feeding tubes increase upper airway resistance and may compromise gas exchange in infants. The cream may separate if human milk is fed continuously, and the infant may not receive all of the fat (and much of the energy) contained in the feeding. Infants given continuous feedings take longer to achieve full enteral feeding, but there are no significant differences in growth, days to discharge, or incidence of NEC except in the subgroups of infants listed in Advantages (Premji & Chessell, 2003).

- Continuous transpyloric (nasoduodenal) feedings

  Uses: Often used in cases of delayed gastric emptying, severe gastroesophageal reflux and aspiration, and use of continuous positive airway pressure (CPAP), in which the stomach may be distended with air.

  Shortcomings: This method has no conclusive advantage over gastric tube feedings in promotion of energy intake, weight gain, or growth (McGuire & McEwan, 2003). It bypasses the stomach, where lingual (from the mouth) and gastric lipases perform a significant amount of fat digestion in the infant, and thus may result in incomplete fat absorption. Other potential problems are bacterial overgrowth of the upper intestine, intestinal perforation, and difficulty positioning the tube tip beyond the pylorus. The cream may separate if human milk is fed continuously, and the infant may not receive all of the fat (and much of the energy) contained in the feeding.

Monitoring the response to enteral tube feedings

- Include all assessment measures listed above for infants receiving TPN.
- Measure abdominal girth (usually just above the umbilicus) every 2 to 8 hours or as indicated. Girth should not increase more than 2 cm after feedings.
- Evaluate the color of the gastric residual before each intermittent feeding or every 2 to 3 hours during continuous feedings. Bile-stained (green or yellow) fluid usually indicates reduced GI motility and should be reported to the physician. Feedings may need to be decreased or stopped until the problem resolves.
- Position the infant on the right side after feedings, if possible, to promote gastric emptying.
- Note infant's color, respiratory effort, oxygen saturation, and any increase in prevalence of apnea and bradycardia in assessing response to feedings.
- Check stools for occult blood, which may signal NEC. Check for an anal fissure if blood is present in stools.
- Check the pH of the urine regularly. Immature infants have a low renal capacity for acid excretion, and many infant formulas result in a large renal acid load. (Human milk contains a low renal acid load.) The blood pH may be normal, even when the renal acid load is excessive, because of compensatory mechanisms maintaining acid-base balance; however, persistently acid urine may indicate a need for alkali therapy or use of a formula with a reduced renal acid load.

Nipple feedings. Nipple feedings are used in infants with a normal respiratory rate (<60 breaths/min) and the ability to coordinate breathing, sucking, and swallowing. Usually, these infants are at least 33 to 34 weeks' gestational age (either born after that period of gestation, or the combined prenatal and postnatal ages are equivalent to that period).

Monitoring the response to nipple feedings. Monitor the infant as for enteral tube feeding. In addition, the infant should be closely observed for signs of distress (cyanosis, bradycardia, apneic episodes, excessive fatigue) during and after feedings. Weigh the breastfed infant on an electronic scale before and after breastfeeding if there is concern about whether intake is adequate. The number of grams gained is approximately equal to the milliliters of milk consumed.

Milk and formulas for low-birth-weight infants

Human milk is an excellent source of antiinfective factors, long-chain fatty acids, and growth factors. Milk from mothers of preterm infants (preterm milk) has higher levels of minerals and protein than milk of mothers delivering at term (term milk). Nevertheless, levels of calcium, phosphorus, energy, zinc, and sodium in preterm milk are likely to be too low for rapidly growing premature infants. Fortifiers containing protein, carbohydrates, lipid, minerals, and vitamins are available for addition to human milk. A simple creamatocrit measurement (measuring the size of the fat layer in milk centrifuged in a capillary tube, just as a hematocrit is obtained on blood) provides a useful approximation of the energy content of the milk and the amount of energy fortification needed (Meier et al., 2002). Infants who receive human milk have a reduced incidence of infection, compared with infants receiving a formula designed for preterm infants. Because of this, and because providing breast milk can strengthen the bond between the mother and her hospitalized infant, mothers of LBW infants should be encouraged to breastfeed. Most mothers of LBW infants will need to pump or hand-express milk for some period of time after birth until the infant is well and strong enough to suckle.

Specially prepared formulas with greater protein, mineral, vitamin, and energy content than formulas for term infants are available for preterm infants whose mothers cannot or do not wish to provide breast milk. The formulas are usually used until the infant's weight is about 1800 g (approximately 4 lb). Characteristics of these formulas are as follows:

- Carbohydrate is provided by corn syrup solids or glucose oligosaccharides in addition to lactose because lactose digestion is not mature.
- Fat includes medium-chain triglycerides (MCTs; approximately 20% to 50% of total fat) in addition to long-chain triglycerides (LCTs). Use of MCTs helps to compensate for low intestinal lipase activity and bile salt release.
- Energy is concentrated into a smaller volume than in formulas for term infants (24 kcal/oz rather than 20 kcal/oz).
- Levels of minerals and protein are increased in comparison to formulas for term infants to promote growth.
- Protein is predominately in the form of whey, a more readily digestible protein than the other major milk protein, casein. Whey protein is less likely than casein to cause formation of a lactobezoar (a coalescence of indigestible material in the gastrointestinal tract, usually the stomach, causing partial or complete obstruction of the tract).
- Taurine, an amino acid needed for retinal and brain development and for optimal formation of bile salts, is included.
- Very-long-chain polyunsaturated fatty acids are included. These fatty acids (arachidonic acid and docosahexaenoic acid) are normally transferred to the fetus via the placenta during gestation and are found in human milk, but are not abundant in cow's milk, which is used to make many infant formulas. These fatty acids are believed to be important in development of the central nervous system and vision.
- Carnitine, which facilitates entry of long-chain fatty acids into the mitochondria for metabolism, is included. Although adults can synthesize carnitine, the immature enzyme systems in preterm infants may result in deficiency.
- Nucleotides are added to promote tissue synthesis.

Supplementation

If receiving unfortified human milk, the infant may be prescribed 2 to 3 mg/kg/day of elemental iron as ferrous sulfate drops. Iron-fortified formula usually provides enough iron to meet needs. Vitamin A supplementation of VLBW infants reduces the risk of death and chronic lung disease; it can be given mixed with intravenous lipid emulsions or via repeated intramuscular injections, but the relative benefits and risks of these two routes have not been determined (Darlow & Graham, 2002).

Bronchopulmonary dysplasia (BPD)

Infants with BPD often exhibit delayed growth. BPD increases the work of breathing and thus increases energy needs. Hypoxia may impair intestinal absorption, as well as nutrient metabolism. Gastroesophageal reflux, oral aversion, fluid and caloric restriction, recurrent infections, and rehospitalizations are common and interfere with adequate nutrition. "Catch-up" growth in infants with BPD is more rapid when feedings are supplemented with more protein, energy, zinc, calcium, and phosphorus than are available in standard infant formulas. Using a formula designed for preterm infants or a human milk fortifier for 9 to 12 months may result in improved growth.

Cleft Lip or Palate
Pathophysiology

Cleft lip and palate are two separate disorders but they are often found together. Cleft lip varies in severity from a small notch in the lip margin to a complete separation extending into the floor of the nose. Cleft palates may be unilateral or bilateral and may involve the soft and/or hard palate. Deformed or absent teeth are common, especially with cleft palate. A submucous cleft is a defect in the hard palate that is covered by an intact soft palate. It may be missed at birth because the signs are subtle. Possible causes of clefts include maternal drug or alcohol exposure, nutritional factors (e.g., inadequate folate), or genetic factors. Pierre Robin sequence (or complex) is a syndrome associated with cleft palate, in which the lower jaw is unusually small or is set back from the upper jaw. The tongue is displaced backward, with a risk of obstruction of air passage.

Treatment

Treatment needs depend on the severity of the defect. The complete treatment program for the child with a cleft lip or palate may require years of special treatment by a team consisting of a pediatrician, plastic surgeon, otolaryngologist, pediatric dentist, prosthodontist, orthodontist, speech therapist, geneticist, medical social worker, psychologist, nurse, and dietitian. The initial surgical repair of cleft lip usually occurs at about 2 to 3 months of age, and this repair may be revised one or more times later.

A cleft palate is usually closed by 9 to 12 months of age to aid in development of normal speech.

Nutritional Care

Assessment

The primary problem of an infant with cleft lip or palate is inefficient feeding, caused by difficulty making an adequate seal so that efficient sucking can be accomplished and regurgitation of the milk through the nose. Delayed growth may be seen (see Table 20-2), especially in infants with larger defects. Infants with Pierre Robin sequence are especially likely to have difficulty sucking because of difficulty in maintaining an open airway while feeding.

Intervention and teaching

Feeding problems

Breastfeeding is usually successful with a cleft lip, because the soft tissue of the breast helps to block the defect in the lip. Many children with cleft palate can also be breastfed. For those infants who are not breastfed, special feeding equipment is available to facilitate feeding. An obturator (soft plastic shield) may be used to cover a cleft palate during feeding, but most clinicians prefer the use of a soft nipple with an enlarged feeding hole on a pliable bottle. Several versions of the nipple and bottle are available commercially (e.g., Haberman feeder, Mead Johnson cleft palate feeder, and Pigeon bottle; information is available from the Cleft Palate Foundation at www.cleftline.org). The individuals involved in feeding the infant need instruction on safe feeding practices:

- Be patient in feeding the infant. Do not rush, leave the infant alone with a propped bottle, or put an older infant to bed with a bottle. Do not place an infant with Pierre Robin sequence in a horizontal position during feeding. Infants with cleft palates are at risk for pulmonary aspiration during feeding. Observe the infant carefully for choking, difficulty breathing, or cyanosis during a feeding.
- Squeeze the bottle gently and rhythmically (not continuously), trying to follow the infant's sucking rhythm. The Pigeon bottle has an adjustable regulator for milk flow.
- Try angling the nipple to the side of the mouth to allow the infant to use the gum to help compress the nipple.

■ Burp the infant often because the defect causes more air swallowing than in the normal infant. Even older infants will need to stop during the feeding and burp.

Sickle Cell Disease

Although sickle cell disease (SCD) is not only a pediatric illness, the topic is included in this chapter because children with SCD are especially likely to have nutritional deficits and growth failure.

Pathophysiology

SCD is a genetically transmitted disorder in which the person has an abnormal form of hemoglobin (Hgb S). This disorder is found predominantly among individuals with African ancestry. Hgb S causes the red blood cell (RBC), which is normally a flexible biconcave disk, to form a rigid sickle shape. The RBCs are prone to hemolysis, and their rigid shape also causes them to occlude the small vessels. Many of the complications associated with SCD (e.g., retinopathy, necrosis of the femoral head, splenic infarction with resulting impaired immune function, liver and kidney dysfunction, stroke) are related to ischemia caused by these occlusions. Infections and chronic pain are common problems in SCD. Acute chest syndrome (development of a new pulmonary infiltrate, fever, and respiratory symptoms) can result from viral or bacterial infection, but it is frequently associated with vascular occlusion in the lung. It can progress to adult (acute) respiratory distress syndrome. Episodes of acute anemia can be life threatening. Acute anemia results either from increased hemolysis, pooling of large amounts of blood cells and platelets in the spleen (splenic sequestration), or aplastic crisis (shortened red blood cell lifespan without a compensatory increase in reticulocyte formation, usually resulting from a viral infection).

Treatment

Hydroxyurea, an antineoplastic agent, is used to decrease hemolysis and the need for transfusion in adult patients, but its safety and effectiveness in children has not been established. Pharmacologic therapy is given as needed for infections and pain relief. RBC transfusions are administered in acute anemia, and splenectomy is frequently carried out if splenic sequestration has occurred or the spleen is markedly enlarged. Individuals who have had splenectomy remain on long-term prophylactic antibiotic treatment. Organ damage (liver or kidney failure) is treated as appropriate. Cholecystectomy may be required for bilirubin gallstones (caused by excessive hemolysis) and hip replacement for femoral head necrosis. Bone marrow transplantation is currently the only curative form of treatment.

Nutritional Care

Assessment

Assessment is summarized in Table 20-2. Children with SCD are especially likely to have height and weight below average for age and decreases in subcutaneous fat and muscle mass. These nutritional problems may contribute to delayed puberty.

Intervention and teaching

Fluid needs

Maintaining adequate hydration is the most important measure to reduce the risk of vascular occlusion. Fluids should be consumed or infused at 1 to 1.25 times the maintenance requirements (see Table 8-3). The family (and the child, as he/she becomes old enough) should be taught what normal fluid intake should be, based on weight, as well as the need to avoid vigorous physical activity; increase fluid intake during (moderate) physical activity and fever; replace fluid losses promptly during episodes of vomiting or diarrhea (contact the health care provider immediately if oral fluid replacement is unsuccessful); and avoid exposure to the sun or excessive heat. In addition, they should be taught to recognize signs of dehydration (thirst, dry mucous membranes, poor skin turgor, and sunken eyes and fontanel in infants). The family should keep oral rehydration solutions available and should be taught to give them frequently in small amounts if fluid deficits occur.

Energy and protein needs

Resting energy needs are increased in SCD. This may be related to tissue hypoxia from the impairment in circulation, because anaerobic metabolism (used when oxygen is not readily available) yields less energy than aerobic metabolism does. Protein needs are also slightly increased (approximately 10% greater than the DRI [see Table 1-1]), but adequate amounts of protein are readily obtained if energy needs are met. Energy intake should be adequate to maintain a normal rate of growth and development (see standardized growth charts in Appendix D). The biologic parents' heights should be obtained and used as a guide to the growth expected from the child. Frequent assessment of length or height, weight, head circumference (in children less than 3 years), and pubertal status (of children over 10 years) is a guide to determining whether nutritional needs are met or the energy intake goal needs to be higher. Intensive nutrition counseling and follow-up may be adequate to improve intake for many children. Modular products supplying protein and/or energy can be added to foods and beverages if necessary to increase nutrient density (see Table 8-2). Some children may benefit from use of age-appropriate oral supplements (see Table 8-1).

Micronutrient needs

Numerous micronutrient deficits have been observed in children with SCD, including zinc, folate, copper, and vitamin B_6. These may be related to increased needs for RBC formation, since RBC lifespan is decreased by ongoing hemolysis. A multivitamin supplement providing the DRI for the child's age, and supplementation of zinc and copper at the level of the DRI, is appropriate. However, iron supplements, including multivitamin-multimineral supplements containing iron, should be used only if iron deficiency is documented (i.e., low serum ferritin levels and increased total iron binding capacity). There is a risk of iron overload in these patients with continual release of iron from RBC.

REFERENCES

Darlow BA, Graham PJ: Vitamin A supplementation for preventing morbidity and mortality in very low birthweight infants, *Cochrane Database Syst Rev* 4: CD000501, 2002.

Fanaroff AA, Martin RJ: *Neonatal-perinatal medicine: diseases of the fetus and infant*, ed 7, St Louis, 2002, Mosby.

Kleinman RE, ed: *Pediatric nutrition handbook*, ed 5, Elk Grove Village, IL, 2004, American Academy of Pediatrics.

McGuire W, McEwan P: Transpyloric versus gastric tube feeding for preterm infants, *Cochrane Database Syst Rev* 3: CD003487, 2003.

Meier PP et al: Mothers' milk feedings in the neonatal intensive care unit: accuracy of the creamatocrit technique, *J Perinatol* 22:646-649, 2002.

Premji S, Chessell L: Continuous nasogastric milk feeding versus intermittent bolus milk feeding for premature infants less than 1500 grams, *Cochrane Database Syst Rev* 2: 2004.

SELECTED BIBLIOGRAPHY

Barden EM et al: Body composition in children with sickle cell disease, *Am J Clin Nutr* 76:218, 2002.

Buchowski MS et al: Equation to estimate resting energy expenditure in adolescents with sickle cell anemia, *Am J Clin Nutr* 76:1335, 2002.

Pandya AN, Boorman JG: Failure to thrive in babies with cleft lip and palate, *Br J Plast Surg* 54:471, 2001.

Vaucher YE: Bronchopulmonary dysplasia: an enduring challenge, *Pediatrics in Review* 23:349, 2002.

APPENDIXES

Appendix A
Functions and Dietary
Sources of Some
Important Nutrients

Appendix A   Functions and Dietary Sources of Some Important Nutrients

Function	Signs and Symptoms of Deficiencies/ Individuals at Increased Risk of Deficiencies (if Applicable)	Food Sources
Water Solvent for many chemical reactions in metabolism, participant in some chemical reactions (e.g., sugar digestion), temperature regulation, removal of wastes, lubrication and cushioning, transport of nutrients throughout the body	Dehydration, or fluid volume deficit: thirst, flushed skin, sense of apprehension, nausea, heat exhaustion, increased pulse rate and temperature, mental confusion, cyanosis, poor skin turgor, loss of body weight *At risk:* infants and young children with diarrhea or vomiting, elderly	Water and other beverages; water contained in foods (esp. fruits, vegetables); metabolic water released from the oxidation of nutrients in the body
Carbohydrates *Glucose and carbohydrates that yield glucose:* energy (4 kcal/g carbohydrate from food, 3.4 kcal/g IV glucose), protein sparing*	Ketosis (excessive production of ketones from incomplete metabolism of fat): increased urination and thirst, dehydration (see above), flushed dry skin, rapid shallow respirations, fruity odor of breath *At risk:* individuals with diabetes	Grain products, vegetables, fruits, milk, yogurt, ice cream, sugar, honey, syrup, jelly, jam, candy, other sweets

Fiber, insoluble[†]: Improve elimination by increasing fecal mass	Constipation, diverticula (herniations that protrude through the musculature of the large intestine and can become inflamed), hemorrhoids; possibly increased risk of colon cancer	Legumes, whole-grain breads and cereals, vegetables, fruits
Fiber, soluble: Delay gastric emptying, slow glucose absorption, inhibit cholesterol absorption	Hyperglycemia; hypercholesterolemia	Citrus fruits, oat bran, legumes
Amino Acids/Nitrogen[‡] Constituents of structural proteins (muscles, bones), enzymes, antibodies, hormones, chromosomes; transport oxygen, nutrients, and wastes in the blood; acid-base balance; energy (provide 4 kcal/g)	Hypoalbuminemia, edema, lymphopenia, hair easily pluckable, skin lesions, poor wound healing *At risk:* Serious acute or chronic disease, elderly	Meats, poultry, fish, eggs, milk, yogurt, cheese, legumes, nuts, grain products

Continued

Function	Signs and Symptoms of Deficiencies/ Individuals at Increased Risk of Deficiencies (if Applicable)	Food Sources
Lipids (Fats and Oils) Energy (9 kcal/g); insulation and protection of body organs; essential fatty acids (EFA): precursors of eicosanoids (hormone-like compounds)—prostaglandins, thromboxanes, prostacyclins, and leukotrienes; linoleic acid, an omega-6 EFA: omega-3 fatty acids are also involved in eicosanoid formation	Essential fatty acid deficiency: dry scaly skin, poor wound healing, delayed growth in children *At risk:* Premature infants, individuals receiving total parenteral nutrition	Nuts, seeds, and their oils; meat, poultry, fish, eggs, whole milk, cream, and their products—butter, yogurt, ice cream, cheese Essential fatty acids: safflower, sunflower, corn, cottonseed, and soybean oils Omega-3 fatty acids: canola and soybean oils, fatty fish such as salmon, tuna, sardines
Fat-Soluble Vitamins *Vitamin A* Formation and maintenance of epithelial tissue, formation of visual rods and cones, anti-	Night blindness, growth retardation, Bitot's spots, corneal drying and damage (xerophthalmia),	Liver, fortified milk; beta-carotenes (vitamin A precursor): deep yellow vegetables and fruits, e.g., carrot,

oxidant (a substance that prevents damage to cells from "free radicals"—oxygen-containing compounds that can disrupt proteins and lipids in cells, possibly contributing to aging and development of cancers)	follicular hyperkeratosis *At risk:* individuals with fat malabsorption, poor vegetable intake	sweet potato, butternut squash, apricot, cantaloupe; deep leafy vegetables, e.g., spinach, broccoli, greens
Vitamin D Forms the hormone calcitriol, which increases calcium and phosphorus absorption in the intestine, decreases urinary loss of calcium, and regulates bone calcium	Rickets (children): bowed legs, enlarged joints, knobby deformities on rib cage Osteomalacia (adults): weakness of bones, bony pain *At risk:* people with little sun exposure (institutionalized elderly or children, cultural clothing practices that cover most skin), dark-skinned individuals	Nondiet sources: sun exposure Fortified milk, fatty fish (tuna, salmon, sardines), fortified cereals

Continued

Function	Signs and Symptoms of Deficiencies/Individuals at Increased Risk of Deficiencies (if Applicable)	Food Sources
Vitamin E		
Antioxidant, protects cell membranes from free radical damage	Anemia due to red blood cell hemolysis, neuropathy, and myopathy *At risk:* premature infants, individuals with fat malabsorption	Plant oils and margarine made from them, whole grains, wheat germ, nuts, peanuts, sweet potato, avocado
Vitamin K		
Activation of clotting factors II (prothrombin), VII, IX, and X	Increased prothrombin time, ecchymoses, bleeding *At risk:* newborns, individuals receiving prolonged courses of antibiotics (rare)	Egg yolk, liver, green leafy vegetables, synthesized by gut bacteria, green tea
Water-Soluble Vitamins (Vitamin C and the B Complex)		
Vitamin C (ascorbic acid)		
Formation of collagen, thyroxine, epinephrine,	Scurvy: petechiae, easy bruising, bleeding gums, painful joints, poor wound healing	Citrus fruits, strawberries, kiwi fruit, broccoli, peppers (red, green, or chili), cantaloupe,

		brussels sprouts, cauliflower, papaya, tomatoes, potatoes
norepinephrine, steroid hormones; antioxidant	*At risk:* smokers, individuals with poor fruit and vegetable intake, oral contraceptive users, alcoholism, increased stress of illness, surgery, trauma	
Thiamin (B₁) Component of coenzyme (thiamin pyrophosphate or TTP) in carbohydrate metabolism	Beriberi: weakness, irritability, peripheral neuropathy, deep muscle pain; wet beriberi: enlarged heart, tachycardia, congestive heart failure; Wernicke-Korsakoff syndrome: confusion, ataxia, eye muscle paralysis *At risk:* alcoholics	Pork, whole-grain and enriched breads and cereals, legumes, liver, nuts
Riboflavin (B₂) Component of coenzymes (flavin mononucleotide [FMN] and flavin adenine dinucleotide [FAD]) in carbohydrate, protein, and fat metabolism	Cheilosis (cracking at mouth corners), glossitis (inflamed tongue), seborrheic dermatitis (scaly, greasy skin) *At risk:* alcoholics	Milk, yogurt, enriched breads and cereals, liver

Continued

Appendix A   Functions and Dietary Sources of Some Important Nutrients—cont'd

Function	Signs and Symptoms of Deficiencies/ Individuals at Increased Risk of Deficiencies (if Applicable)	Food Sources
Niacin (B₃) Components of coenzymes (nicotinamide adenine dinucleotide [NAD] and nicotinamide adenine dinucleotide phosphate [NADP]) in energy production from carbohydrates, fats, and protein and fat synthesis	Pellagra: anorexia, skin lesions in areas exposed to sunlight, confusion; classic symptoms, "4 Ds," are dermatitis, diarrhea, dementia, death *At risk:* alcoholics, poverty causing corn and rice to be major protein sources in the diet	Meats, peanuts, enriched breads and cereals, potato with skin
Pantothenic acid Component of coenzyme A, involved in fatty acid and cholesterol	Rarely seen; occurs only experimentally or with other B vitamin deficiencies:	Widespread, especially in organ meats, meat, poultry, fish, mushrooms, avocado, milk

synthesis and lipid, protein, and carbohydrate synthesis	burning sensation in feet, fatigue *At risk:* alcoholics	
Pyridoxine (B6) Component of coenzyme (pyridoxal phosphate [PLP]) involved in transamination reactions, synthesis of hemoglobin	Neuropathy, microcytic anemia *At risk:* alcoholics, oral contraceptive users, pregnant women, people receiving isoniazid (for tuberculosis)	Whole grains, meat, poultry, fish, bananas, potatoes
Biotin Cofactor for enzymes in synthesis of fat and purines (DNA, RNA), glucose metabolism	Rarely seen; dermatitis, atrophy of papillae on tongue, hypercholesterolemia *At risk:* usually high regular intake of raw egg white, alcoholics, prolonged use of antibiotics	Liver, egg yolk, cauliflower, cheese, whole grains, synthesized by gut bacteria
Folic acid (folacin, folate) One-carbon transfer reactions, e.g., DNA and RNA synthesis, amino acid synthesis	Megaloblastic (macrocytic) anemia, glossitis, diarrhea *At risk:* alcoholics, pregnant women	Green leafy vegetables, liver, orange juice, legumes, enriched grain products

Continued

Appendix A   Functions and Dietary Sources of Some Important Nutrients—cont'd

Function	Signs and Symptoms of Deficiencies/ Individuals at Increased Risk of Deficiencies (if Applicable)	Food Sources
Cobalamin (B₁₂) Methylation reactions (e.g., synthesis of DNA and RNA, folate metabolism)	Megaloblastic (macrocytic) anemia, especially pernicious anemia caused by lack of intrinsic factor produced in the stomach, neuropathy, glossitis *At risk:* elderly, postgastrectomy patients, strict vegetarians, individuals taking >10 times the RDA of vitamin C	Animal products only: liver, meat, fish, poultry, milk, egg, cheese
Major Minerals (More Than 100 mg Needed/Day)		
Calcium Component of bones and teeth, blood clotting, nerve transmission, muscle contraction, enzyme activation	Osteoporosis (thinning of bones with long-term deficiency), tetany (muscle excitability because of decreased serum calcium, usually caused	Milk, yogurt, cheese, canned fish with bones eaten, green leafy vegetables except spinach and Swiss chard, fortified juices, foods made

Phosphorus
Component of bones, teeth, cell membranes; involved in all energy-producing reactions as ATP

by hypoparathyroidism, not dietary Ca deficiency)
At risk: white and Asian women with poor calcium intake, people with fat malabsorption

with milk (e.g., pancakes)

Muscle weakness, cardiorespiratory failure, red blood cell hemolysis
At risk: individuals with rapid tissue synthesis after starvation (refeeding syndrome)

Milk, cheese, yogurt, meats, whole grains, legumes, nuts, food additives, carbonated beverages

Magnesium (Mg)
Component of bones, cofactor in many enzyme systems (glucose, fat, nucleic acid metabolism), involved in nerve

Paresthesias, tremor, muscle spasms, tetany, seizures, coma
At risk: alcoholics, those using diuretic therapy

Nuts, legumes, whole grains, dried fruits

Continued

Appendix A   Functions and Dietary Sources of Some Important Nutrients—cont'd

Function	Signs and Symptoms of Deficiencies/Individuals at Increased Risk of Deficiencies (if Applicable)	Food Sources
transmission and muscles contraction		
Sodium (Na)		
Major cation in extracellular fluid, water balance, nerve transmission	Muscle cramps, nausea, vomiting, dizziness, shock, coma *At risk:* people with excessive perspiration or other fluid loss replaced with plain water	Table salt, processed foods, salted snack foods, condiments, meats, milk, cheese, breads
Potassium (K)		
Major cation in intracellular fluid, water balance, nerve transmission, protein synthesis	Weakness, diminished reflexes, confusion, ileus, cardiac dysrhythmia (heart block) *At risk:* severe diarrhea or vomiting; thiazide diuretics, diabetic ketoacidosis treated with insulin and glucose	Fruits, vegetables, legumes, nuts, whole grains, meats, milk

Chloride (Cl) Major anion in extracellular fluid, water balance, hydrochloric acid in stomach	Hypochloremic alkalosis *At risk*: prolonged vomiting, nasogastric suction	Table salt, salt added in food processing
Trace Minerals or Elements (Less Than 100 mg Needed/Day)		
Chromium (Cr) Cofactor for insulin in glucose metabolism	Glucose intolerance, neuropathy, weight loss, hypercholesterolemia and hypertriglyceridemia *At risk*: heavy users of highly processed foods	Whole grains, brewer's yeast, meats
Copper (Cu) Hemoglobin synthesis, cofactor for many enzymes (e.g., in protein synthesis)	Microcytic anemia, low neutrophil count *At risk*: excessive supplementation with Zn	Liver, meat, shellfish, legumes, nuts, cocoa, copper cookware or water pipes
Fluoride (F) Makes tooth enamel resistant to decay	Dental caries *At risk*: people not receiving	Fluoridated water, toothpaste, dental treatments, tea

Continued

Function	Signs and Symptoms of Deficiencies/ Individuals at Increased Risk of Deficiencies (if Applicable)	Food Sources
	fluoridated water or dental treatments	
Iodine (I) Component of thyroid hormones	Goiter: enlarged thyroid, hypothyroidism Cretinism: infant with short stature and mental retardation born to woman I-deficient during pregnancy *At risk:* none in United States	Iodized salt, seafood, food colorings, bread (from dough conditioner), milk (from cleaning agent in dairies)
Iron (Fe) Oxygen transport in hemoglobin and myoglobin, cytochrome enzyme system	Microcytic anemia *At risk:* infants, children, adolescents, pregnant women, some endurance athletes, individuals with blood loss, postgastrectomy, vegetarians	Liver, meats, eggs, whole and enriched grains, legumes, dark green leafy vegetables, iron cookware

Manganese (Mn) Cofactor in protein, carbohydrate, and fat metabolism	Rare and symptoms uncertain: weight loss, hypocholesterolemia, dermatitis *At risk:* long-term TPN without supplementation		Whole grain, legumes, nuts, leafy vegetables
Molybdenum (Mo) Cofactor in oxidase enzymes	Very rare: tachycardia, stupor, central scotomas (loss of vision), coma *At risk:* long-term TPN without supplementation		Legumes, whole grains
Selenium (Se) Component of glutathione peroxidase, an antioxidant	Cardiomyopathy, sudden death *At risk:* people eating food grown in Se-deficient soil (Keshan province of China, New Zealand), long-term TPN without supplementation		Seafood, whole grains, meats, legumes, milk (meat, milk, and plant Se depend on soil content)

Continued

Appendix A   Functions and Dietary Sources of Some Important Nutrients—cont'd

Function	Signs and Symptoms of Deficiencies/ Individuals at Increased Risk of Deficiencies (if Applicable)	Food Sources
Zinc (Zn) Cofactor in more than 70 enzyme systems involved in growth, sexual maturation, reproduction, taste acuity, immune function	Impaired sense of taste and smell, anorexia, dermatitis, growth retardation, delayed sexual maturity, poor wound healing, impaired immune function *At risk:* excessive Fe supplementation or Cu intake, vegetarian diet, severe diarrhea, intestinal drainage	Shellfish, meats, liver, milk, cheese, eggs, whole grains, legumes

*IV, Intravenous.

Protein sparing refers to the fact that protein can be used for glucose formation via gluconeogenesis (formation of glucose from noncarbohydrates). Adequate carbohydrate intake spares protein to be used for vital functions, rather than energy production.

†Insoluble fiber does not dissolve in water; soluble fiber forms a gel or swells when combined with water.

‡We usually speak of a requirement for protein, but the requirement is actually for nitrogen in the form of amino acids, which are essential (needed in the diet because the body does not produce a sufficient amount) or nonessential (not necessary in the diet because the body synthesizes it). Essential amino acids are histidine, isoleucine, leucine, lysine, methionine, phenylalanine, threonine, tryptophan, valine, and possibly glutamine. In addition, infants require dietary arginine, cysteine (cystine), and taurine.

Appendix B
Dietary Fiber in Common Foods

An adequate intake of fiber is approximately 14 g/1000 kcal consumed. Based on this average, the following estimates can be made for life stage groups.

Table B-1   Dietary Reference Intakes for Total Fiber by Life Stage Group

Life Stage Group	Total Fiber Intake (g/Day)
Young children:	
1-3 years	19
4-8 years	25
Males:	
9-13 years	31
14-50 years	38
>50 years	30
Females:	
9-13 years	26
14-18 years	36
19-50 years	25
>50 years	21
Pregnancy	28
Lactation	29

Reference: Food and Nutrition Board, Institute of Medicine—National Academy of Sciences. *Dietary reference intakes for energy, carbohydrate, fiber, fat, fatty acids, cholesterol, protein, and amino acids (macronutrients)*. Washington, DC, 2002, National Academies Press. Used with permission.

Table B-2 Dietary Fiber in Common Foods

Dietary Fiber (g per Serving)	Foods			
	Grain Products	Fruits	Dried Beans and Peas	Vegetables
10 or more	All Bran (⅓ c) Fiber One (½ c) Wheat bran (½ c)	Figs, dried (10) Peaches, dried (10 halves)		
5 to 9	Bran Buds (⅓ c) Bran flakes (¾ c) Raisin bran (¾ c)	Prunes, dried (10) Prunes, dried, cooked (½ c)	Beans, cooked: great northern, kidney, lima, red, or refried (½ c) Bean soup (1 c)	
3 to 5	English muffin, whole grain or bran (1) Crackling Oat Bran (⅓ c)	Apple with skin (1 med) Apricots, dried (10 halves)	Beans, baked (½ c) Beans or peas, cooked: garbanzos, lentils, navy,	Brussels sprouts, cooked (½ c) Corn, cooked (½ c)

	Fruit & Fiber (½ c) Mueslix (⅔ c) Muffin, bran (1) Nutri-Grain (⅔ c) Ry-Krisp (2) Waffle, frozen (2) Wheat Chex (⅔ c) Wheat germ (¼ c)	Avocado (1 med) Blackberries (½ c) Dates, dried (10) Orange (1 med) Papaya (1 med) Pear, raw (1)	pinto, white, blackeye (½ c) Pea soup (1 c)	Peas, green, canned or frozen (½ c)
1 to 2	Bread: cracked wheat, whole-wheat, mixed grain, rye, oat bran, oatmeal (1 slice)	Applesauce (½ c)		Broccoli, raw or cooked (½ c)
	Brown rice, cooked (1 c)	Apricots (3 med)		Carrot, cooked (½ c)

Continued

Table B-2 Dietary Fiber in Common Foods—cont'd

Dietary Fiber (g per Serving)	Foods			
	Grain Products	Fruits	Dried Beans and Peas	Vegetables
	Cornbread (1 piece)	Blueberries, raw (½ c)		Carrot, raw (1 med)
	Cornflakes (1 c)	Cantaloupe (1 c)		Cauliflower, raw or cooked (½ c)
	Cheerios (1¼ c)	Cherries, sweet, raw (10)		Green beans, frozen, canned, or fresh (½ c)
	French Toast (2 slices)	Grapes (1 c)		
	Granola (¼ c)	Kiwifruit (1 med)		Mushrooms, raw or canned (1 c)
	Grape-Nuts (¼ c)	Mango (1 med)		Olives (10)
	Muffin, all except bran (1)	Nectarine (1 med)		Onions, raw (½ c)
	Pancakes (2)	Peaches, canned (1 c)		Peppers, sweet, raw (½ c)

Ry-Krisp (1)
Shredded Wheat (1 large biscuit)

Peach, raw (1 med)
Pear, canned (½ c)
Pineapple, raw or canned (1 c)
Raisins (2 tbsp)
Strawberries, raw or frozen (½ c)
Watermelon, raw (1½ c)

Potato, baked or boiled without skin (1 med)
Potato salad (½ c)
Soups: minestrone or vegetable (1 c)
Spinach, cooked (½ c)
Squash, summer or winter, cooked (½ c)
Sweet potatoes, cooked (½ c)
Tomato, raw (1 med)
Turnip, cooked (½ c)

Appendix C
Healthy Weight Ranges for Men and Women of All Ages

Height (ft-in)	Weight Range (lb)	Height (cm)	Weight Range (kg)
4'10"	90-120	147	41-54
4'11"	96-125	150	44-57
5'0"	97-128	152	44-58
5'1"	101-133	155	46-60
5'2"	105-136	157	48-62
5'3"	108-141	160	49-64
5'4"	111-145	162	50-66
5'5"	114-150	165	52-68
5'6"	117-155	168	53-70
5'7"	120-160	170	54-73
5'8"	125-164	173	57-75
5'9"	129-169	175	59-77
5'10"	132-174	178	60-79
5'11"	136-179	180	62-81
6'0"	140-184	183	64-84
6'1"	144-189	185	65-86
6'2"	148-195	188	67-89
6'3"	152-200	191	69-91
6'4"	156-205	193	71-93
6'5"	160-211	196	73-96
6'6"	164-216	198	75-98

Adapted from *Nutrition and your health: dietary guidelines for Americans*, ed 5, Washington, DC, 2000, U.S. Department of Agriculture, U.S. Department of Health and Human Services.

Appendix D
Growth Charts
(United States)

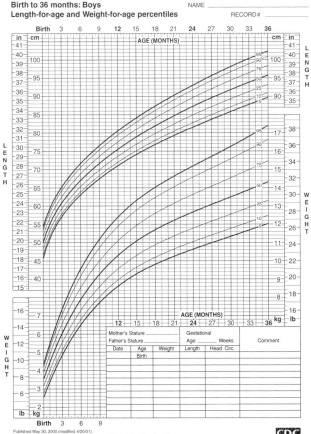

Birth to 36 months: Boys
Length-for-age and Weight-for-age percentiles

NAME _____
RECORD# _____

Published May 30, 2000 (modified 4/20/01).
SOURCE: Developed by the National Center for Health Statistics in collaboration with
the National Center for Chronic Disease Prevention and Health Promotion (2000).
http://www.cdc.gov/growthcharts

CDC
SAFER · HEALTHIER · PEOPLE™

Birth to 36 months: Boys
Head circumference-for-age and
Weight-for-length percentiles

NAME _____

RECORD# _____

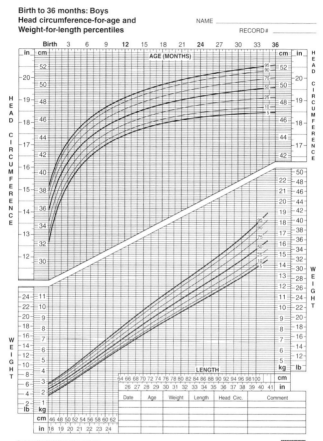

Published May 30, 2000 (modified 10/16/00).
SOURCE: Developed by the National Center for Health Statistics in collaboration with
the National Center for Chronic Disease Prevention and Health Promotion (2000).
http://www.cdc.gov/growthcharts

Birth to 36 months: Girls
Length-for-age and Weight-for-age percentiles

NAME _____

RECORD # _____

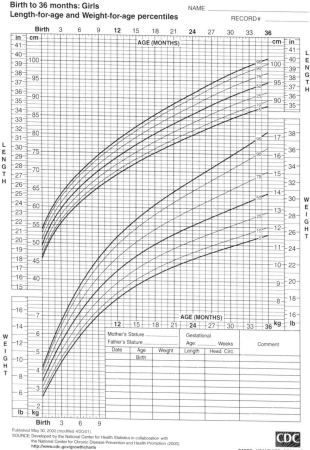

Published May 30, 2000 (modified 4/20/01).
SOURCE: Developed by the National Center for Health Statistics in collaboration with
the National Center for Chronic Disease Prevention and Health Promotion (2000).
http://www.cdc.gov/growthcharts

SAFER · HEALTHIER · PEOPLE™

Birth to 36 months: Girls
Head circumference-for-age and
Weight-for-length percentiles

NAME _____

RECORD# _____

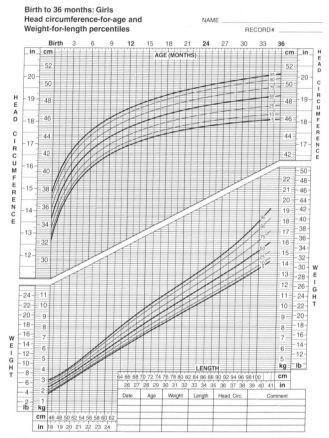

Published May 30, 2000 (modified 10/16/00).
SOURCE: Developed by the National Center for Health Statistics in collaboration with
the National Center for Chronic Disease Prevention and Health Promotion (2000).
http://www.cdc.gov/growthcharts

CDC
SAFER · HEALTHIER · PEOPLE™

2 to 20 years: Boys
Stature-for-age and Weight-for-age percentiles

NAME _____

RECORD# _____

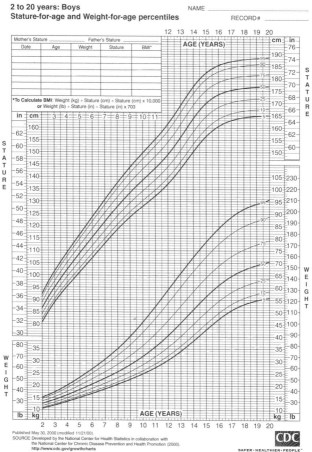

*To Calculate BMI: Weight (kg) ÷ Stature (cm) ÷ Stature (cm) x 10,000
or Weight (lb) ÷ Stature (in) ÷ Stature (in) x 703

Published May 30, 2000 (modified 11/21/00).
SOURCE: Developed by the National Center for Health Statistics in collaboration with
the National Center for Chronic Disease Prevention and Health Promotion (2000).
http://www.cdc.gov/growthcharts

SAFER · HEALTHIER · PEOPLE™

2 to 20 years: Boys
Body mass index-for-age percentiles

NAME _____

RECORD# _____

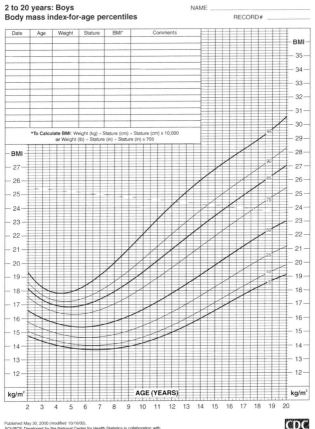

*To Calculate BMI: Weight (kg) ÷ Stature (cm) ÷ Stature (cm) x 10,000
or Weight (lb) ÷ Stature (in) ÷ Stature (in) x 703

Published May 30, 2000 (modified 10/16/00).
SOURCE: Developed by the National Center for Health Statistics in collaboration with
the National Center for Chronic Disease Prevention and Health Promotion (2000).
http://www.cdc.gov/growthcharts

NAME _____

Weight-for-stature percentiles: Boys

RECORD# _____

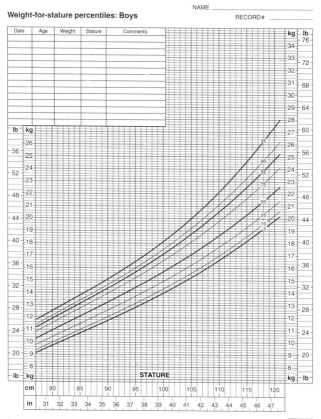

Date	Age	Weight	Stature	Comments

STATURE

cm 80 85 90 95 100 105 110 115 120

in 31 32 33 34 35 36 37 38 39 40 41 42 43 44 45 46 47

Published May 30, 2000 (modified 10/16/00).
SOURCE: Developed by the National Center for Health Statistics in collaboration with
the National Center for Chronic Disease Prevention and Health Promotion (2000).
http://www.cdc.gov/growthcharts

SAFER · HEALTHIER · PEOPLE™

2 to 20 years: Girls
Stature-for-age and Weight-for-age percentiles

NAME _____

RECORD# _____

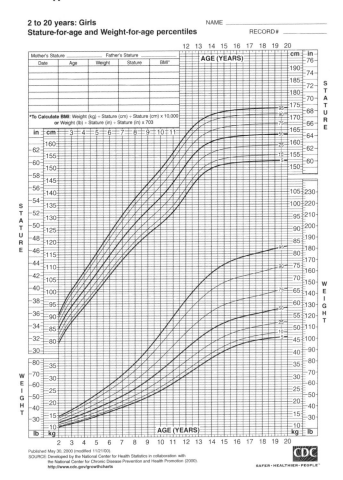

*To Calculate BMI: Weight (kg) ÷ Stature (cm) ÷ Stature (cm) x 10,000
or Weight (lb) ÷ Stature (in) ÷ Stature (in) x 703

Published May 30, 2000 (modified 11/21/00).
SOURCE: Developed by the National Center for Health Statistics in collaboration with
the National Center for Chronic Disease Prevention and Health Promotion (2000).
http://www.cdc.gov/growthcharts

CDC
SAFER·HEALTHIER·PEOPLE™

2 to 20 years: Girls
Body mass index-for-age percentiles

NAME _____

RECORD# _____

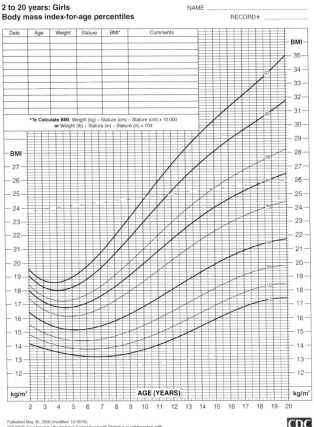

Date	Age	Weight	Stature	BMI*	Comments

*To Calculate BMI: Weight (kg) ÷ Stature (cm) ÷ Stature (cm) x 10,000
or Weight (lb) ÷ Stature (in) ÷ Stature (in) x 703

AGE (YEARS)

Published May 30, 2000 (modified 10/16/00).
SOURCE: Developed by the National Center for Health Statistics in collaboration with
the National Center for Chronic Disease Prevention and Health Promotion (2000).
http://www.cdc.gov/growthcharts

CDC
SAFER·HEALTHIER·PEOPLE™

NAME _____

Weight-for-stature percentiles: Girls

RECORD# _____

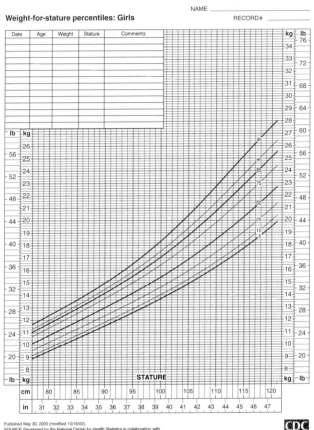

Date	Age	Weight	Stature	Comments

STATURE

Published May 30, 2000 (modified 10/16/00).
SOURCE: Developed by the National Center for Health Statistics in collaboration with
the National Center for Chronic Disease Prevention and Health Promotion (2000).
http://www.cdc.gov/growthcharts

CDC
SAFER · HEALTHIER · PEOPLE™

Appendix E
Triceps Skinfold Percentiles

Appendix E   Triceps Skinfold (TSF) Measurements for White and Blacks (W/B) in Millimeters

Age (Year)	Percentiles for Females (W/B)			Percentiles for Males (W/B)			
	5th	85th	95th	5th	85th	95th
6	6/4	13/11	16/19	5/4	12/9	16/13
7	6/4	14/13	19/21	5/4	12/8	18/15
8	6/4	16/16	21/23	5/4	13/10	20/17
9	7/4	17/17	24/25	5/4	13/11	21/19
10	7/5	18/18	26/27	5/4	16/12	22/20
11	8/5	20/21	28/29	5/4	18/13	23/22
12	8/6	22/23	29/30	5/4	18/14	24/23
13	8/6	24/25	31/32	5/4	18/14	24/24
14	8/7	24/26	31/33	5/4	18/16	24/25
15	9/7	25/27	32/34	5/4	18/18	24/25
16	9/7	26/27	32/34	5/4	17/17	24/26

17	9/7	26/27	33/34	5/4	17/17	23/26
18-20	10/7	27/30	34/35	4/3	17/17	22/23
21-29	10/8	29/33	35/37	5/3	20/17	24/25
30-35	11/9	33/36	38/42	5/4	19/18	24/25
36-41	12/10	33/37	38/45	5/4	19/19	23/24
42-50	12/12	35/38	40/44	5/4	19/18	24/26
51-59	13/13	32/35	39/42	5/4	18/15	24/23
60-69	12/12	31/33	36/39	5/4	17/15	23/23

Note: Because overweight is increasing in prevalence in the United States and other industrialized nations, the 95th percentile is likely to be a very conservative indicator of the presence of overweight/obesity. Therefore, the 85th percentile is included; individuals with skinfolds at the 85th percentile or greater should be carefully assessed for other signs of overweight/obesity. The triceps skinfold measurement correlates more closely with overweight in women than in men.

Appendix F
Laboratory
Reference Values

Appendix F   Laboratory Reference Values

Test	Reference Range	
	Adult	Pediatric
Albumin, serum (g/dl)	3.5-5.0	3.4-5.6
Calcium, serum (mg/dl)		
Total	8.5-10.5	1-3 yr: 8.7-9.8; >3 yr: 8.7-10.7
Ionized or free	4.6-5.3	4.9-5.5
Carnitine, serum (μmol/L)		
Total	24-100	24-89
Free	20-88	
Beta-carotene, serum (μg/dl)	10-85	
Ceruloplasmin, serum (mg/dl)	18-45; ↑ in pregnancy	24-46
Cholesterol, total, serum (mg/dl)	<200	120-170
Chromium		
Blood (μg/L)	2.8-4.5	
Serum (μg/L)	0.12-2	
Urine (μg/day)	0.1-2	
Copper, serum (μg/dl)	M: 70-140 F: 80-155 Preg: 118-302	<6 mo: 20-70; 1-19 yr: 80-170

Appendix F   Laboratory Reference Values—cont'd

Test	Reference Range	
	Adult	Pediatric
C-peptide, serum (ng/ml)	0.78-1.89	
Creatinine		
Serum (mg/dl)	M: 0.7-1.3 F: 0.6-1.1	Infant: 0.2-0.4; child: 0.3-0.7; adolescent: 0.5-1.0
Urine (mg/kg/day)	M: 14-26 F: 11-20 Elderly: >10	Infant and child: 8-22; adolescent: 8-30
Fat, fecal*	2-6 g/day or >95% retention of dietary fat	>95% retention of dietary fat
Ferritin, serum (ng/ml or µg/L)	M: 12-300 F: 10-150	7-140
FIGLU (formimino-glutamic acid), urine (mg/day)	<35[†]	
Folate, serum (ng/ml)	5-25	2-18
Glucose, serum or plasma, fasting (mg/dl)	70-110	65-110
Glucose, plasma, 2 hr postload[‡] (mg/dl)	<140	
Glycated or glycosylated hemoglobin (HbA$_{1c}$), blood (%)	<7	<7

Continued

Appendix F   Laboratory Reference Values—cont'd

Test	Reference Range	
	Adult	Pediatric
Hematocrit (%)	M: 42-50 F: 37-44	Infant: >32; 2-12 yr: 32-42; adolescent: 34-44
Hemoglobin, total, blood (g/dl)	M: 14-18 F: 12-16	11-15
Insulin, fasting, serum (μU/ml)	2-25	
Insulin-like growth factor–1 or somatomedin C, plasma (ng/ml)	42-110	0-8 yr: M: 0-103; F: 0-128 9-10 yr: M: 15-148; F: 24-158 11-13 yr: M: 55-216; F: 65-226 14-15 yr: M: 114-232; F: 124-242 16-17 yr: M: 84-221; F: 94-231
Iron, serum (μg/dl)	M: 65-170 F: 50-170	50-120
Iron-binding capacity, total, serum (μg/dl)	250-460	268-570
LDL cholesterol, serum or plasma (mg/dl)	<130 (<100 for individuals at high risk for heart disease)	
Magnesium, serum (mEq/L) (mmol/L)	1.3-2.1 0.65-1.05	1.4-1.8 0.70-0.91
Niacin, urine (mg/day)	2.4-6.4	

Appendix F   Laboratory Reference Values—cont'd

Test	Reference Range	
	Adult	Pediatric
Nitrogen, total, fecal (g/day)	<2	Infants: 0.1-0.5
Osmolality, serum (mOsm/kg H_2O)	280-295	275-296
Phosphorus, serum (mg/dl)	2.7-4.5	10 day-2 yr: 4.5-6.7; >2 yr: 4.5-5.5
Prealbumin or transthyretin or thyroxine-binding prealbumin, serum (mg/dl)	15-36, ↑ in pregnancy	14-36
Selenium (μg/dl)		
Blood	58-234	
Serum	46-143	
Transferrin, serum (mg/dl)	M: 215-365 F: 250-380	200-440
Transthyretin, see Prealbumin		
Triglycerides, serum, fasting (mg/dl)	M: 40-160 F: 35-135	0-15 yr: 30-138
Urea nitrogen, urine (g/day)	12-20	
Vitamin A (retinol), serum or plasma (mg/L)	0.3-1.2	1-12 yr: 0.20-0.50; 13-17 yr: 0.26-0.70
Vitamin B_{12}, serum (pg/ml)	160-950	74-385
(pmol/L)	118-701	100-520
Vitamin C, plasma (mg/dl)	0.5-1.5	

Continued

Appendix F   Laboratory Reference Values—cont'd

Test	Reference Range	
	Adult	Pediatric
Vitamin D$_3$, 1,25-dihydroxy, serum (pg/ml)	18-64	15-80
Vitamin E (α-tocopherol), serum (mg/L)	5.0-18.0	2-13 y: 5.5-9.0; >14 y: 5.0-18.0
Xylose absorption test[§]		
Blood (mg/dl)	>30 (2 hr postingestion)	>15 (1 hr postingestion)
Urine (g/5 hr)	>3.5-4 (or >14% of ingested dose)	>4 g (or >16% of ingested dose)
Zinc, serum (μg/dl)	70-150	70-150

Values compiled from Burtis CA, Ashwood ER. *Tietz textbook of clinical chemistry*, ed 3. Philadelphia, 1999, WB Saunders; Pagana KD, Pagana TJ. *Mosby's diagnostic and laboratory reference*, ed 6. St. Louis, 2003, Mosby; Soldin SJ et al. *Pediatric reference ranges*, ed 4. Washington, DC, 2003, American Association for Clinical Chemistry.

[*]Usually adults are instructed to consume 100 g fat/day for 3 days before the test; calculating dietary retention of fat requires keeping a diet diary for at least 1 day.

[†]Elevated values occur in folate deficiency.

[‡] Test requires ingestion of a 75 g glucose load.

[§]Adults ingest 25 g xylose; pediatric dose usually adjusted for body weight.

Appendix G
Caffeine Content
of Selected Beverages
and Foods*

Appendix G   Caffeine Content of Selected Beverages and Foods*

Beverage or Food	Caffeine (mg)
Coffees, 240-ml (8-oz) Servings	
Coffee, brewed	135
Orange Cappuccino[†]	102
Coffee, instant	95
Café Vienna[†]	90
Mocha[‡] or Swiss Mocha[†]	55-60
Amaretto[‡]	30
Coffee, decaffeinated	5
Teas, 240-ml (8-oz) Servings Unless Otherwise Specified	
Bigelow Raspberry Royale	83
Tea, leaf or bag; black, pekoe or oolong	50
Snapple iced tea, all varieties, 480 ml (16 oz)	48
Nestea Pure Sweetened Iced Tea, 480 ml (16 oz)	34
Tea, green	30
Arizona iced tea, assorted varieties, 480 ml (16 oz)	15-30
Tea, instant	15
Tea, decaffeinated	<5
Tea, herbal	0

Continued

Appendix G   Caffeine Content of Selected Beverages and Foods*—cont'd

Beverage or Food	Caffeine (mg)
Soft Drinks, 360-ml (12-oz) Servings	
Jolt	72
Mountain Dew, Surge	51-55
Coca-Cola, Diet Coke	45-47
Dr. Pepper, regular or diet; Sunkist Orange Soda; Pepsi-Cola	37-41
Barq's Root Beer	23
7-Up or Diet 7-Up, Barq's Diet Root Beer, caffeine-free colas (all types, regular or diet), Minute Maid Orange Soda, Mug Root Beer, Sprite or Diet Sprite	0
Caffeinated Waters, 0.5-L (16.9-oz) Servings	
Java Water	125
Aqua Blast	90
Water Joe, Aqua Java	50-70
Other	
Ben & Jerry's No Fat Coffee Fudge Frozen Yogurt, 1 cup	85
Coffee ice creams, 240 ml (1 cup)	30-60
Dannon coffee yogurt, 240 ml (1 cup)	45
Cappuccino or café au lait yogurts, 180-240 ml (6-8 oz)	<5
Dark chocolate, 1 bar (1.5 oz)	31
Milk chocolate, 1 bar (1.5 oz)	10
Cocoa, hot chocolate, or chocolate milk, 240 ml (8 oz)	5

Information from *Caffeine content of foods and drugs*, press release from the Center for Science in the Public Interest. Available at *www.cspinet.org*. Accessed December 20, 2003; Barone JJ, Roberts HR. Caffeine consumption: food. *Chem Toxicol* 34:119, 1996; and beverage and food manufacturers.

*Many over-the-counter and some prescription medications contain higher levels of caffeine than these beverages and foods. Consult the product label or a pharmacist about the caffeine content of drugs.

†General Foods International Coffee.

‡Maxwell House Cappuccino.

Appendix H
Drug-Nutrient
Interactions

Box H-1   Drugs Affecting Appetite

Appetite Depressants
    Amphetamines and related compounds
        Benzphetamine (Direx)
        Phenylpropanolamine (Dexatrim,
          Dimetapp, Triaminic)
    Antibiotics/antivirals/antifungals
        Amphotericin B (Fungizone)
        Gentamicin (Garamycin)
        Metronidazole (Flagyl)
        Zidovudine (AZT)
    Carbonic anhydrase inhibitors
        Acetazolamide (Diamox)
        Dichlorphenamide (Daranide)
    Digitalis preparations
    Methylphenidate
    Serotonin reuptake inhibitors: all, including
      fluoxetine, fluvoxamine, sertraline
Appetite Stimulants
    Antidepressants
        Amitriptyline (Elavil)
    Antihistamines
        Astemizole (Hismanal)
        Cyproheptadine (Periactin)
    Tranquilizers
        Lithium carbonate (Lithane)
        Benzodiazepines: all, including:
        Prazepam (Centrax)
        Diazepam (Valium)

Continued

Box H-1 Drugs Affecting Appetite—cont'd

Phenothiazines: all, including:
Chlorpromazine (Thorazine)
Promethazine (Phenergan)
Steroids
Anabolic steroids:
Oxandrolone (Anavar)
Glucocorticoids:
Dexamethasone (Decadron)
Methylprednisolone (Medrol)
Cannabinoids
Tetrahydrocannabinol (marijuana, THC)
Dronabinol (synthetic THC)

Box H-2 Drugs Whose Absorption Is Significantly Affected by Food

Absorption Increased	Absorption Reduced
Atovaquone (high-fat meals)	Amprenavir (high-fat meals)
Carbamazepine	Azithromycin (not tablet)
Cyclosporine	Captopril
Griseofulvin	Ciprofloxacin[*][†]
Lovostatin	Delavirdine
Nelfinavir	Didanosine
Nitrofurantoin	Digoxin (bran fiber)
Ritonavir	Indinavir
Saquinavir	Levodopa (high-protein meals)
Sertraline	Penicillins
Tenofovir (high-fat meals)	Phenytoin[†]
Theophylline (extended	Stavudine (high-fat meals)
release form; do not take	Tetracyclines[*]
less than 1 hour before	Warfarin[†]
a high-fat meal; do not	Zalcitabine
take after the evening meal)	Zidovudine

For drugs whose absorption is improved by food, take with a meal, except as noted.
For drugs whose absorption is decreased by food, take at least 1 hour before or 2 hours after a meal.
[*]Especially dairy products.
[†]Enteral tube feedings.

Table H-1   Nutritional Effects of Selected Drugs

Drug	Effect on Nutrition
Antiinflammatory Agents	
Aspirin	↑ Urinary loss of vitamin C; Fe deficiency caused by GI blood loss
Colchicine	↓ Absorption of vitamin B_{12}; fat, carotene, lactose, protein, Na, K^+
Indomethacin	↑ Urinary loss of vitamin C; Fe deficiency caused by GI blood loss
Antineoplastic drugs	See Chapter 12
Carbonic Anhydrase Inhibitors	
All	Hyperglycemia; ↑ excretion of K^+
Cardiac Drugs	
Digitalis, digoxin, digitoxin, etc.	Diarrhea, malabsorption of all nutrients
Chelating Agents	
Penicillamine	↓ Absorption of Cu, Zn, Fe
Corticosteroids	
All	↑ Protein catabolism; ↓ protein synthesis; hyperglycemia; ↑ serum triglycerides and cholesterol; ↓ absorption of Ca, P, K^+; ↑ requirements for vitamins C, B_6, D, folic acid, Zn; osteopenia
Diuretics	
All	↑ Urinary excretion of Mg, Zn, K^+, thiamin (some greater than others)
Ethacrynic acid	Hypomagnesemia, hypokalemia; ↑ loss of urinary Ca
Furosemide	↓ Glucose tolerance; hyperglycemia; ↑ loss of urinary Ca

Continued

Table H-1   Nutritional Effects of Selected Drugs—cont'd

Drug	Effect on Nutrition
Thiazides	↓ Glucose tolerance; hyperglycemia; hypokalemia
H₂-Receptor Antagonists	
All (cimetidine, famotidine, nizatidine, ranitidine)	↓ Fe and Ca absorption caused by ↑ gastric pH
Hypocholesterolemics	
Cholestyramine, clofibrate, colestipol	↓ Absorption of fat, carotene, vitamins A, E, D, K, B₁₂, Fe
Laxatives	
Cathartics (e.g., senna, cascara)	↑ Fecal loss of Ca and K⁺ (clinically significant only with laxative abuse)
Mineral oil	Potential for ↓ absorption of vitamins A, D, E, K, Ca²⁺; recent evidence indicates that effects on vitamin absorption are probably not clinically significant
Levodopa	↑ Requirements for vitamin B₆

Opiates

Heroin — $\downarrow$ Glucose tolerance, $\downarrow K^+$

Oral contraceptive agents — $\downarrow$ Serum vitamin C; possible $\downarrow$ serum vitamin B_{12}, B_6, B_2, folate, Mg, Zn; $\uparrow$ Hct, Hgb, serum Fe, Cu, vitamins A, E

Parasympatholytic Agents

Atropine — $\downarrow$ Fe absorption caused by $\uparrow$ gastric pH

Uricosuric agents (for gout) — $\uparrow$ Excretion of Ca, Mg, Na, K^+, P, Cl, vitamin B_2, amino acids

Urinary Antiseptics

Nitrofurantoin — $\downarrow$ Serum folate; megaloblastic anemia

Table H-2 Foods, Food Components, or Nutrients with Specific Effects on Drug Action

Food, Food Component, or Nutrient	Drugs Affected
Diet Factors That Decrease Drug Effectiveness	
Vitamin K sources; liver, cabbage, spinach, kale, olive oil, soybean oil and margarines and salad dressings made with it	Coumarin
Caffeine	Guanadrel
Folic acid supplement	Methotrexate
High-protein diet	Levodopa
Pyridoxine (vitamin B_6) supplement*	Levodopa
Supplements of Fe, Mg, Zn, and Ca	Fluoroquinolones
Diet Factors That Increase Risk of Drug Toxicity	
Caffeine	Lithium
Sodium-restricted diet	Lithium
Folate deficiency	Methotrexate
Potassium deficit	Digitalis and related drugs
Diet Factors with Other Drug Interactions	
Alcohol—decreases drug elimination and thus increases levels	Abacavir

Grapefruit juice—decreases first pass extraction and causes elevated blood drug levels; avoid taking grapefruit juice with these drugs	Many drugs, including cyclosporine; felodipine, nifedipine, nimodipine, and other calcium antagonists (calcium channel blockers); saquinavir; triazolam
Imported (natural) licorice—can cause excessive potassium losses, cardiac dysrhythmia, sodium and water retention	Thiazides: chlorothiazide, hydrochlorothiazide, chlorthalidone
Salt substitutes (potassium-containing)—drug can elevate potassium levels	ACE (angiotensin converting enzyme) inhibitors
Tyramine and dopamine sources: liver, hard salami and other dry sausages; any pickled, aged, fermented, or smoked protein foods such as pickled herring, aged cheese, yogurt; commercial gravies; meat extracts; alcoholic beverages; sour cream; soy sauce; Italian broad (fava) beans; raisins; figs; bananas—can cause headache, hypertensive crisis, potential intracranial hemorrhage	Monoamine oxidase (MAO) inhibitors: phenelzine, isocarboxazid, tranylcypromine, procarbazine

*>5 mg/day.

REFERENCES

Anderson KE, Greenblatt DJ. Assessing and managing drug-nutrient interactions. *J Am Pharm Assoc (Wash)* 42:S28, 2002.

Chan LN. Drug-nutrient interaction in clinical nutrition. *Curr Opin Clin Nutr Metab Care* 5:327, 2002.

Lourenco R. Enteral feeding: drug/nutrient interaction. *Clin Nutr* 20:187, 2001.

Sanford MG et al. Protocols for identifying drug-nutrient interactions in patients: the role of the dietitian. *J Am Diet Assoc* 102:729, 2002.

Appendix I
Selected Nutrition Resources

Because of space limitations, this list cannot be complete; however, it provides some of the major sources of nutrition information and a starting point for finding additional resources.

General Information about Nutrition and Food Safety

(Includes sources of information about a wide variety of nutrition topics in health and disease.)

American Dietetic Association
120 S. Riverside Plaza, Suite 2000
Chicago, IL 60606-6995
Consumer information line: (800) 366-1655
www.eatright.org

Center for Food Safety and Applied Nutrition
U.S. Food and Drug Administration
5100 Paint Branch Parkway
College Park, MD 20740-3835
(800) SAFEFOOD
www.cfsan.fda.gov/

Center for Nutrition Policy and Promotion
U.S. Department of Agriculture
3101 Park Center Drive, Room 1034
Alexandria, VA 22302-1594
(703) 305-7600
www.usda.gov/cnpp/

Center for Science in the Public Interest
1875 Connecticut Avenue, NW

Suite 300
Washington, DC 20009
(202) 322-9110
www.cspinet.org

Centers for Disease Control and Prevention
Public Inquiries/MASO
Mailstop F07
Atlanta, GA 30333
www.cdc.gov/health/

Food and Nutrition Information Center
Agricultural Research Service, USDA
National Agricultural Library, Room 105
10301 Baltimore Avenue
Beltsville, MD 20705-2351
(301) 504-5719
www.nal.usda.gov/fnic/

Gateways to U.S. government food safety and nutrition information
online:
www.FoodSafety.gov
http://chid.nih.gov (combined health information database)
http://health.nih.gov
www.nutrition.gov

Local dietitians or nutritionists (registered dietitians or RDs)

Medem
www.medem.com

National Institutes of Health Center for Complementary and
Alternative Medicine
NIH
Bethesda, MD 20892
(888) 644-6226
www.nccam.nih.gov

Nutritional Analysis Tool
www.nat.uiuc.edu

Aging

National Institute on Aging
Building 31, Room 5C27
31 Center Drive, MSC 2292

Bethesda, MD 20892
(301) 496-1752
www.nia.nih.gov

National Policy and Resource Center on Nutrition and Aging
Dept. of Dietetics and Nutrition
Florida International University
University Park, OE200
Miami, FL 33199-1517
www.fiu.edu/~nutreldr

Nutrition Screening Initiative
1010 Wisconsin Avenue, NW
Suite 800
Washington, DC 20007
www.aafp.org/nsi/

AIDS and HIV Infection

AIDS Nutrition Services Alliance
1030 15th Street, NW
Suite 86
Washington, DC 20005-1511
(202) 289-5650
www.aidsnutrition.org

Centers for Disease Control and Prevention National AIDS
  Prevention Information Network
CDC NPIN
3401 Colesville Road, Suite 200
Silver Spring, MD 20910
(800) 458-5231
http://cdcnpin.org

Cancer

American Cancer Society
PO Box 102454
Atlanta, GA 30368-2454
(800) ACS-2345
www.cancer.org

Cancer Information Service
National Cancer Institute
(800) 422–6237
http://cis.nci.nih.gov/ or http://cancer.gov/cis/

Children's Health

National Institute of Child Health and Human Development
NICHD Clearinghouse
PO Box 3006
Rockville, MD 20847
(800) 370-2943
e-mail: NICHDClearinghouse@mail.nih.gov
www.nichd.nih.gov

Diabetes

American Diabetes Association
Attention: National Call Center
1701 North Beauregard Street
Alexandria, VA 22311
(800) 342-2383
www.diabetes.org

Juvenile Diabetes Research Foundation International (JDRF)
120 Wall Street
New York, NY 10005-4001
(800) 533-CURE (2873)
www.jdrf.org

National Diabetes Information Clearinghouse
1 Information Way
Bethesda, MD 20892-3560
(800) 860-8747
email: ndic@info.niddk.nih.gov

National Institute of Diabetes, Digestive, and Kidney Diseases
National Institutes of Health
www.niddk.nih.gov/

Eating Disorders

Anorexia Nervosa and Related Eating Disorders, Inc.
www.anred.com

National Eating Disorders Association
603 Stewart Street, Suite 803
Seattle, WA 98101
(800) 931-2237
www.nationaleatingdisorders.org

Fraud and Quackery

Center for Food Safety and Applied Nutrition
U.S. Food and Drug Administration
5100 Paint Branch Parkway
College Park, MD 20740-3835
(800) SAFEFOOD
www.cfsan.fda.gov/

National Council Against Health Fraud
119 Foster Street
Peabody, MA 01960
(978) 532-9383
www.ncahf.org

Quackwatch
PO Box 1747
Allentown, PA 18105
www.quackwatch.org

Gastrointestinal Diseases

Celiac Sprue Association/USA
PO Box 31700
Omaha, NE 68131-0700
(402) 558-0600
www.csaceliacs.org

Crohn's and Colitis Foundation of America
386 Park Avenue South, 17th Floor
New York, NY 10016-8804
www.ccfa.org

Cystic Fibrosis Foundation
6931 Arlington Road
Bethesda, MD 20814
(800) FIGHTCF
www.cff.org

National Digestive Diseases Information Clearinghouse
2 Information Way
Bethesda, MD 20892-3570
(301) 654-3810 or (800) 891-5389
www.digestive.niddk.nih.gov

Heart Disease

American Heart Association National Center
7272 Greenville Avenue
Dallas, TX 75231-4596
(800) 242-8721
www.americanheart.org

National Center for Cardiac Information
8180 Greensboro Dr., #1070
McLean, VA 22182
www.cardiacinfo.org

National Heart, Lung, and Blood Institute Information Center
Attention: Website
PO Box 30105
Bethesda, MD 20824-0105
(301) 592-8573
e-mail: NHLBIinfo@rover.nhlbi.nih.gov
www.nhlbi.nih.gov/health/infoctr/

Kidney Disease

National Kidney and Urologic Disease Information
    Clearinghouse
3 Information Way
Bethesda, MD 20892-3580
(301) 654-4415 or (800) 891-5390
e-mail: nkudic@info.niddk.nih.gov
www.kidney.niddk.nih.gov

National Kidney Foundation, Inc.
30 East 33rd Street, #1100
New York, NY 10016
(212) 889-2210 or (800) 622-9010
www.kidney.org

Neurologic Disorders

American Stroke Association National Center
7272 Greenville Avenue
Dallas, TX 75231
(888) 478-7653
www.americanheart.org

National Stroke Association
9707 East Easter Lane
Englewood, CO 80112-3747
(800) 787-6537
www.stroke.org

NIH Neurological Institute
PO Box 5801
Bethesda, MD 20824
(800) 352-9424 or (301) 496-5751
www.ninds.nih.gov

United Cerebral Palsy Association
1660 L Street, NW
Suite 700
Washington, DC 20036
(800) 872-5827
www.ucpa.org

Nutrition Support

American Society for Parenteral and Enteral Nutrition
8630 Fenton Street, Suite 412
Silver Spring, MD 20910
(301) 587-6315
www.nutritioncare.org

Oley Foundation for Home Parenteral and Enteral Nutrition
Albany Medical Center
214 Hun Memorial, A-28
Albany, NY 12208-3478
(800) 776-OLEY
www.c4isr.com/oley/

Obesity and Overweight

North American Association for the Study
   of Obesity (NAASO)
8630 Fenton Street, Suite 918
Silver Spring, MD 20910
(301) 563-6526
www.naaso.org

Overeaters Anonymous
6075 Zenith Court, NE

Rio Rancho, NM 87114-6424
(505) 891-2664
e-mail: info@overeatersanonymous.org
www.oa.org

Weight-Control Information Network
1 WIN Way
Bethesda, MD 20892-3665
(877) 946-4627 or (202) 828-1025
www.niddk.nih.gov/health/nutrition

Pregnancy, Lactation, and Women's Health

La Leche League International
1400 North Meacham Road
Schaumburg, IL 60173-4808
(847) 510-7730
www.laleche.org

March of Dimes Birth Defects Foundation
1275 Mamaroneck Avenue
White Plains, NY 10605
(800) 996-2724
www.modimes.org

National Maternal and Child Health Information Center
Health Resources and Services Administration
Maternal and Child Health Bureau
Parklawn Building, Room 18-05
5600 Fishers Lane
Rockville, MD 20857
(301) 443-2170
www.ask.hrsa.gov

National Women's Health Information Center
U.S. Department of Health and Human Services Office on
    Women's Health
8550 Arlington Boulevard, Suite 300
Fairfax, VA 22031
(800) 994-WOMAN
www.4women.org

National Women's Health Resource Center
120 Albany Street, Suite 820

New Brunswick, NJ 08901
(877) 986-9472
www.healthywomen.org

Pulmonary Disease

Cystic Fibrosis Foundation
6931 Arlington Road
Bethesda, MD 20814
(800) FIGHTCF
www.cff.org

National Heart, Lung, and Blood Institute Information Center
PO Box 30105
Bethesda, MD 20824-0105
(301) 592-8573
e-mail: NHLBIinfo@rover.nhlbi.nih.gov
www.nhlbi.nih.gov/health/infoctr

Selected Journals, Magazines, and Newsletters

American Journal of Clinical Nutrition
Consumer Reports on Health
Diabetes Care
Diabetes Forecast
FDA Consumer
Harvard Health Letter, Harvard Heart Letter, Harvard Men's Health Watch, and *Harvard Women's Health Watch* (all can be accessed at www.health.harvard.edu)
Journal of the American Dietetic Association
Journal of the American Medical Association
Journal of Nutrition Education
Journal of Parenteral and Enteral Nutrition
Nutrition and the MD
Nutrition in Clinical Practice
Nutrition Reviews
Nutrition Today
Tufts Health & Nutrition Letter (http://navigator.tufts.edu)

Appendix J
Modified Diets*

Diets Modified in Texture or Consistency

Clear Liquid Diet
Common uses/rationale: Early postoperative period; provides fluids and some electrolytes with little residue (indigestible food).
Diet modification/comments: Includes only broth, gelatin, clear fruit juices, popsicles, tea and other clear beverages, low-residue supplements; usually does not provide the RDA for any nutrients except perhaps vitamin C and should not be used more than 2 to 3 days without supplementation.

Full Liquid Diet
Common uses/rationale: Facial trauma or mandibular fractures, esophageal stricture, postoperative patients; supplies protein and carbohydrate for healing and energy in an easily swallowed form.
Diet modification/comments: Foods that are liquid at room temperature; milk, ice cream, strained soups, pudding, all juices, enteral feeding products; many allowed foods contain lactose and are not well tolerated by lactose-intolerant individuals; low in iron unless commercial liquid supplements are used.

Soft Diet
Common uses/rationale: Postoperative period, dental problems, hiatal hernia; avoids foods that are difficult to chew and digest; low in residue.
Diet modification/comments: Includes tender, low-fiber foods: cooked vegetables, cooked or canned fruits, tender meats, no fried foods or coarse whole grains; can be nutritionally complete, except perhaps for fiber.

Mechanical Soft, Pureed, or Ground Diet
Common uses/rationale: Dysphagia or dental problems; little chewing required.
Diet modification/comments: Same as soft diet except meats, fruits, and vegetables are ground or pureed.

High-Fiber Diet
Common uses/rationale: Constipation, diverticulosis, hemorrhoids; increases stool bulk and stimulates intestinal elimination.
Diet modification/comments: No food excluded; emphasize whole grains (oatmeal, whole-wheat breads and cereals, brown rice), raw or lightly cooked vegetables; raw or dried fruits, legumes; bran may be added; encourage at least 8 cups of fluid a day to hydrate fiber and create soft stool; nutritionally complete.

Diets with Protein or Amino Acid Modifications

High-Protein Diet
Common uses/rationale: Burns, trauma, major surgery, corticosteroid therapy, hepatitis; provides protein for healing or tissue formation; steroids increase conversion of protein to glucose, which creates increased needs.
Diet modification/comments: Increased serving sizes of meat, dairy products, eggs, legumes; ensure that carbohydrate and fat intake is adequate for protein sparing (providing energy so that protein is not used to meet energy needs); nutritionally adequate.

Low-Protein Diet
Common uses/rationale:
Liver or renal failure, when there is limited ability to metabolize or excrete the nitrogen release by breakdown of protein.
Diet modification/comments: Intake of meats, poultry, fish, eggs, nuts, dry beans, dairy products, grain products, and starchy vegetables is limited; see Chapters 11 and 16; nutritional status must be carefully monitored.

Continued

Gluten-Free Diet
Common uses/rationale: Celiac disease (gluten-sensitive enteropathy or nontropical sprue); intake of gluten, a protein in most grains, causes damage to the intestinal mucosa in individuals with this disorder.

Diet modification/comments: Eliminate wheat, rye, barley and possibly oats from the diet; see Table 11-3 for more detail.

Low-Phenylalanine Diet
Common uses/rationale: Phenylketonuria (PKU), an inborn error of metabolism affecting the conversion of phenylalanine to tyrosine, results in severe retardation if a low-phenylalanine diet is not begun in infancy; intellectual function is best if the individual continues on the diet indefinitely; women with PKU should follow a low-phenylalanine diet before conception (optimally) and throughout pregnancy to avoid damage to fetus.

Diet modification/comments: Restrict meat, milk, eggs, breads, and other sources of dietary protein; low-phenylalanine infant formulas (Lofenalac [Mead Johnson] or PKU 1 [Milupa]) and milk replacements (Phenyl-free [Mead Johnson] or PKU 2 [Milupa]) are available, as are low-protein breads and pastas; avoid the sugar substitute aspartame; blood levels of phenylalanine are monitored to determine the amount of phenylalanine allowed in the diet and the success of dietary restrictions.

Low-Tyramine Diet or Monoamine Oxidase Inhibitor (MAOI) Diet
Common uses/rationale: Used for as long as an individual is receiving an MAOI, a class of antidepressant medication including phenelzine, isocarboxazid, tranylcypromine; tyramine and dopamine formed by aging, protein breakdown, and putrefaction in foods could cause headache and hypertensive crisis.

Diet modification/comments: Avoid liver; alcohol; any aged, pickled, fermented, or smoked protein foods (all cheese, smoked or dried meats, salted dried or smoked fish, pickled herring, aged game); meat extracts; commercial gravies; yeast extracts; sour cream; yogurt; soy sauce, chocolate; homemade yeast bread; bananas; avocados; figs; raisins; Italian broad (fava) beans; eggplant; limit to 1 small orange/day; limit to ½ cup tomato/day; nutritionally adequate.

Diets with Carbohydrate Modifications

Diabetic Diet
Common uses/rationale: Diabetes, controls hyperglycemia by regulating the amount of dietary carbohydrate consumed at any time and distributing the carbohydrate throughout the day.
Diet modification/comments: Amount of carbohydrate, protein, and fat in diet is calculated and is divided into 3 to 6 (or more) meals and snacks during the day; diet is also low in cholesterol and saturated fat to reduce the risk of heart disease, a common complication in diabetes; nutritionally adequate.

Low-Sugar Diet
Common uses/rationale: Corticosteroid therapy, which can cause glucose intolerance.
Diet modification/comments: Restrict simple sugars (sweets and fruits); nutritionally adequate.

Lactose-Restricted or Lactose-Free Diet
Common uses/rationale: Lactase deficiency (which may be either primary or genetically determined, or secondary to intestinal mucosal damage in gastroenteritis, radiation therapy of the bowel, celiac disease, etc.); deficiency of lactase, the enzyme that digests milk sugar (lactose), results in cramping, bloating, and diarrhea after lactose consumption.
Diet modification/comments: Restrict milk and milk products except hard cheeses; most individuals tolerate small amounts of milk, ice cream, and cultured milk products (e.g., yogurt, buttermilk, acidophilus milk); lactase is available for consumption with milk products; can be nutritionally adequate; assess calcium intake.

Galactose-Free Diet
Common uses/rationale: Galactosemia, an inborn error of metabolism, results from inability to metabolize galactose to glucose; sequelae of galactosemia include cataracts (in galactokinase deficiency) and vomiting, failure to thrive, hepatomegaly, jaundice, cataracts, learning disorders, and ovarian dysfunction in deficiencies of galactose-1-phosphate uridyltransferase. Galactose and lactose (which is composed of galactose and glucose) must be omitted from the diet permanently.

Continued

Diet modification/comments: Avoid all dairy products, commercial products to which lactose is added (frankfurters, margarine, instant mashed potatoes, etc.), medications containing lactose as a filler; soy formula, soy milk fortified with calcium, or a calcium supplement should be used daily.

Diets with Fat or Cholesterol Modifications

Low-Fat Diet

Common uses/rationale: Decrease discomfort or pain in steatorrhea or gallbladder disease.

Diet modification/comments: Limit intake of fats (oils, margarine, butter, bacon, avocado, olives, salad dressings, egg yolk) to no more than 5 servings/day; use lean cuts of meat, poultry without skin, and skim milk and dairy products made with skim milk; avoid chocolate candy; coconut, breads made with fat, peanut butter, pastry; see Table 11-2; nutritionally adequate.

Low-Cholesterol, Low-Saturated-Fat diet

Common uses/rationale: Decrease risk or progression of arteriosclerotic heart disease.

Diet modification/comments: Limit intake of egg yolks to 2/week; limit meat intake to about 5-6 oz/day; use lean meats, poultry without skin, skim milk, and dairy products made with skim milk; use corn, cottonseed, soybean, canola, olive, sunflower, and safflower oils; avoid coconut and palm oils and butter or foods containing these products; avoid organ meats (liver, kidney, brains, sweetbreads); see Chapter 14; nutritionally adequate.

Diets Used in Diagnostic Testing

5-Hydroxyindoleacetic Acid (5-HIAA) Test Diet

Common uses/rationale: Used for about 3 days before and during 24-hour urine collection for 5-HIAA. Used in diagnosis and monitoring of carcinoid tumors, which secrete serotonin (metabolized in the liver to 5-HIAA).

Diet modification/comments: Omit foods containing serotonin: avocado, banana, eggplant, pineapple, plums, tomatoes, and walnuts.

300 g Carbohydrate Diet
Common uses/rationale: Used for approximately 3 days before a glucose tolerance test, since low-carbohydrate diet can result in a falsely abnormal result.
Diet modification/comments: Includes 300 g or more of carbohydrate/day in a balanced diet.

Vanillymandelic Acid (VMA) Test Diet
Common uses/rationale: Used for 2 to 3 days before and during 24-hour urine collection for VMA; the test is used in diagnosis of pheochromocytoma, an adrenal tumor that secretes high levels of epinephrine and/or norepinephrine; VMA is a metabolic product of these substances, and some foods increase VMA levels.
Diet modification/comments: Eliminate caffeine (coffee, tea, cola beverages, chocolate), apples, bananas, citrus fruits, vanilla and vanilla-containing foods, tomatoes, and squash.

100 g Fat Diet

Common uses/rationale: Used for about 3 days before and 3 days during 72-hour stool collection for fat analysis; used in assessing steatorrhea and malabsorption; adults should not excrete more than 5 g fat/day in feces; children should not excrete more than 5% to 7% of fat consumed.
Diet modification/comments: Include 100 g fat/day in diet by consumption of margarine, butter, oil, meats, whole milk, eggs, etc.; most young children cannot consume 100 g fat/day; a record of their intake is kept, and fecal fat is expressed as a proportion of the intake.

---

*In some instances, the rationale for using the diet is not well supported by empirical evidence; nevertheless, these diets are often used in clinical practice. Certain modified diets are thoroughly described in the text; consult the appropriate chapters for more information. These include the diabetic or "ADA" (American Diabetes Association) diets (see Chapter 17); low-sodium diets (see Chapter 14); low-protein diets (see Chapters 11 and 16); low-fat and/or low-cholesterol diets (see Chapters 11 and 14); and gluten-free diets (see Chapter 11).

Appendix K
Food Safety
Guidelines

Common or Especially Serious Food-Borne Illness

Campylobacteriosis (*Campylobacter jejuni*)
Symptoms: Abdominal pain, diarrhea, nausea, headache, muscle pain, and fever; rare: Guillain-Barré syndrome (acute paralysis).
People most at risk: This is the most common foodborne illness, but children under 5 years and individuals 15-29 years of age are most frequently affected. Arthritis, a rare complication, occurs primarily in people who have human lymphocyte antigen B27.
Common food sources: Raw and undercooked meat and poultry, unpasteurized milk, untreated water.
Prevention: Cook food thoroughly; use pasteurized milk and cheese; use water from a safe source.

Botulism (Toxin from *Clostridium botulinum*)
Symptoms: Generalized muscle paralysis—double vision, inability to swallow, speech difficulty, respiratory insufficiency.
People most at risk: All are at risk from disease caused by ingesting the toxin; infants less than 12 months may develop infant botulinism from ingesting *C. botulinism* spores in honey.
Common food sources of toxin: Home-canned or prepared low-acid foods (e.g., corn, green beans, soup, spinach, chicken, mushrooms, peppers, low-acid tomatoes, garlic-in-oil mixtures); bulging or leaking commercial canned foods; smoked or dried fish.
Prevention: Use proper canning methods for low-acid foods (consult U.S. Department of Agriculture or state agricultural extension service publications); garlic-in-oil mixtures must be acidified or treated with antimicrobials; avoid commercially

canned foods from bulging or leaking cans. *Discard any food that is suspect; never taste it*. Never let infants less than 12 months old eat honey.

Enterohemorrhagic *Escherichia coli* Infection (*E. coli*)
Symptoms: Abdominal cramping, diarrhea (watery progressing to bloody).
People most at risk: All.
Common food sources: Meats, especially raw or undercooked ground meat; unpasteurized milk, apple cider, or apple juice; vegetable sprouts.
Prevention: Cook all meat to an interior temperature of 160° F (72° C); use pasteurized milk, cider, and juice and cheese made with pasteurized milk; wash uncooked raw fruits and vegetables in clean drinking water; avoid raw sprouts even if they have been washed.

Listeriosis (*Listeria monocytogenes*)
Symptoms: Flulike symptoms initially—chills, fever, headache, and sometimes nausea and vomiting; can progress to bacteremia, meningitis, and encephalitis, and these complications may occur as much as 3 weeks after initial infection; spontaneous abortion or stillbirth.
People most at risk: Pregnant women, newborns, people with impaired immunity, and people taking cimetidine or antacids.
Common food sources: Unpasteurized milk and cheese; raw or undercooked meat, poultry, and fish.
Prevention: Use pasteurized milk and cheese made from pasteurized milk; use hard cheeses rather than soft cheeses (soft cheeses include Mexican queso blanco, fresco, de hoya, de crema, or asadero; brie; Camembert; feta; Roquefort and other blue-veined cheese) or cook soft cheeses until bubbling if pregnant or immunosuppressed; if unpasteurized hard cheeses are consumed, choose those aged at least 60 days; cook all meat, fish, and poultry thoroughly.

Salmonellosis (*Salmonella* Bacteria)
Symptoms: Abdominal cramping, nausea, vomiting, diarrhea, fever, headache; chronic: arthritic symptoms.
People most at risk: Elderly, infants, and individuals with immune suppression; AIDS patients are ~20 times more likely than the general population to contract salmonellosis.

Continued

Common or Especially Serious Food-Borne Illness—cont'd

Common food sources: Raw or undercooked eggs, poultry, and meat; seafood; dairy products; salad dressing; cream-filled desserts and toppings; dried gelatin.

Prevention: Cook eggs, poultry, meats, and seafoods thoroughly; avoid foods made with raw or undercooked eggs (Caesar salad, chiffon-type pies, some meringues, royal icing); use pasteurized milk and cheese; avoid cross-contamination of foods or cooking utensils (see p. 603).

Shigellosis or Bacillary Dysentery (*Shigella* Bacteria)

Symptoms: Abdominal pain; cramps; diarrhea; fever; vomiting; blood, pus, or mucus in stools.

People most at risk: Infants, elderly, and immunosuppressed; especially those with AIDS and AIDS-related complex.

Common food sources: Salads (potato, tuna, shrimp, macaroni, and chicken), raw vegetables, milk and dairy products, poultry.

Prevention: Refrigerate salads as soon as they are prepared; use pasteurized dairy products; wash raw produce thoroughly; cook poultry thoroughly.

Staphylococcal Food Poisoning (*Staphylococcus aureus*)

Symptoms: Nausea, vomiting, abdominal cramping, and prostration.

People most at risk: All.

Common food sources: Raw or undercooked meat, poultry, and egg products; salads such as egg, tuna, chicken, potato, and macaroni; bakery products such as cream-filled pastries and cream pies; sandwich fillings; milk and dairy products.

Prevention: Cook meats, poultry and eggs thoroughly; refrigerate salads and susceptible bakery products; keep sandwiches cool until serving.

Toxoplasmosis (*Toxoplasma gondii*)

Symptoms: Central nervous system disorders, particularly mental retardation and visual impairment.

People most at risk: Young children, fetus (if mother becomes infected).

Common food sources: Meat, especially pork.

Prevention: Cook all meats thoroughly.

Vibrio vulnificus Infection

Symptoms: Gastroenteritis—abdominal cramping, diarrhea, nausea; primary septicemia—septic shock, bulbous skin lesions.

People most at risk: Gastroenteritis—all; primary septicemia—all individuals with diabetes, cirrhosis, leukemia, AIDS, or those who take immunosuppressive drugs or steroids.

Common food sources: Raw or undercooked shellfish.

Prevention: Cook all shellfish thoroughly.

Yersiniosis (*Yersinia* Bacteria, Especially *Y. enterocolitica*)

Symptoms: Fever, abdominal pain, diarrhea, and/or vomiting; symptoms may mimic appendicitis; the bacteria may also cause infections of wounds, joints, and the urinary tract.

People most at risk: Young children, debilitated people, elderly, those with AIDS, and persons undergoing immunosuppressive therapy.

Common food sources: Meats (pork, beef, lamb, etc.), oysters, fish, raw milk, and produce.

Prevention: Cook all meats and fish thoroughly; use pasteurized milk; wash produce well, especially if eaten raw.

Reducing the Risk of Food-Borne Illness

Purchasing Food

- Choose only pasteurized milk and dairy products and hard cheeses. If hard cheese made with unpasteurized milk is consumed, be sure that it was aged at least 60 days. If soft cheeses are purchased, plan to cook them until they are bubbling.
- Make sure that any "sell by" or "use by" date on the food label has not passed.
- Avoid purchasing any food that shows evidence of cross-contamination by another product (e.g., cooked seafood), and bag fresh or frozen meats, poultry, and fish separately from produce or other foods that could become contaminated.
- Quickly get foods that need refrigeration into the freezer or refrigerator. On hot days, an ice chest may be needed during transport of foods.

Continued

Reducing the Risk of Food-Borne Illness—cont'd

- Some foods (e.g., produce, spices) are irradiated. This process is approved by the Food and Drug Administration as a method for reducing or eliminating pathogenic bacteria, insects, and parasites from foods. It does not leave any radioactivity in the food.
- Avoid cracked eggs.

Food Storage
- Keep refrigerator set at 40° F (4° C) or less. This is sufficient to halt the growth of most common bacteria.
- Use fresh shell eggs within 4 to 5 weeks and eggs cooked in the shell within 1 week.
- Use fresh refrigerated poultry, seafood, and ground meat within 1 to 2 days or freeze. Use refrigerated fresh whole cuts of meat (beef, pork, lamb, etc.) within 3 to 5 days.
- Refrigerate leftovers as soon as possible (within 2 hours or less). If there is a large amount, divide it into smaller units so that they will chill quickly. Use leftovers within 3 to 4 days. When in doubt, throw it out.

Food Handling and Preparation
- Wash hands before preparing any food.
- Wash hands and any used utensils after preparing one food and before starting preparation of another. This reduces the risk of cross-contamination (e.g., contamination of raw salad vegetables from raw meat cut on the same cutting board).
- A bleach solution (5 ml [1 teaspoon] bleach in 1 liter of water) is effective in cleaning countertops and cutting boards used in food preparations. It can be kept in a spray bottle in the kitchen for convenience.
- Thaw frozen foods in the refrigerator, in cold water, or in the microwave.
- Marinate foods in the refrigerator, not out on the counter.
- When taking foods off the grill, do not put the cooked items on the same platter that held the raw meat. Raw meat juices can contain bacteria that could cross-contaminate cooked foods.

- Use a meat thermometer to check the internal temperature of meats, fish, and poultry for doneness (145° F [63° C] for 15 seconds for seafood, 160° F [72° C] for meats, and 180° F [82° C] for the interior of the thigh on whole poultry). Internal color is not an accurate guide to doneness of meats.
- Avoid raw or undercooked eggs, which may be found in items such as Caesar salad, homemade ice cream, eggnog, some meringues, and chiffon-type pies. Undercooked eggs have runny, rather than firm, yolks or whites.
- Wash fresh fruits and vegetables thoroughly with drinking water. Use of detergent may leave a residue on the food, and detergents are not approved for human consumption by the Food and Drug Administration.
- Clean cutting boards thoroughly with hot soapy water after use and rinse well; sanitize with dilute bleach solution (15 ml [1 tablespoon] in 4 liters [1 gallon] water) or by washing in a dishwasher. Avoid cross-contamination of foods; for example, do not use the same knife and cutting board to cut up meat and to dice raw vegetables without cleaning the utensils between the foods. Plastic cutting boards are easier to clean than wooden ones.
- Cook stuffing in a separate dish, outside the bird. If you choose to cook a stuffed bird, use a meat thermometer and be sure that the middle of the stuffing reaches 165° F (74° C). Do not buy prestuffed birds or prestuff them for later cooking; stuff them immediately before cooking.
- Reheat leftovers until they reach at least 165° F (74° C).

Serving Foods
- Keep hot foods above 140° F (61° C) and cold foods below 40° F (4° C).
- Serve cooked foods on clean dishes with clean hands and clean utensils. Never put cooked foods on a dish that has held raw products unless the dish is first washed with soap and water.
- Perishable foods used for picnics should be kept in an ice chest chilled with ice or frozen gel packs to a temperature of 40° F (4° C) or less until they are consumed. Keep the ice

Continued

Reducing the Risk of Food-Borne Illness—cont'd

chest closed as much as possible to keep the temperature from rising. Leftovers should be discarded if they cannot be maintained at 40° F (4° C) or less until they reach home.

- Perishable items packed in lunches for school or lunch should be kept chilled with a frozen juice box or frozen gel pack until lunch. Any perishable items not eaten at lunch should be discarded and not brought home and reused.

Glossary

achalasia: incomplete relaxation of the lower esophageal sphincter after swallowing.

acute-phase reactant: a protein synthesized and released by the liver in increased quantities in response to injury, trauma, inflammation, or infection, e.g., C-reactive protein, fibrinogen, serum amyloid A, and α_1-acid glycoprotein.

Adequate Intake (AI): a recommendation for the level of intake of a nutrient. The AI is assigned, rather than a Recommended Dietary Allowance (RDA), when the nutrient intake recommended is believed to cover the needs of almost all of the population, but nutrient needs cannot be quantified as precisely as those for an RDA.

alcohol abuse: heavy drinking with an increasing tolerance for ethanol but no withdrawal symptoms when drinking stops.

alcoholism: a strong craving for ethanol, associated with increasing tolerance to alcohol's intoxicating effects and symptoms of withdrawal when drinking is discontinued.

alternative medical therapies: a group of diverse medical and health care systems, practices, and products that are not presently considered to be part of conventional medicine but are used in place of conventional therapies. An example is the use of diet and meditation to treat cancer rather than conventional surgical, radiation, and chemotherapy treatments.

anabolism: formation of new body tissue.

anemia of chronic disease: an anemia observed in some patients affected by cancer, renal failure, and other chronic illnesses in which the bone marrow fails to produce adequate red blood cells, even though iron stores may be normal. The anemia is often normocytic (normal-sized cells), rather than microcytic, as in iron deficiency.

anorexia nervosa: a psychiatric eating disorder often resulting in extreme thinness. The affected person usually has a strong aversion to food intake and a distorted body image (perceiving himself or herself as fat when the opposite is the case).

anthropometric measurements: measurements of the designated aspects of the human body, such as height and weight.

antioxidant: any of various substances (such as beta-carotene, vitamin C, and vitamin E) that inhibit oxidation or reactions promoted by oxygen and peroxides and apparently protect the living body from the deleterious effects of free radicals.

attention deficit/hyperactivity disorders (ADHDs): a set of related disorders characterized by focusing on irrelevant stimuli, impulsive behavior, inconsistency, and lack of persistence. Overactivity may be a feature of the disorder in some children.

basal energy expenditure: amount of energy required to maintain the critical life processes (e.g., breathing, beating of the heart) in an individual at rest, in a comfortable thermal environment, and after an overnight fast. Usually used as a synonym for *basal metabolic rate* and *resting metabolic rate*.

body mass index (BMI): an indication of the appropriateness of a person's weight for height, which correlates relatively well with measures of body fat. BMI is usually calculated as the person's weight (in kg) divided by the height (in meters) squared.

bronchopulmonary dysplasia (BPD): lung damage almost always found in infants who have required oxygen therapy and mechanical ventilation. BPD is characterized by a persistent requirement for supplemental oxygen beyond 36 weeks of gestational age.

bulimia nervosa: a psychiatric eating disorder characterized by repeated episodes of bingeing on large amounts of foods, followed by efforts to rid the body of the food by self-induced vomiting or abuse of laxatives and diuretics. Also known as the *binge-purge syndrome*.

cancer cachexia: a severe form of cancer-related malnutrition associated with a poor prognosis and characterized by anorexia, early satiety, weight loss, anemia, weakness, and muscle wasting.

carbohydrate counting: a technique for planning the diet in diabetes that focuses on the carbohydrate content of foods consumed.

carotenes: another term for carotenoids.

carotenoids: a group of pigments (yellow, orange, or red) found in plant and animal products. Beta-carotene, lutein, cryptoxanthin, and zeaxanthin are examples of carotenoids. All carotenoids have some vitamin A activity, but beta-carotene is the primary vitamin A precursor.

catabolism: breakdown of body tissues.

celiac disease (nontropical sprue or gluten-sensitive enteropathy): a disorder characterized by impaired absorption and steatorrhea. It results from intestinal mucosal damage caused by an immune reaction to the gliadin fraction of the gluten protein or closely related proteins.

chylomicron: a lipoprotein formed in the intestine after consumption of fat. It transports the fat from the intestinal cell into the lymph and from there into the blood.

colostrum: the milk produced for about the first 3 to 5 days after birth. Colostrum is yellowish, rich in immunoglobulins and lymphocytes, and higher in protein than mature human milk.

complementary medical therapies: a group of diverse medical and health care systems, practices, and products that are not presently considered to be part of conventional medicine but are used together with conventional therapies. An example is the use of aromatherapy to relieve discomfort following surgery.

complete protein: a protein that contains all of the essential amino acids in sufficient amounts and in proportion to one another so that it can support growth and maintenance of tissues.

Crohn's disease: a form of inflammatory bowel disease that can affect any portion of the gastrointestinal tract and can extend through all layers of the bowel. It is often associated with severe chronic diarrhea, nutritional deficits, and weight loss.

cystic fibrosis (CF): a disease resulting from a defect in the cystic fibrosis transmembrane conductance regulator (CFTR) gene. This defect prevents the formation of CFTR, a protein involved in chloride transport across cell membranes in the body. It results in several problems, including thickened mucous secretions in the lungs, interfering with lung function and promoting respiratory infections, and pancreatic insufficiency.

cytokines: immunoregulatory proteins such as the interleukins, tumor necrosis factor, and interferon that are secreted by cells, especially those of the immune system.

Daily Value (DV): a reference value used in nutrition labeling of foods. The DV, which is based on the Recommended Dietary Allowance (RDA), provides a guideline to the amount of a particular nutrient that the daily diet should contain. On the label, information for most nutrients is expressed in both units of weight (g or mg) and %Daily Value (DV).

dehydration: a deficit of body fluid.

Dietary Guidelines for Americans: guidelines written in lay language that are intended to help Americans optimize their health and reduce nutrition-related health risks.

Dietary Reference Intakes (DRIs): guidelines for nutrient intake for the healthy population. The DRIs contain two types of measures, the Recommended Dietary Allowances (RDAs) and Tolerable Upper Intake Levels. The DRIs do not focus merely on preventing deficiency diseases but quantify the relationship between nutrients and risk of disease, e.g., calcium and osteoporosis. The DRIs include important nonnutrients found in food, such as fiber.

dumping syndrome: a common side effect of gastric bypass or gastrectomy. It occurs because stomach contents pass into the small bowel rapidly. Nutrients that raise the osmotic concentration within the small bowel substantially, such as simple carbohydrates, draw fluid into the bowel and cause a reduction in the circulating blood volume. The symptoms include dizziness, sweating, nausea, weakness, tachycardia, and diarrhea.

dysphagia: difficulty in swallowing.

elemental formulas: liquid diets containing nutrients in a form easy to digest, absorb, and assimilate (e.g., hydrolyzed protein and/or free amino acids). These are commonly used for individuals with digestive or absorptive disorders. Also known as *predigested* or *oligomeric formulas.*

enteral feedings: feedings delivered into any part of the gastrointestinal tract. Enteral feedings are given either by mouth or by tube.

erythropoietin: a hormone produced by the kidney that stimulates red blood cell formation.

essential amino acids (EAAs): amino acids that cannot be synthesized in the body in the amounts needed for the building of tissues and therefore must be provided by the diet.

Estimated Average Intake (EAR): the average daily nutrient intake that is believed to meet the requirements of half the healthy individuals in a life stage or gender group.

extremely low birth weight (ELBW): weighing less than 1000 g at birth.

failure to thrive: failure of an infant to regain his or her birth weight by 3 weeks of age, or continuous weight loss or failure to gain weight at the appropriate rate during infancy or childhood.

fetal alcohol syndrome (FAS): a constellation of congenital abnormalities that results from alcohol intake during pregnancy. Features of FAS may include microcephaly (abnormally small head circumference), prenatal and postnatal growth failure, mental retardation, facial abnormalities, cleft palate, skeletal-joint abnormalities, abnormal palmar creases, cardiac defects, and behavioral abnormalities. The only known preventive measure is to avoid drinking alcohol during pregnancy.

Food Guide Pyramid: a schematic tool to help individuals plan a varied diet. The pyramid has six components. The base is made up of the grain group, emphasizing the importance of this group as a foundation to good nutrition. The next layer is composed of two groups, vegetables and fruits. The third layer from the bottom is composed of milk products and meat, poultry, fish, eggs, and nuts. The apex of the pyramid, the smallest part, is devoted to fats and sweets, as a reminder to use these products only sparingly.

food hypersensitivity: an immunologic (allergic) reaction to ingestion of a food or food additive. Symptoms can include anaphylaxis, failure to thrive (in infants and children), vomiting, abdominal pain, diarrhea, rhinitis, sinusitis, otitis media, cough, wheezing, rash, urticaria, and atopic dermatitis.

food jags: periods during which young children consume only one or two foods for several days. This behavior is normal unless it lasts more than a few days.

functional food: a foodstuff (such as a fortified food or a dietary supplement) that is held to provide health or medical benefits in addition to its basic nutritional value; also known as a *nutraceutical*.

gastroesophageal reflux disease (GERD): reflux of stomach contents into the esophagus.

gastroparesis: partial paralysis of the stomach; the condition is common among individuals with diabetes and is associated with postprandial nausea, vomiting, and abdominal distension.

gestational diabetes mellitus: diabetes that first becomes evident during pregnancy.

gliadin: a part of the gluten protein, found in wheat. Closely related proteins (prolamins) are found in rye and barley. An immune reaction to the prolamins causes damage to the intestinal mucosa in susceptible individuals.

gluten: a protein found especially in wheat that gives dough a sticky texture.

glycemic index: ratio between the change in the blood glucose concentration produced by consuming some food, compared with the change produced by some reference carbohydrate (usually white bread or glucose).

glycosylated hemoglobin (HbA_{1c}): hemoglobin with glucose molecules attached; it is increased by elevated blood glucose over the life span of the red blood cells and serves as an indicator of blood glucose concentrations over a period of several weeks to a few months.

hemochromatosis: a genetic disorder in which excessive iron is stored in various organs—especially the liver, pancreas, heart, gonad, skin, and joints—disrupting organ function.

hepatic encephalopathy: a disorder resulting from accumulation of toxic substances in the blood as a result of liver failure. It is characterized by memory loss, personality change, tremors, and a decrease in the level of consciousness. The affected person may progress to stupor and coma.

hepatic steatosis (nonalcoholic fatty liver disease [NAFLD]): a condition characterized by vesicles of fat deposited in the hepatocytes (liver cells) and more common among obese than normal-weight individuals. NAFLD may be associated with necrosis of the hepatocytes and fibrosis of liver tissue. Cirrhosis and liver failure are possible sequelae.

hepatitis: an inflammation of the liver caused by a virus, toxin, obstruction, parasite, or drug.

high biologic value (HBV) proteins: proteins of high quality that promote positive nitrogen balance; believed to be effective in maintenance and synthesis of tissues.

high-density lipoprotein (HDL): a lipoprotein formed in the liver to transport cholesterol from the tissues to the liver for metabolism. This function makes HDL protective against heart disease, and thus the HDL-cholesterol is considered "good" cholesterol.

hydrogenated fat: fat to which hydrogen atoms have been added to remove some of the double bonds. Hydrogenation converts the fats from liquids to solids (e.g., shortening or margarine) and increases the number of *trans* molecules in the fat.

hyperemesis gravidarum: severe nausea and vomiting that may continue throughout pregnancy.

hypermetabolism: abnormally increased energy expenditure, as occurs in sepsis or following injuries such as burns.

hyperoxaluria: excessive loss of oxalates in the urine.

impaired glucose tolerance (IGT): having a glucose concentration ≥140 mg/dl (7.8 mmol/L) and <200 mg/dl (11.1 mmol/L) 2 hours after ingestion of a 75-g glucose load; a risk factor for later development of diabetes mellitus.

incomplete protein: a protein lacking in one or more essential amino acids and therefore lacking in the ability to maintain normal growth and maintenance of tissues.

inflammatory bowel disease (IBD): two types of inflammatory processes, Crohn's disease and ulcerative colitis, that affect the gastrointestinal tract. Crohn's disease can affect any part of the gastrointestinal tract and can extend through all layers of the bowel. Ulcerative colitis is primarily a disease of the large bowel, and it affects only the intestinal mucosa and the submucosal layer. The most common symptom is chronic bloody diarrhea. Nutritional deficits are common, especially in Crohn's disease, where malabsorption and weight loss may be severe.

insulin resistance: impaired response of cells (primarily those in the skeletal muscle and adipose tissue) to insulin.

insulin resistance syndrome: see *metabolic syndrome*.

isoflavones: compounds found in soy that appear to lower low-density lipoprotein (LDL) cholesterol concentrations.

ketogenic diet: a high-fat diet that stimulates ketone production.

leptin: the product of the *ob* gene. Leptin is released by adipose (fat) tissue, and it appears to provide a mechanism for the adipose tissue to communicate with the central nervous system and contribute to the control of food intake and energy metabolism.

lipodystrophy syndrome: a group of side effects of antiretroviral therapy for HIV infection that include high triglyceride levels in the blood, diabetes, and redistribution of fat in the body resulting in changes in bodily conformation and that are believed to result especially from treatment with protease inhibitors.

lipoproteins: the major carriers of lipids (fats) in the plasma. They are formed of lipids bound to proteins.

low birth weight (LBW): weighing less than 2500 g (5.5 lb) at birth.

low-density lipoproteins (LDLs): lipoproteins that have a very high content of cholesterol, which the LDL deposit in the tissues. The cholesterol in LDL is considered to be the main cause of elevated cholesterol levels, making LDL-cholesterol the so-called "bad" cholesterol in causation of heart disease.

malnutrition: poor nutritional status (either undernutrition or overnutrition). It can result from inadequate intake, disorders of digestion or absorption, or excessive intake of nutrients.

medium-chain triglyceride (MCT): a triglyceride (consisting of glycerol bound to three fatty acids) in which the fatty acids are 8 to 12 carbons in length. MCTs are most often used in the nutritional care of people with limited digestive and absorptive ability.

medical nutrition therapy: nutrition assessment, planning, intervention, and guidance provided by a nutrition professional.

metabolic equivalent (MET): One MET is the energy required while sitting quietly—for example, while reading a book.

metabolic syndrome: a condition characterized by insulin resistance and defined as having three or more of the following characteristics: (1) waist circumference >102 cm (men) or 88 cm (women), (2) blood pressure of at least 130/85 mm Hg, (3) fasting serum glucose level of at least 110 mg/dl (6.1 mmol/L); (4) serum triglyceride level of at least 150 mg/dl, and (5) high-density lipoprotein (HDL) cholesterol level of less than 40 mg/dl in men and 50 mg/dl in women. The metabolic syndrome is a risk factor for cardiovascular disease. Also known as the *insulin resistance syndrome* or *syndrome X*.

micelle: a combination of bile salts and fat in which the bile emulsifies fat into very small particles to increase its exposure to digestive enzymes and to enhance its solubility so that it can be absorbed by the intestinal mucosa.

monounsaturated fatty acid: a fatty acid with one carbon-carbon double bond.

necrotizing enterocolitis (NEC): an intestinal disorder most often occurring in preterm infants. On x-ray, gas can be seen between the layers of the intestine; in severe cases, intestinal perforation and peritonitis are present.

nephrolithiasis: formation of calculi (stones) in the kidney.

nephrotic syndrome: a condition in which there is damage to the basement membrane of the nephrons. The syndrome is characterized by loss of protein in the urine, edema, and decreased serum albumin concentrations.

nitrogen balance: the relationship between the amount of nitrogen (from proteins or amino acids) consumed and the amount excreted. Balance is positive if more nitrogen is consumed than excreted and negative if more nitrogen is excreted than consumed.

nonessential amino acid: an amino acid that can be synthesized in the body in amounts sufficient to maintain tissue and sustain growth.

nonnutritive feeding: sucking a pacifier. It develops muscle tone needed for feeding by nipple and may be soothing for infants in stressful situations.

nutraceutical (also nutriceutical): a foodstuff (such as a fortified food or a dietary supplement) that is held to provide health or medical benefits in addition to its basic nutritional value; also known as a *functional food.*

nutritional quackery: promotion of misconceptions about food and nutrition. Examples include the idea that certain foods or dietary supplements have "fat-burning" properties and the belief that nutritional supplements are necessary to maintain health.

nutrition assessment: the process used to evaluate nutritional status, identify malnutrition, and determine which individuals need aggressive nutritional support.

nutrition support: the provision of specially formulated and/or delivered parenteral or enteral nutrients to maintain or restore optimal nutritional status.

omega-3 fatty acid (n-3 fatty acid): a fatty acid with a carbon-carbon double bond three carbons from the omega (methyl group) end of its chain. These fatty acids have been reported to reduce serum triglyceride concentrations and to reduce the aggregation of platelets, resulting in a reduced risk of myocardial infarction (heart attack). Fish from cold waters are generally rich in omega-3 fatty acids; canola oil is another source.

osmolality: the property of a solution that depends on the concentration of solute (the number of osmotically active particles) per kilogram of solvent (usually water).

pancreatitis: inflammation, edema, and necrosis of the pancreas as a result of digestion of the organ by pancreatic enzymes.

parenteral feedings: delivery of nutrients via the intravenous route.

phytochemical: a chemical component of a plant, especially one having health-protective effects.

pica: the consumption of substances usually considered nonfoods (e.g., clay) or of excessive amounts of food products low in nutrients (e.g., ice, cornstarch).

polymeric formulas: liquid diets used for oral supplementation or enteral tube feeding. Polymeric formulas contain intact (not predigested) carbohydrates, proteins, and fats.

polyunsaturated fatty acid: a fatty acid containing more than one carbon-carbon double bond.

prebiotic: a food ingredient that beneficially affects the host by selectively stimulating the growth or the activity of one or a limited number of nonpathogenic bacteria in the colon.

preeclampsia: a syndrome characterized by hypertension, albuminuria, and excessive edema. Also called *pregnancy-induced hypertension* or *toxemia*.

pregnancy-induced hypertension (PIH): a syndrome characterized by hypertension, albuminuria, and excessive edema. Also called *preeclampsia* or *toxemia*.

probiotic: live microorganisms that confer a health benefit on the host, improving immune and nonimmune mechanisms of resistance to infection in the intestine.

protein-energy malnutrition (PEM): undernutrition resulting from inadequate intake, digestion, or absorption of protein or calories. There are two forms, kwashiorkor and marasmus, and it is possible to have a combined form, referred to as *marasmic kwashiorkor*. PEM is also known as **protein-calorie malnutrition (PCM)**.

Recommended Dietary Allowance (RDA): an amount of a nutrient estimated to meet the biological needs of almost all (97% to 98%) of the healthy population. The RDA is one of the measures included in the Dietary Reference Intakes (DRIs).

refeeding syndrome: a potential complication of refeeding of the severely malnourished individual. During refeeding, especially with high-carbohydrate feedings, insulin levels rise and cellular uptake of glucose, water, phosphorus, potassium, and other nutrients is stimulated. Serum levels of phosphorus, potassium, magnesium, and other minerals or electrolytes subsequently fall, if close attention is not paid to their replacement. Refeeding syndrome is characterized by cardiac dysrhythmias, congestive heart failure, hemolysis, muscular weakness, seizures, acute respiratory failure, and a variety of other complications, including sudden death.

respiratory quotient (RQ): the ratio of the carbon dioxide produced to the oxygen consumed in a given unit of time.

resting energy expenditure (REE): amount of energy required to maintain the vital life processes (e.g., breathing, circulation) at rest in an overnight-fasted condition and in a comfortable environmental temperature.

sensitivity: the probability that a test indicates a nutrient deficiency, given that the person actually does have a deficiency.

short-bowel syndrome: varying degrees of impaired digestion and absorption resulting from surgical removal of parts of the intestines.

small for gestational age (SGA): exhibiting intrauterine growth failure; low birth weight and length for the infant's gestational age.

specificity: the probability that a test indicates no nutrient deficiency, given that the person does not have a deficiency.

steatorrhea: loss of excess fat in the stools.

syndrome X: see metabolic syndrome.

systemic inflammatory response syndrome: a severe systemic response to a condition (such as trauma, an infection, or a burn) that provokes an acute inflammatory reaction.

therapeutic lifestyle changes (TLC): a systematic approach to correction of dyslipidemia and reduction of risk of heart disease including dietary changes to reduce saturated and *trans* fat intake to <10% of total energy intake and cholesterol intake to <200 mg/day; adjustment of energy intake to maintain or reduce weight; regular physical activity; and recommendations to consider consuming increased viscous fiber, plant sterols/stanols, and soy protein.

thermic effect of food (TEF): production of body heat as a result of food intake; the energy required to digest and absorb food and transport nutrients to the cells. TEF accounts for approximately 10% of daily energy needs. Also referred to as *diet-induced thermogenesis*.

Tolerable Upper Intake Level (UL): the upper limit of intake associated with a low risk of adverse effects in almost all members of a given population. The UL is one of the measures included in the Dietary Reference Intakes (DRIs).

trans fatty acid: a fatty acid (component of fats) formed when unsaturated oils are partially hydrogenated to make them harder. The fatty acid molecules usually bend at the remaining carbon-carbon double bonds, and in the *trans* fatty acid the two ends of the fatty acid are arranged so that they are on opposite sides of the double bond. (In naturally occurring *cis* fatty acids, the two ends are on the same side of the double bond.)

type 1 diabetes mellitus: previously known as *insulin-dependent diabetes*; characterized by insulin deficiency, which results from destruction of the beta cells of the pancreas, usually by an autoimmune process. Classic symptoms include excessive hunger and thirst and weight loss.

type 2 diabetes mellitus: previously known as *non-insulin-dependent diabetes*; characterized by insulin resistance, or decreased tissue uptake of glucose in response to insulin, along with inability to secrete enough insulin to compensate for the insulin resistance.

ulcerative colitis: a form of inflammatory bowel disease that usually involves only the large bowel and primarily affects the mucosal and submucosal layers of the intestine.

unsaturated fatty acid: a fatty acid (component of fats) that does not contain the maximum possible number of hydrogen atoms, allowing it to have carbon-carbon double bonds. There are two types of unsaturated fatty acids, monounsaturated (having one double bond) and polyunsaturated (having more than one double bond).

very low birth weight (VLBW): weighing less than 1500 g at birth.

very-low-density lipoprotein (VLDL): lipoprotein formed in the liver to transport lipids made in the liver to other body cells. Most of their lipid content is in the form of triglycerides, but they also transport cholesterol.

visceral fat: fat located in proximity to the abdominal visceral organs. Visceral fat lies deeper in the body than the subcutaneous abdominal adipose tissue.

weight cycling: also known as "yo-yo" dieting, occurs when individuals repeatedly lose and regain weight.

Wernicke-Korsakoff syndrome: a serious disorder of the central nervous system that can occur in alcoholism and other thiamin-deficient states. Symptoms are mental confusion, memory loss, confabulation (filling in gaps in memory with fabrication), ataxia, abnormal ocular motility (ophthalmoplegia and nystagmus), and peripheral neuropathy.

Index

Page numbers followed by *b, t,* or *f* indicate boxes, tables, or figures, respectively.